Pediatric Dysphagia

Julina Ongkasuwan • Eric H. Chiou

Editors

Pediatric Dysphagia

Challenges and Controversies

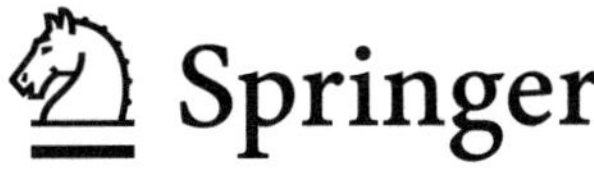 Springer

Editors
Julina Ongkasuwan
Otolaryngology-Head and Neck Surgery
Baylor College of Medicine
Houston, TX
USA

Eric H. Chiou
Pediatric Gastroenterology and Nutrition
Baylor College of Medicine
Houston, TX
USA

ISBN 978-3-030-07286-5   ISBN 978-3-319-97025-7   (eBook)
https://doi.org/10.1007/978-3-319-97025-7

This Springer imprint is published by the registered company Springer Nature Switzerland AG
The registered company address is: Gewerbestrasse 11, 6330 Cham, Switzerland

Preface

Pediatric dysphagia is a clinical problem that crosses disciplines. Children may be seen by numerous medical specialties including pediatric otolaryngology, gastroenterology, pulmonology, speech pathology, occupational therapy, and lactation consultants. The myriad approaches to the diagnosis and management of dysphagia can be confusing for both clinicians and families, resulting in recurrent trips to medical professionals. Feeding is integral to socialization and to bonding between infants and parents. Disruptions in feeding development can be extremely taxing emotionally and economically for families. Children with dysphagia are some of the most challenging patients even for clinicians who specialize in their care.

Given the heterogeneity of causes and manifestations of pediatric dysphagia, this textbook incorporates the perspectives of multiple types of clinicians that care for these patients including otolaryngologists, gastroenterologists, pulmonologists, speech pathologists, occupational therapist, and lactation consultants, which are important to consider according to the individual features and needs of each patient. We also present the advantages as well as potential limitations of various diagnostic modalities. Finally, we highlight current clinical challenges and controversies in the management of pediatric dysphagia. We hope that this book will encourage cross-specialty pollination of ideas and knowledge as well as stimulate further research in the field.

We would like to thank our chapter authors for their time, effort, and erudite contributions. We would also like to thank the Springer editorial staff for their invaluable assistance. Most of all, we would like to thank our spouses, Shirley Chiou and John Anguay, and our children, Sophie, Elyse, Nathan, Dominic, and Christopher, for their continuing love and support.

Houston, TX, USA   Eric H. Chiou
Julina Ongkasuwan

Contents

Contributors

Annie K. Ahn, BA, MD Bobby R. Alford Department of Otolaryngology-Head and Neck Surgery, Texas Children's Hospital, Houston, TX, USA

Joshua R. Bedwell, MD, MS Department of Otolaryngology, Baylor College of Medicine, Texas Children's Hospital, Houston, TX, USA

Andrea M. Begotka, PhD Psychiatry and Behavioral Medicine, Children's Hospital of Wisconsin, Milwaukee, WI, USA

Ryan Belcher, MD Otolaryngology-Head and Neck Surgery, Vanderbilt University School of Medicine, Children's Hospital at Vanderbilt, Nashville, TN, USA

Laura Brooks, MEd, CCC-SLP BCS-S Department of Rehabilitation, Children's Healthcare of Atlanta, Atlanta, GA, USA

Jeffrey Cheng, MD Pediatric Otolaryngology, Division of Head and Neck Surgery and Communication Sciences, Duke University Medical Center, Durham, NC, USA

Eric H. Chiou, MD Department of Pediatrics, Baylor College of Medicine/Texas Children's Hospital, Houston, TX, USA

Shailendra Das, DO Department of Pediatrics, Texas Children's Hospital (Baylor College of Medicine), Houston, TX, USA

Hamdy El-Hakim, FRCS(ED), FRCS(ORL) Department of Surgery, Stollery Children's Hospital, Edmonton, AB, Canada

Lynn Ansley Fordham, MD Department of Radiology, North Carolina Children's Hospital, Chapel Hill, NC, USA

Tsu-Hsin Howe, PhD, OTR, FAOTA Department of Occupational Therapy, New York University, New York, NY, USA

Nancy Hurst, PhD, RN, IBCLC Women's Support Services, Texas Children's Hospital, Houston, TX, USA

Andre Isaac, MD, MSc Otolaryngology-Head and Neck Surgery, Stollery Children's Hospital, Edmonton, AB, Canada

Wendy Johannsen, MSLP, RSLP, SLP (C) Speech and Audiology, Stollery Children's Hospital, Edmonton, AB, Canada

Elton Lambert, MD Pediatric Otolaryngology, Texas Children's Hospital/Baylor College of Medicine, Houston, TX, USA

Chantal Lau, PhD Pediatrics/Neonatology, Baylor College of Medicine, Houston, TX, USA

Deepak K. Mehta, MD, FRCS Department of Otolaryngology, Texas Children's Hospital, Houston, TX, USA

Cheryl Mitchell, OTR, MOT, SCFES Physical Medicine and Rehabilitation, Texas Children's Hospital, Houston, TX, USA

Laura Hinkes Molinaro, MA, CCC-SLP Speech and Language Pathology, Ann and Robert H. Lurie Children's Hospital of Chicago, Chicago, IL, USA

Ellen E. Moore, MA, CCC-SLP Speech, Language and Learning, Texas Children's Hospital, Houston, TX, USA

Mary Frances Musso, DO Bobby R. Alford Department of Otolaryngology-Head and Neck Surgery, Texas Children's Hospital, Houston, TX, USA

Julina Ongkasuwan, MD Department of Otolaryngology Head and Neck Surgery, Baylor College of Medicine/Texas Children's Hospital, Houston, TX, USA

Stacey L. Paluszak, OTR, MS Physical Medicine and Rehabilitation, Texas Children's Hospital, Houston, TX, USA

Priya Raj, MD, MS Department of Pediatric Gastroenterology, Hepatology and Nutrition, Texas Children's Hospital, Houston, TX, USA

Nikhila Raol, MD, MPH Otolaryngology-Head and Neck Surgery, Emory University School of Medicine, Children's Healthcare of Atlanta, Atlanta, GA, USA

Christina A. Rappazzo, CCC-SLP/BCS-S Department of Speech, Language and Learning, Texas Children's Hospital, Houston, TX, USA

Eileen Raynor, MD Pediatric Otolaryngology, Division of Head and Neck Surgery and Communication Sciences, Duke University Medical Center, Durham, NC, USA

Duke University Medical Center, Durham, NC, USA

Rachel Rosen, MD, MPH Division of Gastroenterology and Nutrition, Boston Childrens Hospital, Boston, MA, USA

Tara L. Rosenberg, MD Department of Otolaryngology/Head and Neck Surgery, Baylor College of Medicine/Texas Children's Hospital, Houston, TX, USA

Rinarani Sanghavi, MBBS, MD Department of Pediatrics, UT Southwestern Medical Center/Children's Health Dallas, Dallas, TX, USA

James W. Schroeder Jr, MD Pediatric Otolaryngology, Ann and Robert H. Lurie Children's Hospital of Chicago, Department of Otolaryngology Head and Neck Surgery, Northwestern University, Chicago, IL, USA

Alan H. Silverman, PhD Department of Pediatrics, Medical College of Wisconsin, Milwaukee, WI, USA

William Stoudemire, MD Department of Pediatrics, University of North Carolina at Chapel Hill, Chapel Hill, NC, USA

Prasad John Thottam, DO, FAAP Pediatric Otolaryngology, Beaumont Children's Hospital, Royal Oak, MI, USA

Catherine L. Turk, PhD, CCC-SLP Department of Speech, Language, and Learning, Texas Children's Hospital, Houston, TX, USA

Timothy J. Vece, MD Department of Pediatrics, University of North Carolina at Chapel Hill, Chapel Hill, NC, USA

Susan Willette, MS, CCC-SLP, CLC Speech and Language Pathology, Ann and Robert H. Lurie Children's Hospital of Chicago, Chicago, IL, USA

Jay Paul Willging, MD Department of Otolaryngology, Cincinnati Children's Hospital Medical Center, University of Cincinnati, Cincinnati, OH, USA

Part I
Diagnosis and Treatment of Pediatric Dysphagia

Chapter 1
Embryology and Anatomy

Annie K. Ahn and Mary Frances Musso

Abbreviations

CN   Cranial nerve
CPG   Central pattern generator
LAR   Laryngeal adductor response
LCR   Laryngeal cough reflex
LES   Lower esophageal sphincter
UES   Upper esophageal sphincter

Introduction

The average individual swallows about 500 times per day [1]. Deglutition or swallowing is an essential function for ingestion of nutrition as well as clearance of secretions from the upper aerodigestive tract. This complex process requires the precise coordination of more than 30 muscles located within the oral cavity, pharynx, larynx, and esophagus [2]. The swallowing apparatus is made up of three upper aerodigestive structures: the oral cavity, pharynx, and larynx. These structures function as a hydrodynamic pump with valves that allows food and liquid to be transferred into the stomach without entering the respiratory tract [3]. The act of swallowing is divided into four phases: oral preparatory phase, oral transport phase, pharyngeal phase, and esophageal phase. Dysphagia, or difficulty swallowing, can be secondary to congenital errors or acquired neurologic or anatomic problems. Dysphagia can lead to many negative consequences including malnutrition, dehydration, pneumonia, and reduced quality of life [2]. To effectively treat dysphagia, a comprehensive understanding of deglutition is essential.

A. K. Ahn · M. F. Musso (✉)
Bobby R. Alford Department of Otolaryngology-Head and Neck Surgery, Texas Children's Hospital, Houston, TX, USA
e-mail: annie.ahn@bcm.edu; mxmusso@texaschildrens.org

© Springer International Publishing AG, part of Springer Nature 2018
J. Ongkasuwan, E. H. Chiou (eds.), *Pediatric Dysphagia*,
https://doi.org/10.1007/978-3-319-97025-7_1

Embryology

The neurovascular and musculoskeletal structures of the oral and pharyngeal apparatus of deglutition are formed from branchial arches and pharyngeal pouches. The four pairs of branchial arches are derived from ectodermal and mesodermal tissues and form on the lateral side of the head as outgrowths around 5 weeks of gestation. The mesodermal tissue within each arch remodels to form muscle, connective tissue, cartilage, and bone within the head and neck. The arches derive their motor and sensory innervation from adjacent cranial nerves during development, namely, the trigeminal, facial, vagus, and accessory nerves [3].

The frontonasal prominence leads to the formation of the forehead and nose, and its proper development along with the maxillary and mandibular prominences is necessary for normal craniofacial structures such as the nose, choanae, lips, tongue, palate, mandible, maxilla, and cheeks, which are involved in deglutition and are crucial for an intact swallow [3, 4]. Improper development of these structures can result in problems such as cleft lip and/or palate and velopharyngeal insufficiency.

Incomplete fusion of the posterior cricoid lamina and formation of the tracheoesophageal septum can lead to a laryngeal or laryngotracheoesophageal cleft or a bifid epiglottis. Incomplete separation of the trachea and alimentary tract will lead to a tracheoesophageal fistula, which can present as aspiration [5].

Supporting Structures

Supporting structures including the bones, cartilage, teeth, spaces, salivary glands, and muscles are found within the oral cavity, pharynx, and esophagus that help carry out a normal swallow. The mandible, maxilla, hard palate, hyoid bone, cervical vertebrae, styloid process, and mastoid process of the temporal bone support and stabilize the involved muscles and aid in mastication [2]. Various cartilages including the thyroid cartilage, cricoid cartilage, arytenoids, and epiglottis provide support for several muscles of mastication and help with transferring the lingual and pharyngeal bolus. The teeth are vital to bolus preparation. Two sets of teeth develop in humans, deciduous teeth and permanent teeth. The deciduous teeth erupt between 6 months and 2 years of age [6]. Premolars and third molars are absent in children. The progression of deciduous teeth to 32 permanent teeth begins at about 6 years of age, optimizing mastication and swallowing. Prior to molars erupting, children are able to bite off pieces of food with their incisors but unable to grind it adequately in preparation for swallowing, making them vulnerable to choking with particular food such as nuts, popcorn, grapes, and hotdogs.

The upper aerodigestive tract is divided into four main areas or spaces: the oral cavity, nasopharynx, oropharynx, and hypopharynx. These main spaces are further subdivided into smaller spaces including the piriform sinuses and vallecula, through which a bolus and liquids pass during a normal swallow. This is in comparison to the lateral and anterior sulci, laryngeal vestibule, and laryngeal ventricle which are spaces that normally do not come in contact with the ingested bolus [2]. When residue of liquids or solids is noted in any of these spaces at the conclusion of a swallow, this is indicative of dysphagia. The major salivary glands including the parotid, submandibular, and sublingual glands found in the oral cavity produce 95% of saliva [7]. Minor salivary glands that line the oral mucosa produce additional saliva. Saliva aids with mastication and bolus preparation and transport. Saliva is mostly composed of water; however, the enzymes found within the saliva initiate the digestive process [7].

Neuroanatomy of Swallowing

Swallowing pathways involve a complex neuronal network including portions of the supratentorium (cortical and subcortical), infratentorium (brain stem), and peripheral nervous system (motor and sensory) [2]. Cortical regions including the primary and secondary sensorimotor cortices are active during the voluntary oral preparatory and oral transport phases of swallowing. Several cortical and subcortical sites that are active during the pharyngeal phase of swallowing include the primary and secondary cortices, insula, anterior and posterior cingulate cortices, basal ganglia, amygdala, hypothalamus, and substantia nigra. The medulla oblongata housed within the brain stem is especially active during the involuntary pharyngeal and esophageal phases of swallowing. The regulation of these two phases is aided by a central pattern generator (CPG) found within the medulla oblongata [8]. CPGs are neuronal networks that can produce rhythmic patterned outputs such as respiration and deglutition [8]. Motor neurons that are involved in the swallowing CPG are localized in the brain stem. These motor neurons include the trigeminal, facial, hypoglossal, and motor nuclei, the nucleus ambiguous, and the dorsal motor nucleus of the vagus nerve and two cervical spinal neurons (C1 and C3) [8]. Sensory neurons that regulate the pharyngeal and esophageal phases of swallowing are housed within the brain stem and include the nucleus of the solitary tract and the neighboring reticular formation [2]. Both motor and sensory neurons are found bilaterally within the medulla oblongata and form what is known as the swallowing center (swallowing CPG).

Muscle movements are controlled by several cranial and peripheral nerves and are coordinated within the swallowing center of the brain stem. Oral sensation is transmitted in the trigeminal nerve (CN V). Efferent information in the trigeminal nerve goes to the mylohyoid muscle, the anterior belly of the digastric muscle, and the four muscles of mastication: the masseter, temporalis, and pterygoid muscles. The facial nerve (CN VII) mediates taste sensation from the anterior 2/3 of the tongue. The facial nerve is also responsible for efferent control to the salivary glands, the muscles of facial expression, the stylohyoid, the platysma, and the posterior belly of the digastric muscle. The glossopharyngeal nerve (CN IX) carries taste information from the posterior 1/3 of the tongue. The glossopharyngeal nerve innervates the stylopharyngeal muscle. The most important nerve for swallowing is the vagus nerve (CN X). The pharyngeal and laryngeal mucosae are innervated by the vagus nerve. A branch of the vagus nerve, the recurrent laryngeal nerve, transmits sensation from below the vocal folds and the esophagus. Efferent control in the vagus nerve is facilitated by the ambiguous nucleus (striated muscle) and the posterior nucleus of the vagus (smooth muscles and glands). The intrinsic and some of the extrinsic muscles of the tongue are innervated by the hypoglossal nerve (CN XII).

Muscular Control

Finely tuned coordination of more than 30 muscles located within the oral cavity, pharynx, larynx, and esophagus is necessary for a normal swallow (Table 1.1). The majority of the muscles involved with swallowing are striated, with the exception of the medial and distal esophagus, which have segments that are partially or

Table 1.1 Involved muscles and their innervation and function for the phases of deglutition

Involved muscle	Innervation	Function
Oral preparatory phase		
Orbicularis oris	CN VII	Closes oral fissure; compresses and protrudes lips
Buccinator	CN VII	Presses cheek against teeth
Masseter	CN V_3	Elevates mandible; protrudes mandible
Temporalis	CN V_3	Elevates and retracts mandible
Medial pterygoid	CN V_3	Elevates mandible; protrudes mandible
Lateral pterygoid	CN V_3	Protracts and depresses mandible
Superior longitudinal	CN XII	Curls tongue upward, elevating the tip and sides of tongue
Palatoglossus	CN X	Elevates posterior tongue; pulls soft palate onto tongue
Genioglossus	CN XII	Depresses central part of tongue to form a central trough; tongue protrusion; tongue deviation with unilateral contraction
Oral transport phase		
Genioglossus	CN XII	Depresses central part of tongue to form a central trough; tongue protrusion; tongue deviation with unilateral contraction
Hyoglossus	CN XII	Depresses tongue; retrudes tongue
Styloglossus	CN XII	Retrudes tongue; curls up sides of tongue
Palatoglossus	CN X	Elevates posterior tongue; pulls soft palate onto tongue
Superior longitudinal	CN XII	Curls tongue upward, elevating the tip and sides of tongue

Table 1.1 (continued)

Involved muscle	Innervation	Function
Levator veli palatini	CN X	Elevates soft palate
Musculus uvulae	CN X	Shortens and elevates uvula
Superior pharyngeal constrictor	CN X	Constricts pharyngeal walls
Mylohyoid	CN V	Elevates hyoid bone, floor of mouth, and tongue
Stylohyoid	CN VII	Elevates and retracts hyoid bone
Geniohyoid	CN XII; C1–C2	Moves hyoid bone anteriorly and superiorly
Anterior belly of digastric	CN V_3	Depresses and stabilizes mandible; elevates hyoid bone
Posterior belly of digastric	CN VII	Elevates hyoid bone
Thyrohyoid	CN XII; C1	Depresses hyoid bone; elevates larynx
Stylopharyngeus	CN IX	Elevates pharynx and larynx
Palatopharyngeus	CN X	Tenses soft palate; pulls walls of pharynx superiorly, anteriorly, and medially
Salpingopharyngeus	CN X	Elevates pharynx and larynx
Pharyngeal phase		
Lateral cricoarytenoid	CN X	Adducts true vocal folds
Transverse arytenoid	CN X	Adducts true vocal folds
Thyroarytenoid	CN X	Relaxes vocal ligament; narrows laryngeal inlet
Hyoglossus	CN XII	Depresses tongue; retrudes tongue
Styloglossus	CN XII	Retrudes tongue; curls up sides of tongue
Superior pharyngeal constrictor	CN X	Constricts pharyngeal walls
Middle pharyngeal constrictor	CN X	Constricts pharyngeal walls
Inferior pharyngeal constrictor	CN X	Constricts pharyngeal walls
Mylohyoid	CN V	Elevates hyoid bone, floor of mouth, and tongue
Stylohyoid	CN VII	Elevates and retracts hyoid bone
Geniohyoid	CN XII; C1–C2	Moves hyoid bone anteriorly and superiorly
Anterior belly of digastric	CN V_3	Depresses and stabilizes mandible; elevates hyoid bone
Posterior belly of digastric	CN VII	Elevates hyoid bone
Thyrohyoid	CN XII; C1	Depresses hyoid bone; elevates larynx
Cricopharyngeus	CN IX, X	Constricts pharynx at pharyngoesophageal junction
Proximal esophagus	CN X	Peristalsis
Esophageal phase		
Esophagus	CN X	Peristalsis

CN cranial nerve, *C1* cervical spinal nerve 1, *C2* cervical spinal nerve 2 completely smooth muscle [2] (Figs. 1.1, 1.2 and 1.3). Somatic afferent and efferent feedback is provided mainly by cranial and peripheral nerves for striated musculature and an autonomic enteric system for the smooth muscle [2]. The act of swallowing is divided into four phases: oral preparatory phase, oral transport phase, pharyngeal phase, and esophageal phase. The initial oral stages of deglutition are voluntary and trigger the subsequent involuntary pharyngeal and esophageal phases [10].

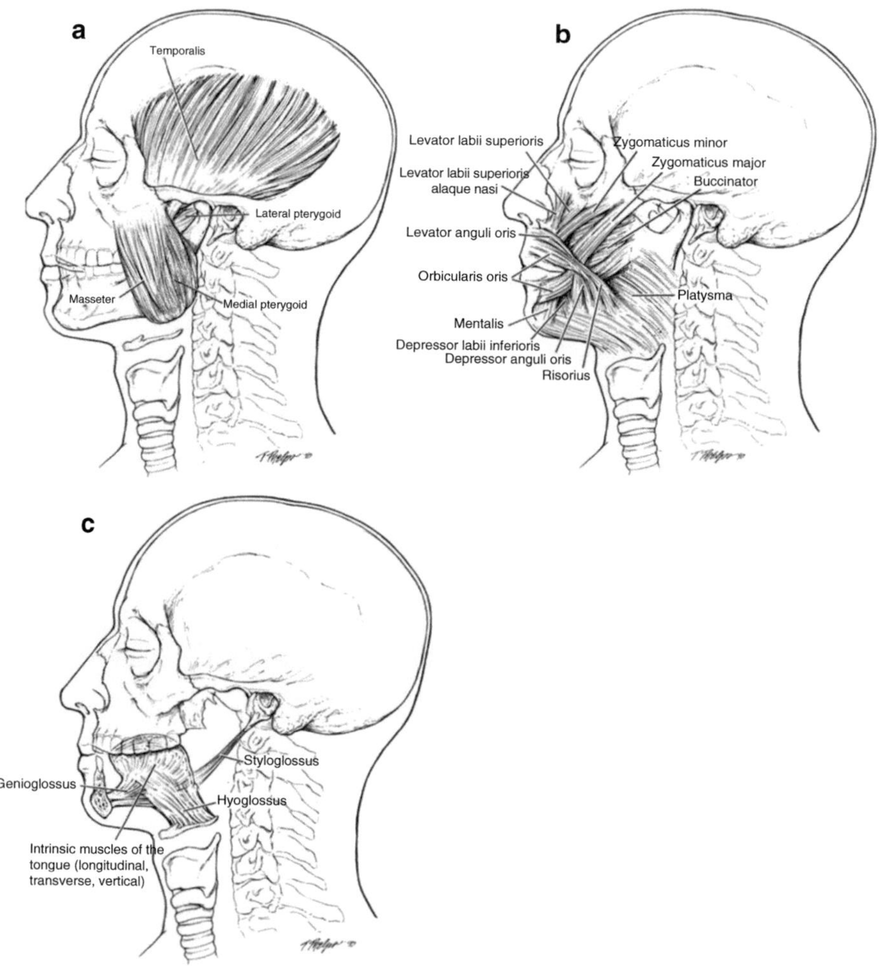

Fig. 1.1 Anatomical relationship of muscles contributing to the oral phase of swallowing. These muscles are controlled by discrete groups of motor neurons in the fifth (**a**), seventh (**b**), and twelfth (**c**) cranial motor nuclei. (From [9]. With permission of Springer)

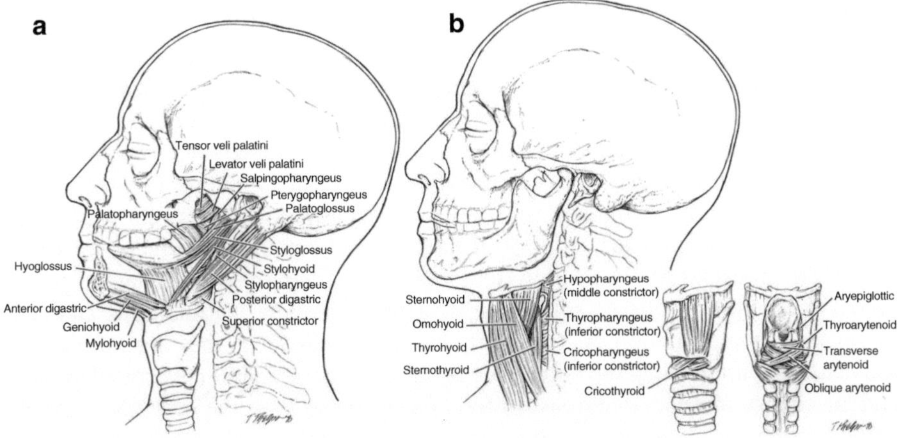

Fig. 1.2 Anatomical relationship of muscles contributing to the pharyngeal phase of swallowing. These muscles are controlled by discrete groups of motor neurons in the fifth, seventh, and twelfth cranial motor nuclei and by motor neurons in the cervical portions of the spinal cord. These muscles are thought of as acting in either the early (**a**) or late (**b**) pharyngeal phase of swallowing. The intrinsic and extrinsic laryngeal muscles also are shown (**b**). (From [9]. With permission of Springer)

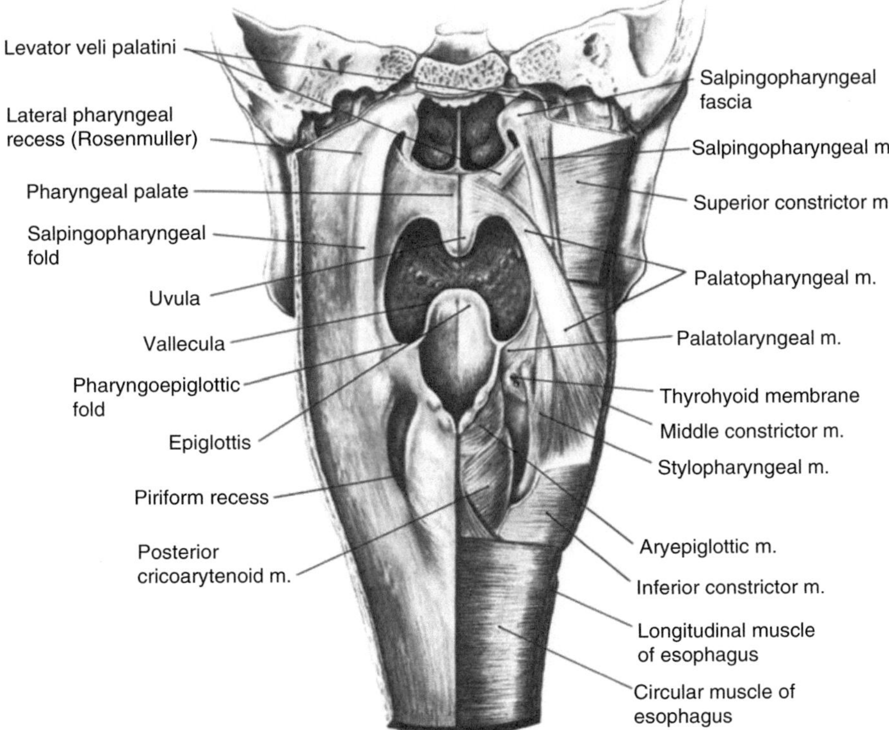

Fig. 1.3 Posterior view of internal pharyngeal musculature and recesses. The mucosa has been stripped from the left half of the preparation to better demonstrate the musculature. (From [9]. With permission of Springer)

Oral Preparatory Phase

The first phase of swallowing, the oral preparatory phase, breaks down food with mastication and forms a bolus in the oral cavity (Fig. 1.4). Bolus formation involves the coordination of lip, buccal, mandibular, and tongue movements. Closure of the upper esophageal sphincter (UES) during this phase is vital to prevent food or liquid from leaving the oral cavity until the individual is ready to initiate swallowing. This phase is under the voluntary control of three cranial nerves. The trigeminal nerve controls the muscles of mastication (temporalis, masseter, medial and lateral ptery-goids) that help break down solid food by actively moving the mandible and also relays sensory information. As food particles are broken down, they are softened by saliva to aid with forming the bolus. The facial nerve coordinates the orbicularis oris and buccinator muscles that assist in food position and keep the oral cavity sealed without premature leakage into the oropharynx. Lateral and vertical tongue move-ments controlled by the hypoglossal nerve help position the food between the teeth. Once the bolus is formed, it is contained between the dorsal surface of the tongue and hard palate. The palatoglossus muscle depresses the soft palate and elevates the posterior tongue, creating a seal against the oropharynx. This prevents premature entry of the bolus into the pharynx. The bolus is captured over the dorsum of the tongue in a spoonlike form, as the genioglossus muscle contracts [2, 12].

Oral Transport Phase

Once a bolus has been formed, it is transitioned into the oropharynx in the oral trans-port phase. The tongue sits partly in the oral cavity and partly in the oropharynx. It is made up of eight pairs of muscles subdivided into intrinsic and extrinsic muscles. The four intrinsic muscles, vertical, transverse, superior longitudinal, and inferior

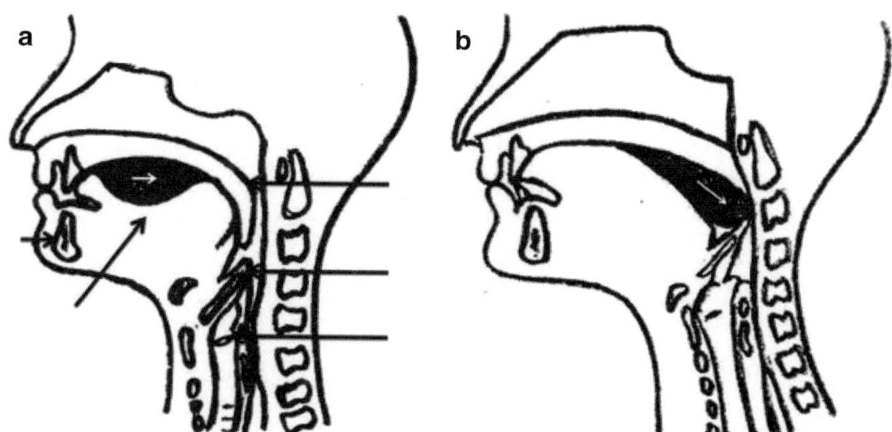

Fig. 1.4 Oral phase of swallowing: (**a**) the bolus is held between the anterior end of the tongue and the hard palate during the initiation of the oral phase, and (**b**) the bolus is propelled into the phar-ynx to trigger the pharyngeal phase. (From [11]. With permission of Springer)

longitudinal muscles, control the shape of the tongue [10]. The extrinsic muscles including the genioglossus, hyoglossus, styloglossus, and palatoglossus control the position of the tongue. The hypoglossal nerve innervates all the muscles of the tongue except the extrinsic palatoglossus muscles, which are innervated by the pharyngeal plexus [13]. These intrinsic and extrinsic muscles of the tongue elevate the tongue in an anterior to posterior fashion to push against the hard palate and propel the bolus toward the oropharynx in a wavelike motion [12]. Simultaneously, the soft palate elevates by contraction of the levator veli palatini and musculus uvulae while the base of tongue moves anteriorly and inferiorly to open the path to the oropharynx [2]. The soft palate also seals off the nasopharynx from the oropharynx, along with the contraction of the superior pharyngeal constrictors, which narrow the nasopharynx to aid with closure and prevent nasal regurgitation. The anterior-superior movement of the base of tongue, hyoid bone, and larynx due to the contraction of the suprahyoid muscles (mylohyoid, stylohyoid, geniohyoid, anterior digastric, and posterior digastric) and the thyrohyoid muscle widens the pharynx. The relaxation of the pharyngeal elevators, stylopharyngeus, palatopharyngeus, and salpingopharyngeus, also widens the pharynx transversely. A ramp is created due to the flattening of the posterior tongue, enabling the bolus to slide into the oropharynx [12].

Pharyngeal Phase

As the bolus is transported into the pharynx, the pharyngeal phase ensues (Fig. 1.5). The pharyngeal phase of swallowing is initiated voluntarily as the bolus crosses the anterior tonsillar pillars by sensory information transmitted by the glossopharyngeal and vagus nerves. Once triggered this complex phase is involuntary and generally lasts 1 second [10]. This pharyngeal swallow response can be affected and modified by food properties such as taste, volume, and texture [2]. When the pharyngeal swallow is triggered, respiration pauses to protect the airway by the contraction of the lateral cricoarytenoid,

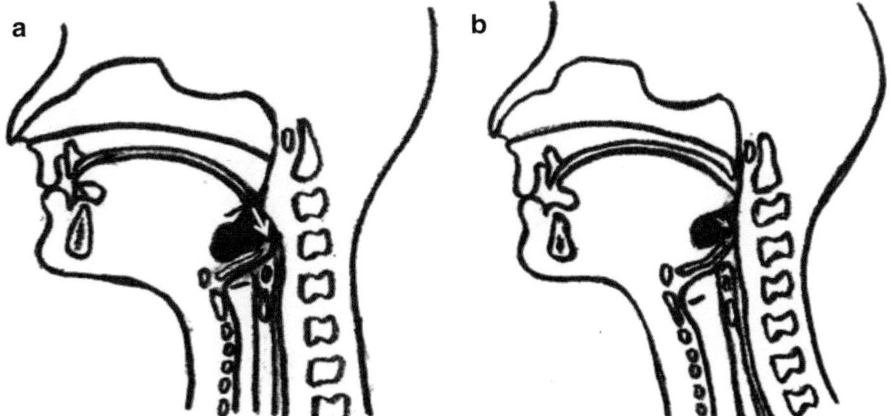

Fig. 1.5 Pharyngeal phase of swallow: the soft palate is elevated and in contact with the pharyngeal wall. The laryngeal inlet is protected by the epiglottis. (**a**) Bolus in the vallecula and (**b**) the tongue base retracted posteriorly toward the pharyngeal wall. (From [11]. With permission of Springer)

transverse arytenoid, and thyroarytenoid muscles, with resultant adduction of the true vocal folds. The pharyngeal muscles including the palatopharyngeus, stylopharyngeus, and salpingopharyngeus then contract to elevate the pharynx superiorly. Simultaneously, the tongue base is retracted toward the posterior pharyngeal wall by the contraction of the hyoglossus and styloglossus muscles activating the contraction of the pharyngeal constrictors (superior, middle, and inferior) in a rostral-caudal direction [2]. The peristaltic contractions induced by the pharyngeal constrictors are known as pharyngeal peristalsis or the pharyngeal stripping wave which squeezes the bolus through the pharynx and into the UES. The anterior and superior movement of the hyoid and larynx by the suprahyoid muscles and thyrohyoid muscles aids in airway protection by tucking the larynx under the base of the tongue and allowing the epiglottis to invert and divert the bolus away from the laryngeal inlet. A negative pressure is also created under the bolus by the elevation of the larynx and hypopharynx, pulling it toward the esophagus [14]. The laryngeal elevation also affects the cricoid cartilage, which aids in pulling open the UES. The UES is composed of the inferior pharyngeal constrictor muscles, cricopharyngeus, and proximal esophagus. At rest the UES is closed by contractions of the cricopharyngeus, and it opens via the relaxation of the cricopharyngeus muscle as signaled by vagal sensory fibers, as well as by distension from the incoming bolus [15, 16]. The resultant negative pressure in the upper esophagus further aids the bolus to move down into the esophagus [14].

Esophageal Phase

The esophageal phase is involuntary and begins once the bolus passes through the UES and enters the esophagus (Fig. 1.6). This is coordinated by the autonomic nervous system through the vagus nerves and the sympathetic ganglia [15]. Relaxation of the UES is very brief lasting approximately 0.5–1.2 s, giving just enough time for the food to

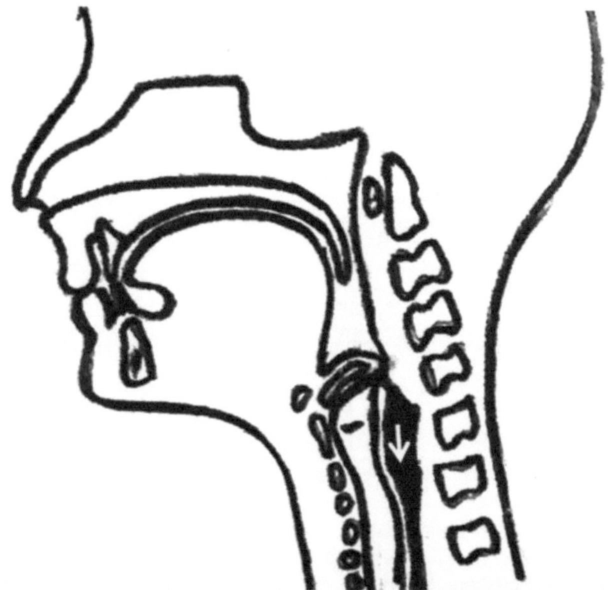

Fig. 1.6 Esophageal phase of swallowing. (From [11]. With permission of Springer)

pass through the UES and into the esophagus [17]. The UES closes again by the contraction of the cricopharyngeus muscle, preventing any retrograde motion of the bolus into the hypopharynx. Once the bolus passes through the UES, it is pushed through the esophagus toward the stomach by peristaltic waves. A primary wave of peristalsis begins in the pharynx and extends down to the stomach [15]. Secondary waves of peristalsis can continue for an hour after the swallow to ensure any residue in the esophagus passes into the stomach [7, 8]. Peristaltic waves in the superior two-thirds of the esophagus progress more rapidly than the inferior one-third secondary to the superior aspect of the esophagus being composed of striated muscle versus the inferior one-third being made up of smooth muscle [10]. The lower esophageal sphincter (LES) consists of a 2–4 cm zone of increased pressure at the lower end of the esophagus. To avoid regurgitation of stomach contents, the LES is contracted at rest from an intrinsic force created by the internal circular muscle fibers of the esophagus and an extrinsic force created by diaphragmatic pressure [10]. Once the bolus passes into the esophagus, these forces relax opening the LES just before the peristaltic wave carrying the bolus reaches it, allowing the bolus to pass through the LES into the stomach.

Infant Swallow

The act of swallowing differs in infants and adults. In infants the teeth have not erupted, the hard palate is flatter, and the hyoid bone and larynx are at a higher position in the neck (C2–C3 level) [6]. As a result, the epiglottis touches the posterior end of the soft palate, and the larynx communicates with the nasopharynx, but the oropharynx is closed away from the airway during swallowing [6] (Fig. 1.7). This protects the infant from aspiration. During the second year of life, the neck elongates and the larynx starts to descend to a lower position.

Swallowing in the infant consists of three components: (1) the suck reflex, which is defined as the delivery system and includes the orobuccal phase of deglutition; (2) the collecting system, the oropharynx; and (3) the transport system defined by the esophagus [18]. Embryologically, swallowing is thought to start in the fetus as early as the 12th week of pregnancy [15]. Sucking and swallowing functions are vital to the newborn infant. Sucking reflexively triggers swallowing in the infant by stimulation of the lips and deeper parts of the oral cavity. The mandible and components of the maxilla including the upper gums, lips, palate, and cheeks allow compression of the nipple and expression of its contents. For the first 3 months of life, the infants fail to differentiate between liquids and solids and attempt to use the same sucking action for both [15]. As the infant develops, the tongue, lips, and mandible are able to achieve the independent functions of biting, chewing, moving food, and forming a bolus.

Airway Protection Mechanisms

Airway protection is a crucial component of swallowing. Respiration and swallowing use similar anatomic pathways, making the coordination of deglutination and respiration necessary to prevent aspiration. Laryngeal penetration is defined as the

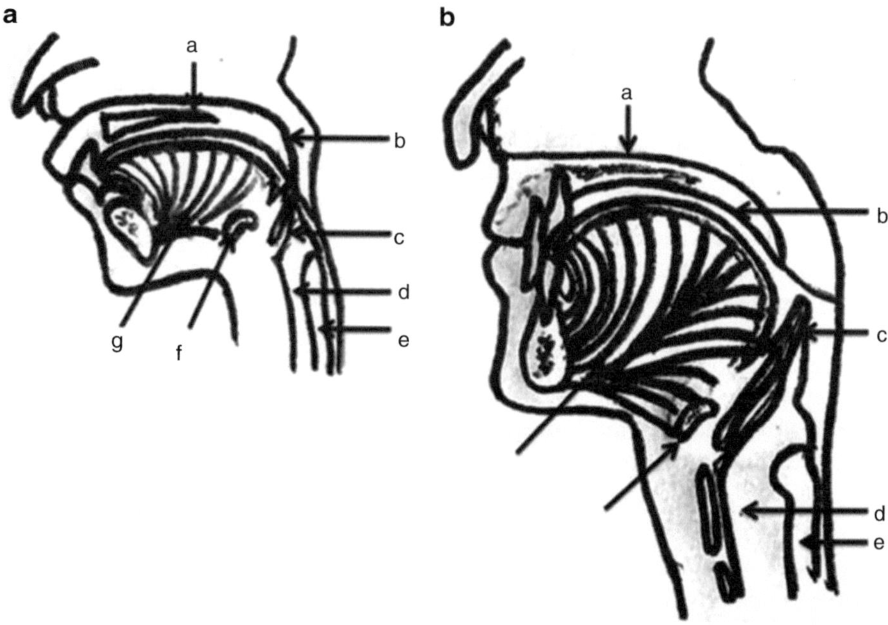

Fig. 1.7 Difference between infant (**a**) and adult (**b**) swallowing passages. In (**a**), the palate is flatter, the epiglottis touches the soft palate, and the hyoid is at a higher position. In (**b**), the palate is more curved, the epiglottis and palate are not in contact, and the oral cavity is larger. *a* hard palate, *b* soft palate, *c* epiglottis, *d* larynx, *e* esophagus, *f* hyoid bone, *g* tongue. (From [6]. With permission of Springer)

passage of material from the mouth or regurgitated from the esophagus that enters into the larynx above the vocal folds [16]. Aspiration is the passage of food, liquid, or secretions past the vocal cords into the trachea. Aspiration can occur before, during, or after swallowing. Laryngeal penetration and microscopic quantities of aspiration can occur in normal individuals. The consequence of aspiration is variable ranging from no effect to aspiration pneumonia or airway obstruction [16].

As described in the pharyngeal phase of deglutition, the airway is protected by glottic closure, epiglottic deflection, and cessation in respiration usually during exhalation. The glottic closure acts as a physical barrier at the laryngeal inlet and temporarily halts respiration until the bolus clears the hypopharynx and enters the esophagus [2]. The epiglottic deflection, secondary to posterior deflection of the epiglottis over the larynx aided by the anterior movement of the arytenoids, creates a physical barrier and allows food or liquid to flow around the airway and into the esophagus [2]. Two laryngeal reflexes also assist in protecting the airway [15]. The sensory innervation of the laryngeal surface is provided by the internal branch of the superior laryngeal nerve (ISLN) of the vagus nerve. The ISLN is essential in ensuring the airway is completely closed during swallowing and in triggering the laryngeal adductor response (LAR) and the laryngeal cough reflex (LCR) that help clear any penetrated or aspirated bolus from the airway. Once the LAR is triggered, the true vocal folds immediately adduct with contraction of the thyroarytenoid muscles to close the airway. The LCR can be triggered not only by tactile but also chemical stimulation of the larynx or trachea and leads to involuntary coughing that aims to clear the airway. Abnormal function of the ISLN places individuals at risk for aspiration and consequent pneumonia [2].

Conclusion

Deglutition is a complex process that involves coordinated movements within the oral cavity, pharynx, larynx, and esophagus. The act of swallowing is divided into four main phases: oral preparatory phase, oral transport phase, pharyngeal phase, and esophageal phase. Precise synchronization between respiration and swallowing is necessary to protect the airway and prevent aspiration. Understanding the normal anatomy and physiology of swallowing is pertinent to successfully diagnosing and treating swallowing dysfunctions.

References

1. Lear CS, Flanagan JB, Moorrees CF. The frequency of deglutition in man. Arch Oral Biol. 1965;10:83–100.
2. Shaw SM, Martino R. The normal swallow: muscular and neurophysiological control. Otolaryngol Clin N Am. 2013;46:937–56.
3. Graney DO, KCY S. Anatomy and developmental embryology of the neck. In: Flint PW, Haughey BH, Lund VJ, Niparko JK, Richardson MA, Robbins KT, et al., editors. Cummings otolaryngology. 5th ed. Philadelphia: Elsevier; 2010. p. 2577–86.
4. Frisdal A, Trainor PA. Development and evolution of the pharyngeal apparatus. Wiley Interdiscip Rev Dev Biol. 2008;3:403–18.
5. Licameli GR, Richardson MA. Diagnosis and management of tracheal anomalies and tracheal stenosis. In: Flint PW, Haughey BH, Lund VJ, Niparko JK, Richardson MA, Robbins KT, et al., editors. Cummings otolaryngology. 5th ed. Philadelphia: Elsevier; 2010. p. 2925–34.
6. Chavan K. Anatomy of swallowing. In: Mankekar G, editor. Swallowing-physiology, disorders, diagnosis, and therapy. New Delhi: Springer; 2015. p. 1–20.
7. Edgar WM. Saliva: its secretion, composition and functions. Br Dent J. 1992;172:305–12.
8. Jean A. Brain stem control of swallowing: localization and organization of the central pattern generator for swallowing. In: Taylor A, editor. Neurophysiology of jaws and teeth. London: Macmillan; 1990. p. 294–321.
9. Cunningham EJ, Jones B. Anatomical and physiological overview. In: Jones B, editor. Normal and abnormal swallowing: imaging in diagnosis and therapy. New York: Springer; 2003.
10. Hennessy M, Goldenberg D. Surgical anatomy and physiology of swallowing. Oper Tech Otolaryngol. 2016;27:60–6.
11. Mankekar G, Chavan K. Physiology of swallowing and esophageal function tests. In: Mankekar G, editor. Swallowing – physiology, disorders, diagnosis and therapy. New Delhi: Springer India; 2015.
12. Dodds WJ, Stewart ET, Logeman JA. Physiology pharyngeal and radiology of the normal phases of swallowing. Am J Roentgenol. 1990;154:953–63.

13. Shah S, Garriano F. Pediatric oral anatomy. Oper Tech Otolaryngol Head Neck Surg. 2015;26:2–7.
14. McConnel FM. Analysis of pressure generation and bolus transit during pharyngeal swallowing. Laryngoscope. 1988;98:71–8.
15. Derkay CS, Schechter GL. Anatomy and physiology of pediatric swallowing disorders. Otolaryngol Clin N Am. 1998;31:397–404.
16. Matsuo K, Palmer JB. Anatomy and physiology of feeding and swallowing: normal and abnormal. Phys Med Rehabil Clin N Am Elsevier Inc. 2008;19:691–707.
17. Indelfinger F. Esophageal motility. Physiol Rev. 1958;38:533–84.
18. Bosma F. Third symposium on oral sensation and perception. Thomas CC, editor. Springfield; 1972.

Chapter 2
Maturation of Infant Oral Feeding Skills

Chantal Lau

Abbreviations

CPG	Central pattern generator
EB	Esophageal body
GA	Gestational age
LES	Lower esophageal sphincter
NICU	Neonatal intensive care unit
NSP	Nutritive sucking pathway
PMA	Postmenstrual age
SLOSR	Swallow-induced lower esophageal sphincter relaxation
TLOSR	Transient lower esophageal sphincter relaxation
UES	Upper esophageal sphincter

Introduction

This chapter reviews our latest understanding of the maturation of infant oral feeding skills. This topic has attracted limited attention from the general public and researchers in the past. However, it gained momentum over the last two decades principally due to the increased survival of infants born prematurely. The majority of infants born term customarily can feed by mouth within hours of birth with no apparent difficulty. Unfortunately, this is not so for those born prematurely. An estimated 380,000 babies are born prematurely each year in the United States (~10% of the annual live births) (www.marchofdimes.org; https://www.cdc.gov/reproductive health/maternalinfanthealth/pretermbirth.htm). While 25–35% of normal children report minor feeding difficulties, 40–70% of infants born prematurely or with chronic medical conditions report more severe problems [1].

C. Lau
Pediatrics/Neonatology, Baylor College of Medicine, Houston, TX, USA
e-mail: clau@bcm.edu

© Springer International Publishing AG, part of Springer Nature 2018
J. Ongkasuwan, E. H. Chiou (eds.), *Pediatric Dysphagia*,
https://doi.org/10.1007/978-3-319-97025-7_2

Once the life-threatening events that these preterm infants encounter are overcome, e.g., intraventricular hemorrhage, necrotizing enterocolitis, bronchopulmonary dysplasia, and periventricular leukomalacia, the medical community caring for these infants and particularly neonatologists in neonatal intensive care units (NICUs) struggle with the difficulties that many of these children face when transitioning from tube to independent oral feeding. Delayed attainment of the latter milestone prolongs these infants' discharge home as their ability to safely and competently feed by mouth is one of the major criteria for hospital discharge [2]. Such occurrence not only increases medical cost but unfortunately also delays mother-infant reunification, an important factor likely aggravating maternal stress, breastfeeding outcome, and mother-infant bonding [3–8]. Unfortunately, such multifaceted consequences may shadow these infants' growth and development, their family, and society over the long term. As such, it is pressing to identify early on the causes impeding their ability to readily attain independent oral feeding as this would facilitate the development of evidence-based therapies that would minimize such long-lasting drawbacks.

The management plan of hospitalized patients for any issue customarily proceeds after a proper analysis of the symptoms and their potential causes. Thus, prior to any recommended treatment, a differential diagnosis is advanced after a systematic review of the potential pathophysiological factors involved. In NICUs, as it pertains to high-risk infants' ability to attain independent oral feeding, the medical team includes attending neonatologists, neonatal nurse practitioners, neonatal nurses, and feeding specialists, i.e., lactation consultants, neonatal nutritionists, occupational therapists (OT), and speech-language pathologists (SLP) (Fig. 2.1). As research into the causes of preterm infants' inability to transition from tube to independent oral feeding is ongoing, realization has grown that

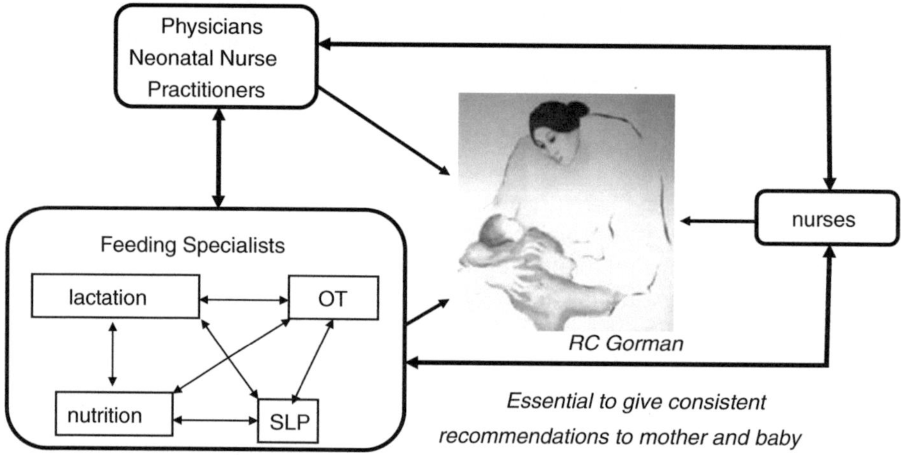

Fig. 2.1 It is important that recommendations provided by the multidisciplinary team members to the mother-infant dyad be consistent throughout their stay in the NICU. OT occupational therapist, SLP speech-language pathologist

caregivers' understanding and approaches to this problem appear constrained by their respective field of expertise. Consequently, consensus for best approach is often debated between the multidisciplinary team members, e.g., best approach to implement oral feeding and importance of qualitative/descriptive vs. quantitative/evidence-based approaches. Any benefit(s) observed following interventions provided by team members is challenged on the basis that it may simply be due to infant normal maturation. Unfortunately, such disagreements often lead to inconsistent messages delivered to the mother-infant dyad by individual caregivers (Fig. 2.1).

Figure 2.2 is a schematic of the "nutritive sucking pathway" (NSP) illustrating the different anatomic and physiologic functions implicated in the transport of a bolus during infant feeding. The corresponding subspecialties implicated if difficulties arise are listed alongside, i.e., occupational therapy, speech-language pathology, pediatric gastroenterology, otolaryngology, and pulmonology. Bolus transport from the oral cavity to the stomach is a continuum of events that must occur swiftly, but in the appropriate *temporal functional* synchrony if it is to be safe and effective. It is essential to know "the feeding physiology during fetal and infant development in order to understand the variety of its disorders and to direct correctly diagnostic and

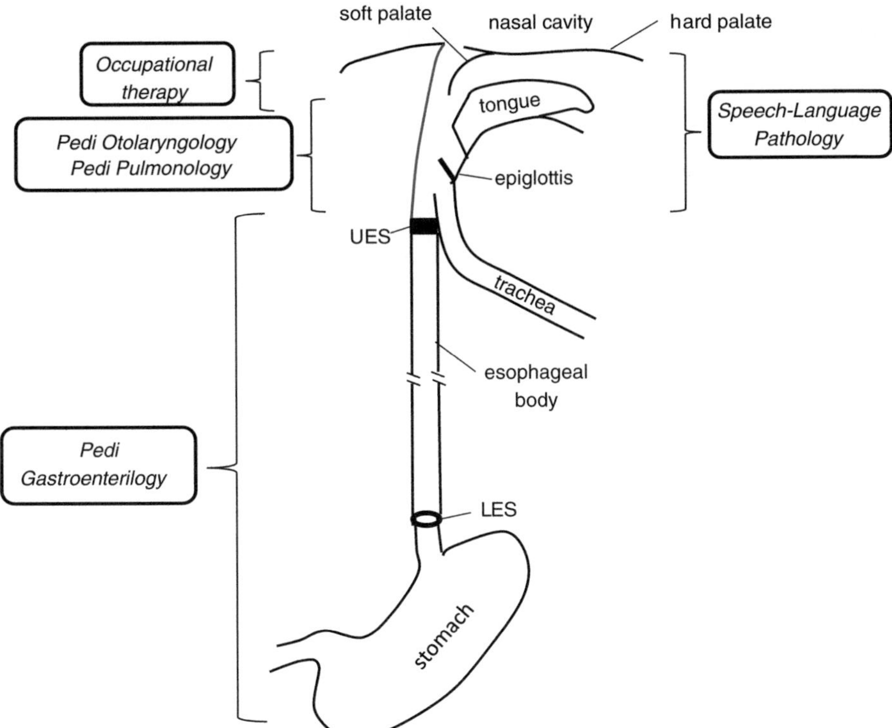

Fig. 2.2 The nutritive sucking pathway – schematic of the physiologic functions implicated in bolus transport from the oral cavity to the stomach and the respective subspecialties commonly involved. UES upper esophageal sphincter, LES lower esophageal sphincter

therapeutic processes" [9]. As such, it is proposed that if the subspecialties involved gain a more integrated understanding of the development/maturation processes of all the functions implicated in the NSP, achieving consensus on the differential diagnosis will be facilitated, followed by determination of most appropriate management. It would naturally flow that compliance to such plan(s) would lead to more consistent feeding approaches and recommendations given to both infants and mothers by team members.

As subsequent chapters describe in greater details treatments and therapies of pediatric dysphagia, this chapter will focus on our current knowledge of the simultaneous maturation of the different physiologic functions involved in *nutritive sucking*. As awareness of the differing timing and rate of maturations of these functions is growing [10], it has become evident that the medical management of these infants needs to continually take into account the ongoing maturation of the individual functions. Indeed, from an observer's perspective, delays/dysfunctions at any level(s) of the NSP will be simply reflected by an overall infant inability to feed such as oxygen desaturation, apnea, and/or bradycardia. Unfortunately, this does not assist in identifying the most likely causes at the root of the feeding problem. The direct visual observation of a rhythmic jaw-lowering pattern during sucking, for instance, is not indicative of the rhythmic functionality of oro-motor musculatures involved in sucking such as the tongue, soft palate, orbicularis oris, masseter, temporal, and suprahyoid muscles [11–15]. Thus assessing infants' "readiness to feed" based only on visual observations is neither reliable nor advisable.

Maturation of Nutritive Sucking

Although sucking has been observed *in utero* as early as 15 weeks gestation (GA), it is uncertain that its functionality is fully developed to face the *ex utero* environment following a premature delivery [16].

A deeper understanding of the development of nutritive sucking has been gained based on the maturation profiles of the *suction* and *expression* component of sucking. As preterm infants transition from tube to independent oral feeding, Fig. 2.3 shows the identification of five descriptive stages of nutritive sucking based on the presence/absence, rhythmicity, and amplitude (mmHg) of the suction and expression components described by Sameroff [17, 18]. *Suction* corresponds to the negative intraoral pressure that draws milk into the mouth in contrast to *expression* which ejects milk into the oral cavity by compression or stripping of the nipple (bottle or breast) between the tongue and the hard palate. Stage 1 with the presence of expression alone is the most immature, and stage 5 with the rhythmic alternation of suction/expression is the most mature which is normally observed in term infants. Expression begins to mature at stage 1, while suction does not appear until stage 2. The maturation profiles of both types of sucking are similar beginning with (1) an arrhythmic appearance, (2) varied amplitudes, (3) rhythmicity attained with varied

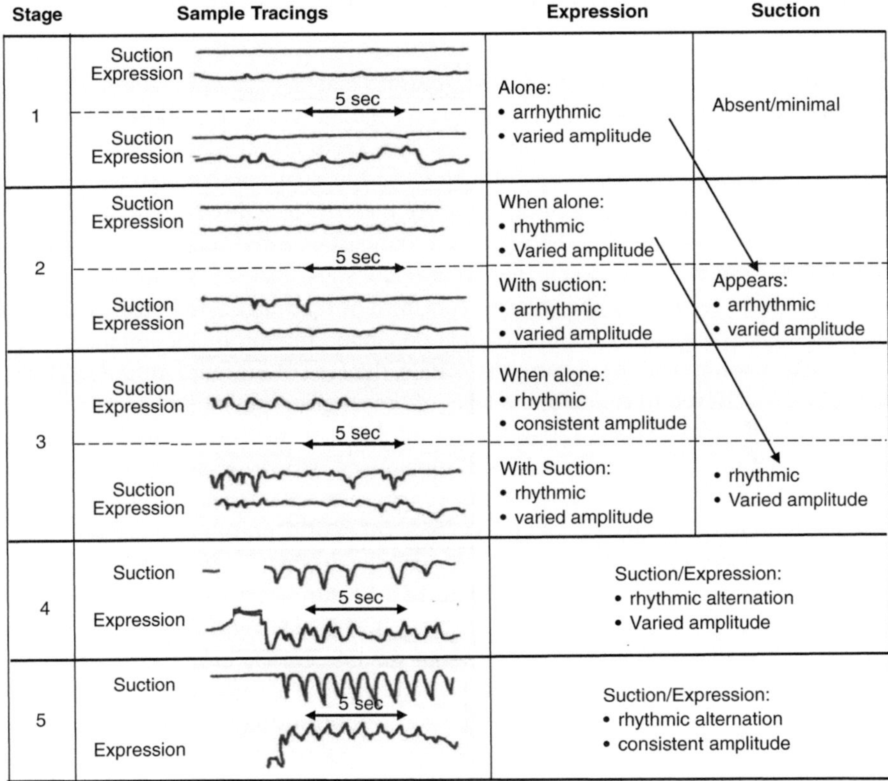

Fig. 2.3 A 5-stage descriptive scale of the maturation process of preterm infants' expression and suction components during nutritive sucking with their respective maturation characteristics

amplitudes, and then (4) rhythmicity attained with consistent amplitude. We observed that these five stages were positively correlated with infants' postmenstrual age (PMA), overall transfer (percent milk taken), and rate of milk transfer (ml/min) over an entire feeding [18]. We further noted that infants using the immature sucking pattern consisting primarily of expression alone can be successful at bottle feeding, albeit not as efficiently as when the more mature stage of alternated suction and expression is used. We speculated that this was likely possible due to the rigidity of the bottle nipple that does not require suction in order to be retained in the mouth during feeding. This contrasts with breastfeeding which, due to the softness of the human breast/nipple, would likely require suction for latching onto the breast and retaining the nipple in the mouth. This may explain why preterm infants perform better at the breast when using a nipple shield when introduced to breastfeeding. As infants within the same gestational age (GA) and PMA can demonstrate a broad range of nutritive sucking aptitude [18, 19], immature nutritive sucking skills may only be one of the reasons an infant feeds poorly.

Maturation of the Oral and Pharyngeal Phase of Deglutition

The swallowing process commonly distinguishes between the oral, pharyngeal, and esophageal phases corresponding to bolus formation and its transport through the pharynx and esophagus, respectively [20]. This section will focus on the oral and pharyngeal phases. The formation of a bolus and its transport through the pharynx require complex sensorimotor interactions followed by executive motor outputs that may not yet be developed in the premature infant. Once an infant latches onto the nipple (breast or bottle) and achieves an efficient suck, the milk bolus is contained in a depression formed by the anterior two third of the tongue and pushed into the oropharyngeal passage by an anterograde peristaltic motion of the tongue against the hard and soft palate. As it currently stands, the area of initiation of the swallowing reflex is believed to reside at the level of the anterior faucial arches, around the epiglottis/vallecular regions [20–22]. The mechanism involved in the pharyngeal transport of a bolus in infants is not well understood. However, taking advantage of technologies developed to obtain kinematic measurements during modified barium swallow studies conducted on adults, two types of contractions have been proposed. A pharyngeal shortening is initiated decreasing the distance between the base of the tongue and the upper esophageal sphincter (UES) during the oropharyngeal phase and is followed by the sequential constriction of the superior, middle, and inferior pharyngeal constrictor muscles that generate an anterograde propulsive contractile wave that carries the bolus toward the UES [23, 24]. This anterograde propulsion parallels the rostro-caudal peristaltic transport of bolus/food observed in the upper and lower gastrointestinal tract.

There is a broad "assortment" of anatomic elements implicated at each step of deglutition. Briefly, the swallow reflex may be hampered by an improper synchronization of the lingual muscles during the bolus formation, its coordination with the closure of the nasal passage by the soft palate to prevent nasal reflux, and its propulsion into the pharynx [25–30]. Once the swallow reflex is generated, safety requires that no penetration/aspiration of liquid into the lungs occurs. However, these adverse events may occur prior to deglutition as a result of poor bolus formation with liquid draining into the pharynx prior to the initiation of the swallow reflex (spillage), during deglutition due to poor or improper closure of the epiglottis as the bolus travels down the pharynx, and/or after deglutition due to residual around the valleculae/pyriform sinuses as a consequence of a weak bolus propulsion from uncoordinated pharyngeal constrictor muscles [20, 31]. In infants, research has shown that with maturation, the swallowing process becomes more adaptable. For instance, formation of the bolus during the oral phase is swifter, there is an increase in the anterograde propulsive contractile wave or "intrabolus pressure" necessary to propel the bolus beyond the UES, infants can handle larger and/or varying bolus sizes, and their ability to increase swallowing rate (swifter deglutition) increases [32–34]. In summary, inappropriate bolus formation, pharyngeal constrictor activity, and/or intrabolus pressure may lead to poor bolus entry into the esophagus. Untimely coordination with epiglottis closure during the swallowing event increases risks of penetration/aspiration into the lungs.

Maturation of Respiration

Nutritive sucking averages one suck per second [35]. Given that clinically stable preterm infants breathe between 40 and 60 breaths/min or 1.5 to 1 breath/s, and pharyngeal swallows may last between 0.37 and 0.7 s, these infants have 0.73–0.3 s left to safely breathe [36]. Additionally, proper oxygenation may be further threatened as minute ventilation is decreased resulting from a decrease in respiratory rate while accompanied with prolonged exhalation and shortened inhalation [37, 38]. It is thus not surprising that many infants do not tolerate oral feeding over an extended time period due to compromise of respiration.

Maturation of the Esophageal Phase of Deglutition

Although the esophagus is a conduit for the transport of the bolus between the pharynx to the stomach, its complex physiology relies on three distinct elements, the upper esophageal sphincter (UES), the esophageal body (EB), and the lower esophageal sphincter (LES), each with differing developmental and functional characteristics. Our understanding has advanced as a result of the continued development of new technologies specially designed to accommodate the fragility and small size of preterm infants, i.e., multichannel esophageal manometry, multichannel intraluminal impedance with/without pH detection(MII/pH-MII), and high-resolution manometry [39–41]. It is expected that technologies currently being developed in children and adults will become available to this infant population in the near future further assisting our understanding of infant oral feeding difficulties, e.g., pressure-flow analysis, integrating pressure, and impedance analysis [42–47].

The UES is a high-pressured zone comprised of the cricopharyngeus, proximal cervical esophagus, and inferior pharyngeal constrictor. The function of the UES during feeding is primarily in preventing esophagopharyngeal reflux during esophageal retrograde activities, as well as decreasing esophageal air insufflation or aerophagia when intrathoracic pressure becomes negative during inhalation (https://www.nature.com/gimo/contents/pt1/full/gimo12.html#).

Jadcherla et al. did not observe any significant difference in UES resting pressure between term and preterm infants (29/9 ± 2.5 weeks GA) monitored at 33–35 weeks PMA [48]. Using high-resolution manometry, Rommel et al. monitored the pharyngoesophageal function of healthy preterm infants (28 ± 1.9 weeks GA) over a 4-week period ranging from 31 to 36 weeks postmenstrual age (PMA), starting from the time they were introduced to oral feeding [49]. Although the UES pressure at relaxation onset and nadir and relaxation duration were not significant between age groups, the UES relaxation *response time* from onset of relaxation to the nadir pressure shortened significantly with age. More specifically, compared to older counterparts (≥ 33 weeks PMA), younger infants (31–32 weeks PMA) took a longer time to reach nadir UES relaxation while demonstrating greater variance in this measure. This would suggest that with maturation, the UES remains at nadir pressure longer, thereby favoring optimal bolus passage across the UES.

As pertaining to esophageal body (EB) activities, premature infants demonstrated greater occurrence of esophageal non-peristaltic patterns, i.e., asynchronous, incomplete, or retrograde waves instead of anterograde peristaltic waves. With maturation, the frequency of these non-peristaltic patterns decreased leading to a greater proportion of anterograde peristaltic waves and improvement in migratory velocity [41, 50–52]. Staiano et al. used high-resolution manometry (HRM) to distinguish between three sequential pressure segments along the EB and observed that only the second pressure segment in the mid-esophagus (proximal smooth muscle region) was well developed before term, while the other two proximal and distal segments continued to improve by term [53]. Such functional immaturity would likely be implicated in infant's oral feeding difficulties and reflux disorder.

The LES is a region of smooth muscle thickening at the esophagogastric junction. There are two primary types of LES relaxation (LESR), namely, swallow-related LESR (SLESR) and transient LESR (TLESR). SLESR allows for the passage of swallowed boluses to properly enter the stomach. Sensorimotor kinetics of LESR appear to depend on the mechanosensitive properties of the stimulus, e.g., media, volume, flow, and type of peristaltic reflex as infants mature [54]. TLESR which occur independently of swallowing typically exhibit a longer and more complete relaxation creating a "common cavity" between esophagus and stomach, thereby facilitating retrograde gastroesophageal reflux as seen in Fig. 2.4 [55, 56]. It is uncertain whether TLESR occur more frequently in preterm than term infants.

In brief, with maturation there is improved synchronization of UES, esophageal body motility, and LES: (i) peak pharyngeal pressure increases above the UES, and UES full relaxation occurs more rapidly implying a more efficient and safe entry into the EB; (ii) esophageal propagating waveforms increase over non-propagating waveforms, concurrently with migratory velocity in the EB, suggesting a faster and safer bolus transport; and (iii) LES relaxation is more timely during transport of luminal contents inferring a more fluent and safer delivery into the stomach.

Simultaneous Maturation of Sucking, Deglutition, Respiration, and Esophageal Function

The information provided above pertains to our current understanding of the maturation profiles of the individual physiologic functions of the NSP. Although we have acquired a better understanding of these individual functions, we do not yet understand how they "interlock" as they mature to ensure the smooth transport of luminal contents from the mouth to the stomach particularly in the case of preterm infants. Caregivers do recognize that immature sucking, delayed swallow, and uncoordinated suck-swallow-respiration are potential causes for

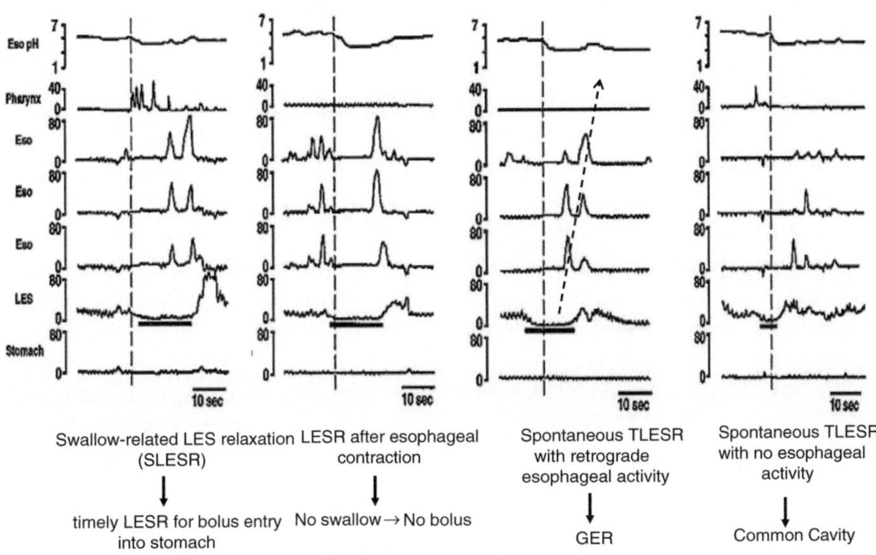

Fig. 2.4 Examples of LES relaxation patterns observed in preterm infants and their potential impact. (Reprinted from Omari et al. [55]. Copyright 1998, with permission from Elsevier)

oral feeding issues and that within each of these functions, there are components that may mature at different times as we have shown in the development of nutritive sucking [10, 57, 58]. Therefore, it is likely that the difficulty encountered by preterm infants to feed by mouth may not only result from individual underdeveloped functions but also from the improper sequential maturation of the coordinated activities of sucking, swallowing, respiration, and esophageal function. All these events are under complex neural control involving sensory afferent and motor efferent branches of cranial nerves V, VII, IX, X, and XII at various levels [20, 59].

In our studies, we hypothesize that such development occurs at two levels: first, appropriate functional maturation needs to occur *within* a physiologic function with the appropriate *synchronization* of the muscles implicated within each function; second, proper *coordination between* functional musculatures of these different functions must follow. Synchronized and coordinated activities necessitate the close interactions between different sets of muscles or functional musculatures, respectively [10, 60]. For instance, at the first level, the synchronization of the "sucking musculature" would require the timely inputs between oral muscles, e.g., the perioral facial and jaw muscles to generate suction, the orbicularis oris to minimize spillage from the mouth, and the lingual muscles for the generation of the expression component (compression/stripping), bolus formation, and its oropharyngeal transport. Swallowing similarly would implicate the synchronization of the "swallowing musculature," e.g., the participation of the soft palate closing the nasal cavity to prevent nasal reflux and the appropriate timing of the epiglottis closure/

opening as the bolus passes through to prevent penetration/aspiration into the lungs and pharyngeal constrictor muscles to rapidly transport the bolus toward the UES. Esophageal transport would require the synchronization of the "esophageal musculature," e.g., the timely sequential UES relaxation and closure upon bolus transfer into the EB, esophageal anterograde peristaltic waves, and LES timely relaxation and closure to allow a smooth bolus transport into the stomach before the next bolus arrives. At the same time, proper activation of the "respiratory musculature," i.e., diaphragm, intercostal muscles, and upper airway musculature from the nose to the glottis, would be required to provide proper oxygen saturation. At the second level, all these differing *functional* musculatures need to work in a proper temporal sequence to ensure the efficient flow of continued luminal contents over an entire feeding session.

We have begun to provide support for this concept as it pertains to the interactions between suction and expression discussed earlier (Fig. 2.3). As oral feeding performance improves, sucking, swallowing frequency, bolus size, and suction amplitude increase, while occurring during a safer phase of respiration, namely away from deglutition apnea and inhalation [18, 34]. As all these functions are rhythmic beginning with infant nutritive sucking at 1 cycle/s [35] and the subsequent functions entrained by the bolus formation, the existence of central neuronal networks or central pattern generators (CPGs) have been advanced as providing the rhythms needed for the appropriate sequential functions to work "in phase" [61–63]. This raises the query as to when the CPGs implicated in oral feeding are formed and mature and "learn to work" in phase with each other. It is speculated that when in phase, safety and efficiency are optimized. Again, if we use the example in Fig. 2.3, one may speculate that within nutritive sucking, the CPG for expression matures before that of suction. When suction appears, both CPGs learn to work in phase, i.e., stages 2–4. During this period, the amplitude of expression and suction demonstrates broad variances. It is not until stage 5 when both CPGs work in phase that amplitude stabilizes. These observations support the concept that synchronization of muscles within a specific function, i.e., expression or suction, needs to mature before coordination with another function can occur, e.g., expression *and* suction [10].

Figure 2.5 shows how early on swallow respirations are "out of phase" when preterm infants swallow most frequently during deglutition apnea and inspiration, thus increasing the risks of oxygen desaturation and penetration/aspiration, respectively. With maturation as observed in term counterparts however, they transition to a safer "in-phase" swallowing-respiration interphase, i.e., during start of inspiration or expiration when minimal air inflow and outflow occur, reducing risks of penetration/aspiration into the lungs.

Therefore, an infant's ability to feed by mouth is a unique example illustrating how varying physiologic functions must be intimately intertwined neurally and functionally before they become safe and efficient. Figure 2.6 is a simple schematic depicting the complexity of this process. Unfortunately, gaps in our

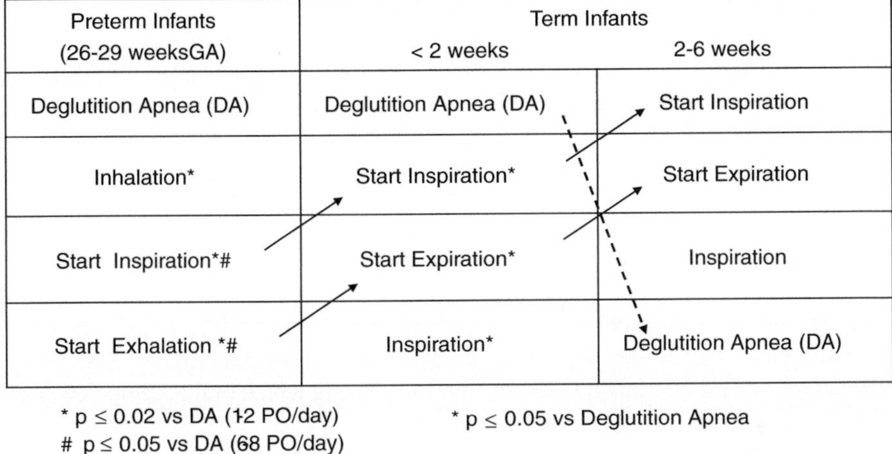

Fig. 2.5 Frequency occurrence of swallow-respiratory interphases: maturational instances of swallow and respiration function being "out of phase" in preterm infants and "in phase" in term counterparts [34]

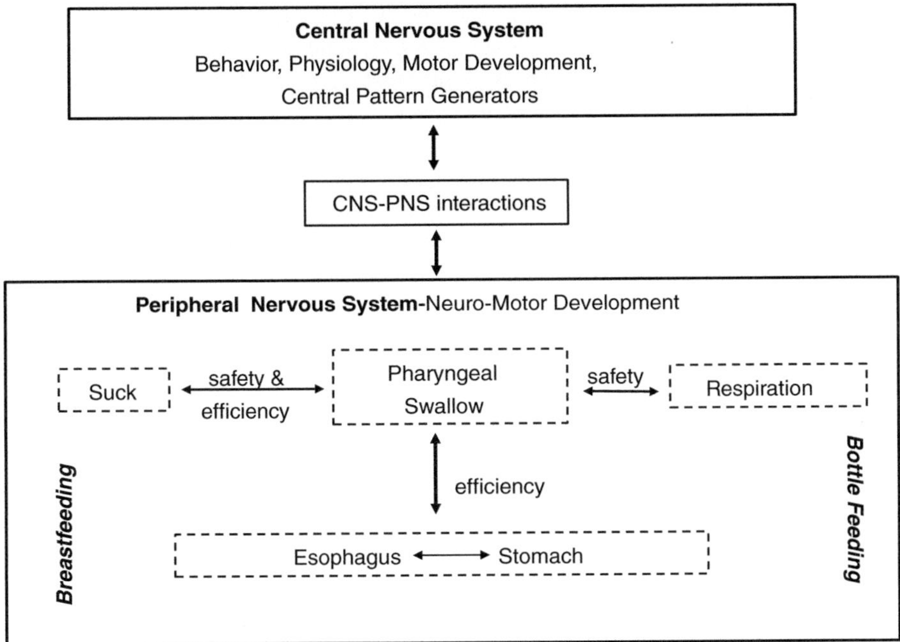

Fig. 2.6 Nutritive sucking pathway (NSP) – schematic presenting the multilevel neuromotor cross-talks required for safe and competent oral feeding. CNS central nervous system, PNS peripheral nervous system

knowledge still hinder the care we provide to our most high-risk infants. Increasing cross-fertilization of ideas and understanding between team members from different subspecialties caring for these infants will hopefully lead to better awareness and recognition of the causes of oral feeding difficulties across all levels of the NPS.

Genes

With the numerous physiologic functions implicated in the NSP and the knowledge that each has different developmental profiles and rate of maturation, it becomes difficult to identify critical and sensitive periods during which oral feeding becomes safe and efficacious.

Do all lives revert back to our genes? Recently, in a landmark study, Maron and colleagues demonstrated that comparative salivary analyses can provide comprehensive and real-time information on nearly all organs and tissues in the developing preterm infant [64]. Using combinations of bioinformatics analyses and a noninvasive salivary collection approach, they monitored a range of down- and upregulated genes on 5 clinically stable preterm infants (28–32 weeks GA) at 5 time points: prior to enteral feeds, at start of feeds, advancing feeds, at introduction of oral feeding, and at full oral feeding. Of the 9286 gene transcripts with statistically significant gene expression changes across subjects over time, 37.9% were downregulated and 62.1% were upregulated. These genes were correlated with developmental pathways (Fig. 2.7). Downregulated genes were associated with development of the embryo, hematologic system, development and function of connective tissue, and survival of the organism. Upregulated genes, in turn, were associated with behavior and the development of the nervous system, organs, and digestive system [64]. From these gene transcripts and using updated and targeted pathway analyses, they narrowed down their search for potential up- and down-regulated candidate genes

Fig. 2.7 Examples of downregulated fetal gene expressions and upregulated postnatal gene expression that potentially may impact the maturation of infant oral feeding around the perinatal period [64, 65]

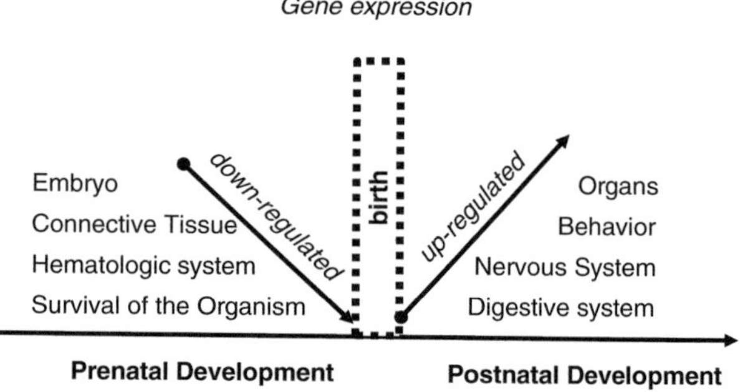

involved with successful oral feeding. Genes were considered if they were associated with "feeding," "digestion," and "development." They identified 2186 genes meeting these criteria highlighting pathways associated with feeding behavior, cranial nerve development, and the development of the nervous, skeletal, and muscular systems, as well as brain, sensory, and facial development relating to oral feeding success [65, 66].

It is evident that the genetic data presented by Maron and collaborators will require further investigation. However, the preliminary data presented are encouraging as they nicely mirror the developmental profiles of the physiologic functions that are of concern for clinicians caring for NICU infants facing difficulty weaning from tube feeding. From these studies, the natural query is raised as to how early upregulation of postnatal developmental genes can be switched on when a premature delivery occurs.

Summary/Conclusion

In reviewing our current understanding of the differing maturational processes that occur along the NSP, it is not surprising that premature infants so frequently encounter difficulties transitioning from tube to independent oral feeding. It is unfortunate, however, that from the caregivers' point of view, deciphering where the causes for these infants' difficulties arise is problematic insofar as infants' response(s) to any feeding problem most often fall into a nonspecific category of behaviors, e.g., feeding refusal, pushing away, disorganization, incomplete feeding, and/or adverse events, e.g., oxygen desaturation, apnea, and bradycardia. For this reason, if the multidisciplinary team members were to conduct a systematic review of the potential culprit(s) that may be implicated along the NSP, they will be reminded that the underlying cause(s) may lie outside of the realm of their respective expertise. Such collective partaking would generate further constructive discussions and analyses that will more readily lead to a differential diagnosis and the development of roadmaps or algorithms for how best to proceed with their young patients' care. Finally, it would be expected that team members' compliance to such collectively agreed-upon management plan will be improved for the benefit of the infants and their family.

Acknowledgments   The author wishes to thank all the mothers and infants who generously participated in her studies, her many collaborators who have supported her work over the years, and the National Institutes of Health for the support (R01 HD-28140; R01 HD 044469; MO1RR000188). The contents of this publication are solely the responsibility of the author and do not necessarily represent the official views of the National Institute of Child Health and Human Development or the National Institutes of Health.

References

1. Rudolph CD, Link DT. Feeding disorders in infants and children. Pediatr Clin N Am. 2002;49:97–112. vi
2. American Academy of Pediatrics. Policy statement. Hospital discharge of the high-risk neonate. Pediatrics. 2008;122:1119–26.
3. Lau C, Hurst N. Oral feeding in infants. Curr Probl Pediatr. 1999;29:105–24.
4. Lau C, Hurst NM, Smith EO, Schanler RJ. Ethnic/racial diversity, maternal stress, lactation and very low birthweight infants. J Perinatol. 2007;27:399–408.
5. Melnyk BM, Crean HF, Feinstein NF, Fairbanks E. Maternal anxiety and depression after a premature infant's discharge from the neonatal intensive care unit: explanatory effects of the creating opportunities for parent empowerment program. Nurs Res. 2008;57:383–94.
6. Premji SS, Currie G, Reilly S, et al. A qualitative study: mothers of late preterm infants relate their experiences of community-based care. PLoS One. 2017;12:e0174419.
7. Gondwe KW, Yang Q, White-Traut R, Holditch-Davis D. Maternal psychological distress and mother-infant relationship: multiple-birth versus singleton preterm infants. Neonatal Netw. 2017;36:77–88.
8. Zanardo V, Gabrieli C, Straface G, Savio F, Soldera G. The interaction of personality profile and lactation differs between mothers of late preterm and term neonates. J Matern Fetal Neonatal Med. 2017;30:927–32.
9. Abadie V, Couly G. Congenital feeding and swallowing disorders. Handb Clin Neurol. 2013;113:1539–49.
10. Amaizu N, Shulman R, Schanler R, Lau C. Maturation of oral feeding skills in preterm infants. Acta Paediatr. 2008;97:61–7.
11. Nyqvist KH, Farnstrand C, Eeg-Olofsson KE, Ewald U. Early oral behaviour in preterm infants during breastfeeding: an electromyographic study. Acta Paediatr. 2001;90:658–63.
12. Tamura Y, Horikawa Y, Yoshida S. Co-ordination of tongue movements and peri-oral muscle activities during nutritive sucking. Dev Med Child Neurol. 1996;38:503–10.
13. Martins CD, Furlan RM, Motta AR, Viana MC. Electromyography of muscles involved in feeding premature infants. Codas. 2015;27:372–7.
14. Gomes CF, Thomson Z, Cardoso JR. Utilization of surface electromyography during the feeding of term and preterm infants: a literature review. Dev Med Child Neurol. 2009;51:936–42.
15. Iida S, Harada T, Okamoto M, Inada Y, Kogo M, Masuda Y. Soft palate movement during sucking behavior. Dysphagia. 2003;18:96–100.
16. Reissland N, Mason C, Schaal B, Lincoln K. Prenatal mouth movements: can we identify co-ordinated fetal mouth and LIP actions necessary for feeding? Int J Pediatr. 2012;2012:848596.
17. Sameroff AJ. The components of sucking in the human newborn. J Exp Child Psychol. 1968;6:607–23.
18. Lau C, Alagugurusamy R, Schanler RJ, Smith EO, Shulman RJ. Characterization of the developmental stages of sucking in preterm infants during bottle feeding. Acta Paediatr. 2000;89:846–52.
19. Lau C, Smith EO. A novel approach to assess oral feeding skills of preterm infants. Neonatology. 2011;100:64–70.
20. Arvedson JC, Lefton-Greif MA. Pediatric videofluoroscopic swallow studies. A profession manual with caregiver guidelines. San Antonio: Communication Skill Builders; 1998.
21. Zancan M, Luchesi KF, Mituuti CT, Furkim AM. Onset locations of the pharyngeal phase of swallowing: meta-analysis. Codas. 2017;29:e20160067.
22. Selley WG, Ellis RE, Flack FC, Brooks WA. Coordination of sucking, swallowing and breathing in the newborn: its relationship to infant feeding and normal development. Br J Disord Commun. 1990;25:311–27.
23. Schwertner RW, Garand KL, Pearson WG, Jr. A novel imaging analysis method for capturing pharyngeal constriction during swallowing. J Imaging Sci. 2016;1:PMC 2017.

24. Thompson TZ, Obeidin F, Davidoff AA, et al. Coordinate mapping of hyolaryngeal mechanics in swallowing. J Vis Exp. 2014;87. doi:https://doi.org/10.3791/51476.
25. Bosma JF, Hepburn LG, Josell SD, Baker K. Ultrasound demonstration of tongue motions during suckle feeding. Dev Med Child Neurol. 1990;32:223–9.
26. Goldfield EC, Buonomo C, Fletcher K, et al. Premature infant swallowing: patterns of tongue-soft palate coordination based upon videofluoroscopy. Infant Behav Dev. 2010;33:209–18.
27. Miller JL, Kang SM. Preliminary ultrasound observation of lingual movement patterns during nutritive versus non-nutritive sucking in a premature infant. Dysphagia. 2007;22:150–60.
28. Goldfield EC, Smith V, Buonomo C, Perez J, Larson K. Preterm infant swallowing of thin and nectar-thick liquids: changes in lingual-palatal coordination and relation to bolus transit. Dysphagia. 2013;28:234–44.
29. Dantas RO, Dodds WJ, Massey BT, Shaker R, Cook IJ. Manometric characteristics of glossopalatal sphincter. Dig Dis Sci. 1990;35:161–6.
30. Wolf LS, Glass RP. Feeding and swallowing disorders in infancy: assessment and management. Tucson: Therapy Skills Builders; 1992.
31. Crompton AW, German RZ, Thexton AJ. Development of the movement of the epiglottis in infant and juvenile pigs. Zoology (Jena). 2008;111:339–49.
32. Omari T, Snel A, Barnett C, Davidson G, Haslam R, Dent J. Measurement of upper esophageal sphincter tone and relaxation during swallowing in premature infants. Am J Phys. 1999;277:G862–6.
33. Buchholz DW, Bosma JF, Donner MW. Adaptation, compensation, and decompensation of the pharyngeal swallow. Gastrointest Radiol. 1985;10:235–9.
34. Lau C, Smith EO, Schanler RJ. Coordination of suck-swallow and swallow-respiration in preterm infants. Acta Paediatr. 2003;92:721–7.
35. Wolff PH. The serial organization of sucking in the young infant. Pediatrics. 1968;42:943–56.
36. Koenig JS, Davies AM, Thach BT. Coordination of breathing, sucking, and swallowing during bottle feedings in human infants. J Appl Physiol. 1990;69:1623–9.
37. Rosen CL, Glaze DG, Frost JD Jr. Hypoxemia associated with feeding in the preterm infant and full-term neonate. Am J Dis Child. 1984;138:623–8.
38. Mathew OP, Clark ML, Pronske ML, Luna-Solarzano HG, Peterson MD. Breathing pattern and ventilation during oral feeding in term newborn infants. J Pediatr. 1985;106:810–3.
39. van Wijk MP, Benninga MA, Omari TI. Role of the multichannel intraluminal impedance technique in infants and children. J Pediatr Gastroenterol Nutr. 2009;48:2–12.
40. Carlson DA, Omari T, Lin Z, et al. High-resolution impedance manometry parameters enhance the esophageal motility evaluation in non-obstructive dysphagia patients without a major Chicago classification motility disorder. Neurogastroenterol Motil. 2017;29:e12941.
41. Omari TI, Miki K, Fraser R, et al. Esophageal body and lower esophageal sphincter function in healthy premature infants. Gastroenterology. 1995;109:1757–64.
42. Rommel N, Omari TI, Selleslagh M, et al. High-resolution manometry combined with impedance measurements discriminates the cause of dysphagia in children. Eur J Pediatr. 2015;174:1629.
43. Ferris L, Rommel N, Doeltgen S, et al. Pressure-flow analysis for the assessment of pediatric oropharyngeal dysphagia. J Pediatr. 2016;177:279.
44. Omari T, Tack J, Rommel N. Impedance as an adjunct to manometric testing to investigate symptoms of dysphagia: what it has failed to do and what it may tell us in the future. United European Gastroenterol J. 2014;2:355–66.
45. Omari TI, Szczesniak MM, Maclean J et al. Correlation of esophageal pressure-flow analysis findings with bolus transit patterns on videofluoroscopy. Dis. Esophagus 2016;29:166–73.
46. Omari TI, Dejaeger E, Van BD, et al. A novel method for the nonradiological assessment of ineffective swallowing. Am J Gastroenterol. 2011;106:1796–802.
47. Omari TI, Dejaeger E, Van BD, et al. A method to objectively assess swallow function in adults with suspected aspiration. Gastroenterology. 2011;140:1454–63.

48. Jadcherla SR, Duong HQ, Hofmann C, Hoffmann R, Shaker R. Characteristics of upper oesophageal sphincter and oesophageal body during maturation in healthy human neonates compared with adults. Neurogastroenterol Motil. 2005;17:663–70.
49. Rommel N, van Wijk M, Boets B, et al. Development of pharyngo-esophageal physiology during swallowing in the preterm infant. Neurogastroenterol Motil. 2011;23:e401–8.
50. Jadcherla SR, Duong HQ, Hoffmann RG, Shaker R. Esophageal body and upper esophageal sphincter motor responses to esophageal provocation during maturation in preterm newborns. J Pediatr. 2003;143:31–8.
51. Omari TI, Barnett CP, Benninga MA, et al. Mechanisms of gastro-oesophageal reflux in preterm and term infants with reflux disease. Gut. 2002;51:475–9.
52. Gupta A, Gulati P, Kim W, Fernandez S, Shaker R, Jadcherla SR. Effect of postnatal maturation on the mechanisms of esophageal propulsion in preterm human neonates: primary and secondary peristalsis. Am J Gastroenterol. 2009;104:411–9.
53. Staiano A, Boccia G, Salvia G, Zappulli D, Clouse RE. Development of esophageal peristalsis in preterm and term neonates. Gastroenterology. 2007;132:1718–25.
54. Pena EM, Parks VN, Peng J, et al. Lower esophageal sphincter relaxation reflex kinetics: effects of peristaltic reflexes and maturation in human premature neonates. Am J Physiol Gastrointest Liver Physiol. 2010;299:G1386–95.
55. Omari TI, Barnett C, Snel A, et al. Mechanisms of gastroesophageal reflux in healthy premature infants. J Pediatr. 1998;133:650–4.
56. Omari T. Lower esophageal sphincter function in the neonate. NeoReviews. 2006;7:e13–8.
57. Lau C. Oral feeding in the preterm infant. NeoReviews. 2006;7:e19–27.
58. Mizuno K, Ueda A. The maturation and coordination of sucking, swallowing, and respiration in preterm infants. J Pediatr. 2003;142:36–40.
59. Shaw SM, Martino R. The normal swallow: muscular and neurophysiological control. Otolaryngol Clin N Am. 2013;46:937–56.
60. Gewolb IH, Vice FL. Maturational changes in the rhythms, patterning, and coordination of respiration and swallow during feeding in preterm and term infants. Dev Med Child Neurol. 2006;48:589–94.
61. Tanaka S, Kogo M, Chandler SH, Matsuya T. Localization of oral-motor rhythmogenic circuits in the isolated rat brainstem preparation. Brain Res. 1999;821:190–9.
62. Jean A. Brain stem control of swallowing: neuronal network and cellular mechanisms. Physiol Rev. 2001;81:929–69.
63. Barlow SM, Estep M. Central pattern generation and the motor infrastructure for suck, respiration, and speech. J Commun Disord. 2006;39:366–80.
64. Maron JL, Johnson KL, Rocke DM, Cohen MG, Liley AJ, Bianchi DW. Neonatal salivary analysis reveals global developmental gene expression changes in the premature infant. Clin Chem. 2010;56:409–16.
65. Maron JL. Insights into neonatal oral feeding through the salivary transcriptome. Int J Pediatr. 2012;2012:195153.
66. Maron JL, Hwang JS, Pathak S, Ruthazer R, Russell RL, Alterovitz G. Computational gene expression modeling identifies salivary biomarker analysis that predict oral feeding readiness in the newborn. J Pediatr. 2015;166:282–8.

Chapter 3
Clinical Evaluation of Breastfed Infants with Dysphagia: A Lactation Consultant's Perspective

Nancy Hurst

Successful breastfeeding requires the infant to remove a sufficient volume of milk from the breast to promote adequate growth and stimulate continued maternal milk production. As such, both the mother and infant have specific roles in the breast-feeding relationship. It is with this perspective that the lactation consultant offers support and instruction to the mother, evaluates the infant's feeding behavior, assesses the maternal lactation status, and develops a plan of care. The scope of practice for the International Board Certified Lactation Consultant (LC) includes the provision of comprehensive maternal, child, and feeding assessments related to lactation and breastfeeding in collaboration with the health-care team in order to deliver coordinated services to women and families [1]. This chapter will describe the role of the LC as an integral member of the health-care team caring for the breastfeeding dyad when infant dysphagia is suspected or confirmed.

The Breastfeeding Mother-Infant Dyad

To say that either the mother or the infant is more vital to establishing breastfeeding would be inaccurate. Each provides a unique set of physiologic, developmental, and behavioral responses to the breastfeeding relationship. To effectively initiate lacta-tion, the mother must receive sufficient breast stimulation, ideally within the first hour following birth and at frequent intervals thereafter. The newborn infant must attach and maintain attachment to the mother's breast – more commonly referred to as latch – to start the cascade of maternal hormonal responses that triggers milk synthesis and ejection. This unique synchrony between mother and infant is funda-mental to the attachment relationship [2]. Early attachment is dependent on the

N. Hurst
Women's Support Services, Texas Children's Hospital, Houston, TX, USA
e-mail: nmhurst@texaschildrens.org

© Springer International Publishing AG, part of Springer Nature 2018
J. Ongkasuwan, E. H. Chiou (eds.), *Pediatric Dysphagia*,
https://doi.org/10.1007/978-3-319-97025-7_3

mother anticipating her infant's needs and recognizing her infant's cues. Conversely, basic infant behaviors such as sucking, crying, and smiling act as stimuli that induce the mother to respond [3].

Critical Periods of Development in Lactation and Breastfeeding

A critical period refers to a time in development during which the brain or target organ is particularly responsive to stimuli or insults followed by an extended period of responsiveness [4]. Such periods exist in lactation and breastfeeding. With the delivery of the placenta following the birth of the infant, progesterone and placental lactogen decrease, thereby removing the suppressive effects of elevated prolactin levels allowing milk synthesis to occur [5]. However, these hormonal changes are not the only component necessary for the onset of lactogenesis II (i.e., secretory phase of lactation), known more commonly as the "coming to volume" stage. The infant's role in this process is to provide the necessary breast stimulation by sucking at the breast early (within the first hour of birth) and at frequent intervals of sustained duration. With each breastfeeding episode, the mother releases the lactogenic hormones – prolactin and oxytocin – which act on the mammary glandular tissue to synthesis and subsequently eject the milk, respectively.

If not interrupted and following an unmedicated labor, newborn infants placed skin to skin with their mothers will begin a cascade of inborn behaviors to seek, find, and attach to the mother's breast [6–8]. These behaviors, such as mouth opening, massaging the breast with their hands, hand to mouth movements, and licking, are associated with maternal oxytocin release [9]. The newborn infant has a distinctive sucking pattern in the first few days after birth that is different from the more mature sucking pattern that will emerge with the onset of lactogenesis II. This sucking pattern is thought to play a key role in initiating the maternal lactation process and is characterized by higher suction pressures [10]. A study of 71 term breastfed infants found that stronger intraoral vacuum was related to earlier onset of lactation when other variables were controlled: maternal age, gestational BMI gain, time to first breastfeeding, formula volume and frequency, and delivery type [11].

Progression of Lactation and Breastfeeding

Lactation post-birth occurs in three stages, namely, initiation, coming to volume, and maintenance. Each stage is distinct in its regulatory mechanisms that influence and impact milk production [12]. Early breast stimulation during the first 72 h postbirth triggers the initiation of milk synthesis. This singular event is critical in launching the "coming to volume" stage, which over the next 4–7 days post-birth will attain a milk volume of 500–750 mL day [5, 13]. Although the surge of prolactin levels during the first few weeks is important in establishing lactation, there is a gradual decline as these levels shift from endocrine to autocrine control of lactation as breastfeeding progresses. Autocrine control is the rate of milk synthesis related to the degree to which the breast has been drained after a feed; the more completely the breast is emptied, the higher milk synthesis [12, 14]. As lactation switches to autocrine control, the maintenance of maternal milk production becomes individualized to the mother-infant breastfeeding dyad. Evidence of this variability was shown in a study of 71 mothers of exclusively breastfed infants where 24-h milk intake measured via test weighing was 788 ± 169 g, with a range of 478–1356 g [15]. Moreover, milk volumes consumed during each feeding (76 ± 12.6, range 0–240 g) and number of feeds in 24 h (11 ± 3, range 6–18) were markedly different among mother-infant dyads. Understanding the various stages of lactation, the regulatory factors at work with each stage, and the unique feeding patterns of the individual dyad as breastfeeding progresses beyond the early weeks is important when developing a plan of care for mothers of infants with feeding problems.

Competent infant feeding behavior requires the coordination of sucking, swallowing, and breathing. Until recently, much of what we know regarding infant oral motor mechanics we have learned by observing bottle-feeding. New technologies (i.e., ultrasound, electromyography, intraoral pressure transducers) have validated the long-standing view that breastfeeding is different from bottle-feeding. These differences, as summarized in Table 3.1, clearly illustrate breastfeeding as a more dynamic endeavor on the part of the infant compared to bottle-feeding. For example, the higher nonnutritive sucking (NNS) pressure may be necessary to stimulate the milk ejection reflex (MER) in the mother to facilitate milk flow during breastfeeding, whereas during bottle-feeding this stimulus is not required to begin milk flow. Interestingly, Moral et al. [16] found that mixed-fed infants – those both

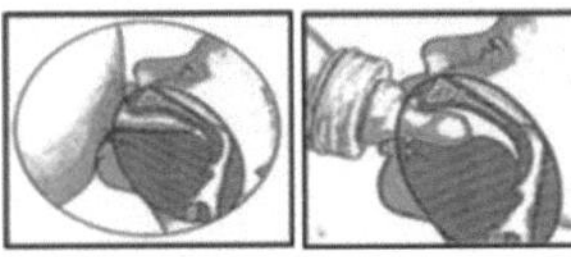

Table 3.1 Differences between breast and bottle-feeding

Measure	Breast	Bottle
NNS pressure [17, 18]	Higher	
NNS frequency [17]	=	=
NS pressure [17]	=	=
NS frequency [16]	Higher	
NS duration (su/min) [17]	Shorter	
NS bursts [18]	Higher	
Feeding efficiency (mL/su) [18]	=	=
Feeding effectiveness (mL/min) [18]		Higher
Feeding pauses [16]	Longer	
Range of facial muscle contractions [19, 20]	Higher	

breastfeeding and bottle-feeding – had similar mean number of nutritive sucking (NS) per minute revealing a modification in mechanics when both methods are practiced.

Ultrasound studies of sucking dynamics indicate that there is a particular position in which the infant positions the nipple within the mouth that is most conducive to effective milk transfer [21–26]. The infant sucking dynamics during breastfeeding observed in these studies reveal the following:

- Infants attach to the breast by creating a baseline vacuum (mean $= -64 + 45$ mmHg) that elongates the nipple and places it within 5–7 mm of the hard-soft palate junction (HSPJ).
- Milk flow occurs with the downward movement of the posterior tongue and soft palate and subsequent decrease in negative pressure (vacuum increased at a mean: -122 to -163 mmHg) during the first half of the suck cycle.
- The entire nipple expands evenly, rather than in a peristaltic motion.
- Tongue motion is reduced at the base of the nipple which is thought to assist in maintaining a baseline vacuum (seal) to the breast.
- During the second half of the suck cycle, the tongue moves up, and the nipple is compressed, vacuum is reduced, and milk clears from the oral cavity under the soft palate to the pharyngeal area.

Whereas these changes in vacuum pressure are key to milk transfer during breastfeeding, the positive pressure created by the maternal MER must occur concurrently to maximize breast emptying and promote continued milk synthesis [17]. As mentioned, NNS with its higher sucking rate compared to NS plays an important role in stimulating the maternal MER. Infant sucking, as well as other cognitive stimuli (i.e., hearing, seeing, thinking of the infant), results in the release of oxytocin in the pituitary and other areas such as the caudate, amygdala, and hippocampus [27]. As the breast empties, the rate of milk flow changes with subsequent milk ejections [28, 29], suggesting that infants may modify their sucking patterns as the breastfeed progresses [26].

Successful coordination of the suck-swallow-breathe reflex requires the segregation of swallowing from breathing. The three phases of swallowing – oral, pharyngeal, and esophageal – are named in relation to the movement of the milk bolus from entry into the mouth to entry into the stomach. During swallowing in the normal breastfed infant, the oral bolus is propelled into the pharynx with the upward movement of the tongue during each suck [21, 30]. Once a sufficient amount of milk accumulates in the pharynx, a swallow is triggered, and the pharyngeal phase begins. With a pause in breathing, the cascade of movements of the soft palate, vocal cords, hyoid, epiglottis, and larynx provides safe passage as the tongue moves the bolus posteriorly toward the upper esophagus [31].

Revelations on swallowing in breastfed infants are coming to light in recent investigations. Goldfield et al. [32] suggested that based on their data, swallowing occurred in a nonrandom distribution in relation to breathing and sucking during breastfeeding. In this and another study [33], breastfed infants swallowed without interfering with sucking, and infants were able to maintain a relatively constant milk flow while continuing to breathe by inserting swallows into particular regions. This may account for the higher oxygen saturation rates measured in breastfed compared with bottle-fed infants [32, 34]. High milk flow rates, size of the bottle teat hole, and compressibility likely influence the variations observed during bottle-feeding when compared with breastfeeding.

Studies designed to measure the suction and expression components of nutritive sucking in preterm infants further clarify our understanding of the development of feeding behavior [35]. Lau's work in describing a 5-stage oral motor developmental scale in bottle-fed preterm infants showed a delay in the maturation of the suction component in relation to that of expression [36]. Their findings reveal that preterm infants using expression only can safely complete a bottle-feeding. However, it is not known whether an infant can breastfeed successfully using expression only given the variability in maternal nipple shape, size, and protractility compared to the firmness of the bottle nipple. The two most common difficulties encountered when preterm infants attempt breastfeeding are slipping off the breast and, if able to latch, falling asleep after a few sucks. An effective intervention for these problems is use of a nipple shield placed over the maternal nipple which provides a more stable nipple shape triggering sucking and increasing milk transfer [37]. Another consideration is as the suction component matures, is there a minimum suction pressure required for the preterm infant to achieve and maintain attachment to the breast? A mean baseline suction pressure of -64 ± 45 mmHg has been measured during pauses in sucking in term breastfed infants whose mothers are not experiencing nipple pain [38]. It is not known if preterm infants need to attain this baseline sucking pressure to breastfeed successfully; however it has been shown that preterm infants using a nipple shield to facilitate milk transfer during early breastfeeding are able to wean from the shield when reaching term-corrected age [37].

The differences in sucking mechanics between breast and bottle-feeding revealed in these studies shed light on the so-called "nipple confusion" issue [39]. Despite the misleading term, some infants have difficulty attaching to the breast after being bottle-fed or offered a pacifier. However, there may be more to this phenomenon than just oral motor mechanics. Mobbs et al. [40] describe the process of imprinting and subsequent latchment as a primary stage of emotional and neurobehavioral development in which the infant recognizes its mother through oral tactile memory. Mobbs proposed that the activation of Merkel cells in the infant's buccal mucosa in response to a tactile stimulus was the first step in oral recognition of the nipple and breast [41, 42]. The main function of the Merkel cells is as a mechanoreceptor of tactile stimuli; information received is passed on as an encoded neural image of the imprinting object to the infant's central nervous system. The encoded messages include shape, edges, and curvatures. Consider in this context the differences in the human breast tissue and nipple with that of the bottle nipple or pacifier. When a decoy (i.e., pacifier, bottle nipple) is given as a replacement of the mother's nipple during the early newborn sensitive period, the distress (confusion) exhibited by the infant is a behavior stemming from the Merkel cell encoding recognition promoting

Table 3.2 Clinical applications of latchment

Optimal	Suboptimal
Providing unrestricted skin-to-skin contact of mother and baby until well after initial latching and baby is asleep	A delay in the introduction of the infant to the breast
Ensuring the mother is aware that introducing a pacifier/bottle nipple should be avoided	Displacement with a thumb, pacifier, or other decoys
Rapid response to distressed infant	Maternal nipple deprivation
Sleeping in close proximity to the infant	Distancing mother and infant during sleep

Adapted from: Mobbs et al. [40]

teat preference fixation. If clinicians and mothers are aware of the evolutionary significance of this newborn sensitive period related to oral tactile input, clinical practices to support optimal latchment could be promoted leading to better outcomes. It should be noted that when a fixation on a pacifier/bottle nipple occurs, an imprinting change can occur – despite emotional distress – by providing skin-to-skin contact with the infant whereby the mother's nipple is the only stimulus available. The following Table 3.2 describes optimal and suboptimal practices related to latchment.

Clinical Breastfeeding Assessment

The LC brings an expertise to the health-care team that includes an assessment of the maternal lactation status coupled with the infant's breastfeeding competence. The mother experiencing problems with breastfeeding may seek assistance from the LC when the infant has been diagnosed with dysphagia of a known cause. When the anomaly or condition is known, the LC can develop a plan that facilitates and/or compensates for any limitations found from the feeding assessment. However, when breastfeeding difficulties are of unknown origin, the LC may be the first to identify problems with dysphagia. One of the most frequent reasons for the mother to seek assistance from the LC is difficulties with the latch. She may report that the infant pulls off the breast frequently during the feed, is fussy at the breast, or refuses to latch at all. Although these behaviors may not be evidence of an underlying dysphagia requiring further diagnostic evaluation, the LC must consider this possibility by conducting a complete feeding assessment and make appropriate referrals to other feeding specialists as needed. The elements of a comprehensive clinical breastfeeding assessment include:

- Maternal and infant history related to initiation/progression of breastfeeding
- Maternal health issues which may delay or prevent normal onset of lactation
- Assessing infant oral sensorimotor responses at rest and via digital suck examination

- Observing general physical, behavioral, neurologic, and physiologic responses of the infant (i.e., tone, symmetry, states of arousal, color, and respirations)
- Maternal breast examination
- Observation of breastfeeding episode
- Measurement of milk transfer during breastfeeding via test weighing

As previously stated, breastfeeding should be viewed as a dyadic relationship. Maternal physiologic responses related to lactation influence milk flow and synthesis and are impacted by early breastfeeding patterns. Obtaining a detailed history from the mother related to lactation sufficiency is useful to identify factors that may indicate a disruption in either the initiation or maintenance of an adequate milk supply [43]. As well, history of the post-birth experience related to the initiation and progression of breastfeeding will inform those factors impacting early breast stimulation and infant behavior.

Readers of this text are likely to be well informed of the general neurologic, physiologic, and oral sensorimotor responses of the infant related to feeding. These responses should be evaluated initially at rest, during a digital suck examination, and when feeding. Genna's text, *Supporting Sucking Skills in Breastfeeding Infants*, provides an excellent stepwise process in performing this assessment [44]. The ability of the infant to perform the work of feeding will be revealed in observing these responses prior to, during, and after feeding.

A mismatch of maternal nipple/areola (i.e., size, shape, protractility) and infant anatomical features/oral motor function (i.e., mouth gap, tongue restriction, weak suck) may result in an ineffective latch. For example, an infant with a small mouth may have difficulty achieving a latch when the mother has a large, broader nipple. A late preterm or hypotonic infant may be unable to maintain attachment to the nipple/areola when the mother has flat or inverted nipples (Fig. 3.1). Infants with ankyloglossia (tongue tie) resulting in restricted tongue range of motion may have

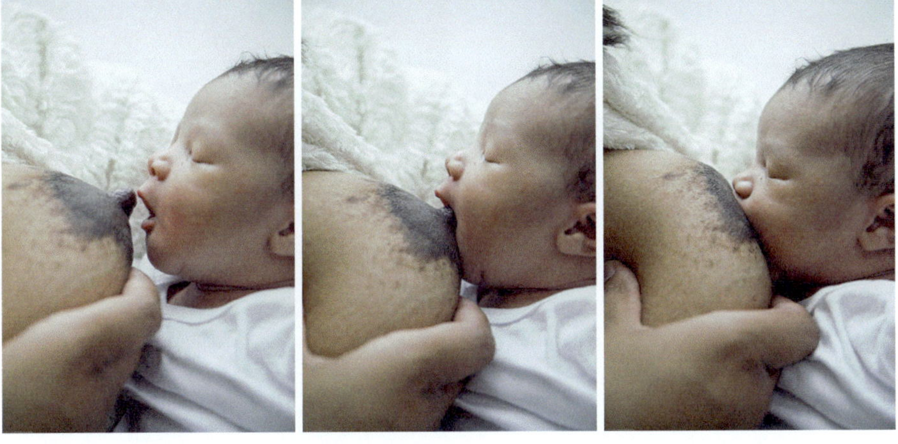

Fig. 3.1 Offering the breast to achieve optimal latch. (© Allen Kramer & Paul Kuntz)

difficulty achieving a sustained deep latch to the breast if able to latch at all [45]. However, depending on the severity of the tongue restriction, an effective latch may be achieved with a mother whose nipples are more elastic and protractile compared to the mother with flat nipples that do not evert easily [21, 46]. Infants of mothers reporting persistent unresolved nipple pain (despite ongoing lactation advice) beyond the first few days/weeks post-birth exert significantly stronger baseline, mean, and peak vacuum pressures during breastfeeding [38, 47]. Even during sucking pauses, these infants exerted significantly stronger vacuum pressures on the breast tissue compared to non-pain control mothers. Identifying any incongruities related to these conditions will help to determine possible interventions to improve outcomes and support the breastfeeding dyad.

Observation of the infant's latch to the breast, suck/swallow/breathing patterns, and behavior before, during, and after the breastfeeding session is key to evaluating the need for interventions to improve feeding. Ideally, the breastfeed begins when the infant cues for readiness to feed. The mother offers the nipple tilted toward the upper lip and nose, waits until the infant drops the jaw to maximum excursion, and draws the infant in close to latch as the mouth opens wide (Fig. 3.1). Note the position of the mother's hand in Fig. 3.1 providing support but placed behind the areolar edge so as to avoid interference with the latch. Once the infant has drawn the nipple/areola tissue deep into the mouth, the rapid sucks associated with a NNS pattern (two or more sucks/sec) characteristic of low milk flow will be observed. Visually, the infant's cheeks will be pressed against the breast, the nose free, and the lips barely visible (Fig. 3.2). The initial maternal MER occurs within the first minute of sucking [48, 49] as characterized by a slowing of one suck per second and usually heard as a soft audible sound. Cervical auscultation with a stethoscope placed over

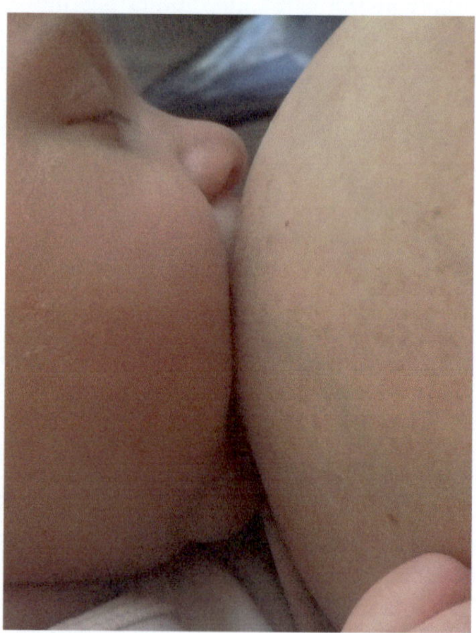

Fig. 3.2 Optimal latch to the breast. (© Nancy Hurst)

the infant's throat may be useful to hear swallowing sounds more distinctly [50, 51]. The rate of swallowing is indicative of milk flow rate. With the first milk ejection, the infant will swallow with every 1–2 sucks; as the milk flow slows, the ratio will range from 1 to 3 sucks per swallow. Watching the infant's behavior as the feeding progresses provides useful information related to milk flow. An assessment of the mother during the feeding should be done concurrently while observing the infant at breast. Objective measures including her posture and responsiveness to infant's cues, as well as subjective measures related to sensations of initial MER and comfort level with latch, will provide useful information in order to provide appropriate interventions.

A definitive measure of milk transfer during breastfeeding is achieved by the test weighing method [52]. Weighing the diapered infant before and immediately after the breastfeeding (without changing the diaper) provides an accurate measure of milk consumed (1 gram infant weight gain equals 1 mL milk intake). Using an electronic scale accurate to 1–2 grams ensures the accuracy of this method [53]. Obtaining milk volume transferred during the feeding provides useful information in order to validate clinical observations and reassure or address maternal concerns regarding adequate milk transfer during feeding [54, 55].

Strategies to Improve Breastfeeding Outcomes

Findings from the clinical breastfeeding assessment will allow the LC to determine an effective plan to improve breastfeeding outcomes for the mother-infant dyad. The importance of a focused, timely management strategy when considering the breastfeeding dyad who is experiencing feeding problems cannot be overstated. The three goals foremost in driving breastfeeding management are attachment at the breast, breast milk production, and caloric intake parameters, with the desired outcome to transfer sufficient milk to the infant to promote optimal growth. A simple ABC mnemonic based on these goals was developed and evaluated by the American Academy of Pediatrics (AAP) and provides an easy stepwise process for the clinician [56, 57].

Initial attachment to the breast and evaluation of infant sucking parameters during feeding provides information to guide the LC in strategies to optimize breastfeeding. When improved attachment to the breast is achieved with facilitative actions such as positioning and oral stimulation, the management plan is fairly straightforward, supports normal development, and requires minimal follow-up to ensure continued progress. When these actions do not result in resolution of the problem, other underlying problems – known or unknown – may exist, and therefore compensatory or so-called second-line strategies are needed to optimize feeding until resolution of the underlying problem. A list of some of these facilitative and compensatory strategies designed to improve breastfeeding are provided in Table 3.3.

Second-line strategies have been so named to include a range of devices and techniques with the goal to reverse the AAP mnemonic from ABC to CBA; that is, ensure the infant is receiving adequate nutrition (calories) concurrently with providing opti-

Table 3.3 Facilitative/compensatory strategies to improve breastfeeding

Infant/maternal finding	Intervention
Poor alignment of infant at breast resulting in shallow latch	Modify infant position to encourage infant self-attachment and place infant where the breast naturally falls
Infant unable to maintain latch (i.e., preterm infant)	Use nipple shield to facilitate attachment and milk transfer
Maternal breast tissue edematous resulting in shallow/difficult latch	Use reverse pressure softening, breast massage, or pumping prior to feeding to soften areola and increase nipple elasticity
Infant not lowering tongue tip and preventing latch	Allow more time for infant to organize and drop tongue; offer finger, tip up, with some expressed breast milk to habituate lowering of the tongue
Infant with ankyloglossia (tongue tie) causing unresolved nipple pain, insufficient milk transfer, and/or poor latch	Use a nipple shield to facilitate latch and milk transfer; referral for frenulotomy if nipple shield does not resolve problem
Infant reluctant to latch and or suck due to slow initial milk flow	Provide at-breast supplementation with supply line feeder to entice latch and continued sucking
Infant gulping, coughing, pulling off the breast due to high milk flow rate due to forceful MER	Breastfeed in prone or side-lying position and/or have mother press on breast to block some ducts and reduce milk flow at onset of initial MER
Infant with cleft lip/palate	Dependent on the extent of the cleft, prone positioning at breast with supply line supplementation may be possible

Adapted from Genna [44]

mal breast stimulation to protect and build milk production while working toward a more effective attachment and feeding behavior at breast. For example, is the inability of the infant to maintain attachment to the breast a result of maturational conditions related to prematurity or a transient issue that will resolve in several hours or days? Knowing when to flip the ABC management strategy is important to maintain infant nutrition and minimize maternal burden. Adding concurrent mechanical milk expression to the breastfeeding regimen is additional work placed on the mother, and a workable plan should be developed in collaboration with the mother and her support network to reduce fatigue and ensure success. That stated, when the infant's condition is such that some or all feedings will have to take place away from the breast, actions need to be taken to protect maternal milk production.

As previously emphasized, the mammary gland is highly sensitive to key lactogenic hormones early post-birth released in response to adequate breast stimulation [5]. In circumstances resulting in a delay and/or decrease in effective breastfeeding, milk expression must be initiated concurrently to either stimulate or maintain full maternal lactation potential. Therefore, early identification and appropriate intervention of breastfeeding problems are crucial in order to avoid insufficient milk production. Several factors should be considered to determine the type of pump to use, including (1) the phase of lactation when mechanical milk expression will be required, (2) the length of time the mother will rely on the pump for maintenance of lactation, and (3) the extent to which the pump will replace the infant for purposes of milk expression and mammary gland stimulation – some feeds or all feeds [58]. Evaluating these factors related to pump dependency will help to determine the most effective plan. Evidence shows that the greater the pump dependency, the more important the pump's effectiveness, efficiency, comfort, and convenience [58–61]. For example, for the mother of a very preterm infant unable to breastfeed at birth and for several weeks thereafter, a hospital-grade breast pump that allows for simultaneous versus sequential pumping and different pump shield sizes to accommodate maternal nipple size is optimal. These pumps are designed to mimic the newborn's unique suction patterns thought to program the mammary gland during the initiation phase of lactation [62]. Due to the critical window of time during this "coming to volume" phase, even partial pump dependency requires these unique features provided by the hospital-grade breast pump in circumstances when the infant is not breastfeeding effectively.

Providing Collaborative, Supportive Multidisciplinary Care

Creating a comprehensive, collaborative health-care team to coordinate care with a common management strategy is essential to reduce maternal/family anxiety and achieve desired outcomes. The lactation consultant can provide expertise within her/his scope of care and should make necessary referrals when findings indicate the need for other opinions and/or treatment modalities. It is equally important to develop a plan that is clear and specific and speaks in terms easily understood by the mother. This requires collaboration with the team as a whole, not as separate providers giving different or conflicting plans of care. It is distressing enough as a mother to experience breastfeeding difficulties; adding to her anxiety confusion over recommendations for treatment will not build her confidence in her ability to feed her infant. For mothers of infants with feeding difficulties, the time will come when total or partial resolution of the problem will occur and the extent to which her infant's feedings are at breast or with expressed breast milk will be known. For those mothers unable to reach their goal of feeding her infant exclusively at breast, the realization will be an emotional one. Health-care providers who anticipate this response and help the mother recognize the tremendous effort she has put forth will find she is less likely to feel a sense of failure and more likely to eventually feel successful.

Finally, breastfeeding self-efficacy and social support are the two most powerful predictors of breastfeeding outcomes. Breastfeeding self-efficacy determines how much effort mothers will expend on breastfeeding, how long they will persevere when confronting challenges, and how resilient they will be in the face of adverse situations [63]. Evidence has shown that mothers with high levels of breastfeeding self-efficacy were more successful in initiating and continuing breastfeeding [64, 65]. As well, women with higher perceived social support are found to have higher levels of breastfeeding self-efficacy [66, 67]. Mothers faced with complex infant feeding situations should be made aware of the importance of recognizing who are active players in their social support network. The LC and other health-care providers will certainly be included in this group; however family and friends are vital to the well-being of the breastfeeding dyad as they work toward an optimal outcome.

References

1. Examiners IBoLC. Scope of practice for International Board Certified Lactation Consultant (IBCLC) Certificants 2008 [updated Sept 15, 2012]. Available from: https://iblce.files.wordpress.com/2017/05/scope-of-practice.pdf

2. Reyna BA, Pickler RH. Mother-infant synchrony. J Obstet Gynecol Neonatal Nurs. 2009;38(4):470–7. PubMed PMID: 19614883.

3. Bowlby J. Attachment. 2nd ed. New York: Basic Books; 1982.

4. Fox SE, Levitt P, Nelson CA 3rd. How the timing and quality of early experiences influence the development of brain architecture. Child Dev. 2010;81(1):28–40. PubMed PMID: 20331653. Pubmed Central PMCID: 2846084.

5. Neville MC, Morton J. Physiology and endocrine changes underlying human lactogenesis II. J Nutr. 2001;131(11):3005S–8S. PubMed PMID: 11694636.

6. Widstrom AM, Lilja G, Aaltomaa-Michalias P, Dahllof A, Lintula M, Nissen E. Newborn behaviour to locate the breast when skin-to-skin: a possible method for enabling early self-regulation. Acta Paediatr. 2011;100(1):79–85. PubMed PMID: 20712833.

7. Brimdyr K, Cadwell K, Widstrom AM, Svensson K, Neumann M, Hart EA, et al. The association between common labor drugs and suckling when skin-to-skin during the first hour after birth. Birth. 2015;42(4):319–28. PubMed PMID: 26463582. Pubmed Central PMCID: 5057303.

8. Ransjo-Arvidson AB, Matthiesen AS, Lilja G, Nissen E, Widstrom AM, Uvnas-Moberg K. Maternal analgesia during labor disturbs newborn behavior: effects on breastfeeding, temperature, and crying. Birth. 2001;28(1):5–12. PubMed PMID: 11264622.

9. Matthiesen AS, Ransjo-Arvidson AB, Nissen E, Uvnas-Moberg K. Postpartum maternal oxytocin release by newborns: effects of infant hand massage and sucking. Birth. 2001;28(1):13–9. PubMed PMID: 11264623.

10. Kent JC, Gardner H, Geddes DT. Breastmilk production in the first 4 weeks after birth of term infants. Nutrients. 2016;8(12). PubMed PMID: 27897979. Pubmed Central PMCID: 5188411.

11. Zhang F, Xia H, Li X, Qin L, Gu H, Xu X, et al. Intraoral vacuum of breast-feeding newborns within the first 24 Hr: cesarean section versus vaginal delivery. Biol Res Nurs. 2016;18(4):445–53. PubMed PMID: 26975780.

12. Kent JC. How breastfeeding works. J Midwifery Womens Health. 2007;52(6):564–70. PubMed PMID: 17983993.

13. Neville MC, Keller R, Seacat J, Lutes V, Neifert M, Casey C, et al. Studies in human lactation: milk volumes in lactating women during the onset of lactation and full lactation. Am J Clin Nutr. 1988;48(6):1375–86. PubMed PMID: 3202087.

14. Daly SE, Kent JC, Owens RA, Hartmann PE. Frequency and degree of milk removal and the short-term control of human milk synthesis. Exp Physiol. 1996;81(5):861–75. PubMed PMID: 8889483.

15. Kent JC, Mitoulas LR, Cregan MD, Ramsay DT, Doherty DA, Hartmann PE. Volume and frequency of breastfeedings and fat content of breast milk throughout the day. Pediatrics. 2006;117(3):e387–95. PubMed PMID: 16510619.

16. Moral A, Bolibar I, Seguranyes G, Ustrell JM, Sebastia G, Martinez-Barba C, et al. Mechanics of sucking: comparison between bottle feeding and breastfeeding. BMC Pediatr. 2010;10:6. PubMed PMID: 20149217. Pubmed Central PMCID: 2837866.

17. Mizuno K, Ueda A. Changes in sucking performance from nonnutritive sucking to nutritive sucking during breast- and bottle-feeding. Pediatr Res. 2006;59(5):728–31. PubMed PMID: 16627890.

18. Taki M, Mizuno K, Murase M, Nishida Y, Itabashi K, Mukai Y. Maturational changes in the feeding behaviour of infants – a comparison between breast-feeding and bottle-feeding. Acta Paediatr. 2010;99(1):61–7. PubMed PMID: 19839957.

19. Gomes CF, Trezza EM, Murade EC, Padovani CR. Surface electromyography of facial muscles during natural and artificial feeding of infants. J Pediatr. 2006;82(2):103–9. PubMed PMID: 16614763.
20. Jacinto-Goncalves SR, Gaviao MB, Berzin F, de Oliveira AS, Semeguini TA. Electromyographic activity of perioral muscle in breastfed and non-breastfed children. J Clin Pediatr Dent. 2004;29(1):57–62. PubMed PMID: 15554405.
21. Geddes DT, Kent JC, Mitoulas LR, Hartmann PE. Tongue movement and intra-oral vacuum in breastfeeding infants. Early Hum Dev. 2008;84(7):471–7. PubMed PMID: 18262736.
22. McClellan HL, Sakalidis VS, Hepworth AR, Hartmann PE, Geddes DT. Validation of nipple diameter and tongue movement measurements with B-mode ultrasound during breastfeeding. Ultrasound Med Biol. 2010;36(11):1797–807. PubMed PMID: 20970028.
23. Jacobs LA, Dickinson JE, Hart PD, Doherty DA, Faulkner SJ. Normal nipple position in term infants measured on breastfeeding ultrasound. J Hum Lact. 2007;23(1):52–9. PubMed PMID: 17293551.
24. Sakalidjs VS, Williams TM, Garbin CP, Hepworth AR, Hartmann PE, Paech MJ, et al. Ultrasound imaging of infant sucking dynamics during the establishment of lactation. J Hum Lact. 2013;29(2):205–13. PubMed PMID: 22965645.
25. Elad D, Kozlovsky P, Blum O, Laine AF, Po MJ, Botzer E, et al. Biomechanics of milk extraction during breast-feeding. Proc Natl Acad Sci USA. 2014;111(14):5230–5. PubMed PMID: 24706845. Pubmed Central PMCID: 3986202.
26. Cannon AM, Sakalidis VS, Lai CT, Perrella SL, Geddes DT. Vacuum characteristics of the sucking cycle and relationships with milk removal from the breast in term infants. Early Hum Dev. 2016;96:1–6. PubMed PMID: 26964010.
27. Neville MC, Morton J, Umemura S. Lactogenesis. The transition from pregnancy to lactation. Pediatr Clin N Am. 2001;48(1):35–52. PubMed PMID: 11236732.
28. Kent JC, Mitoulas LR, Cregan MD, Geddes DT, Larsson M, Doherty DA, et al. Importance of vacuum for breastmilk expression. Breastfeed Med. 2008;3(1):11–9. PubMed PMID: 18333764.
29. Ramsay DT, Mitoulas LR, Kent JC, Cregan MD, Doherty DA, Larsson M, et al. Milk flow rates can be used to identify and investigate milk ejection in women expressing breast milk using an electric breast pump. Breastfeed Med. 2006;1(1):14–23. PubMed PMID: 17661556.
30. Geddes DT, Chadwick LM, Kent JC, Garbin CP, Hartmann PE. Ultrasound imaging of infant swallowing during breast-feeding. Dysphagia. 2010;25(3):183–91. PubMed PMID: 19626366.
31. Mendell DA, Logemann JA. Temporal sequence of swallow events during the oropharyngeal swallow. J Speech Lang Hear Res. 2007;50(5):1256–71. PubMed PMID: 17905910.
32. Goldfield EC, Richardson MJ, Lee KG, Margetts S. Coordination of sucking, swallowing, and breathing and oxygen saturation during early infant breast-feeding and bottle-feeding. Pediatr Res. 2006;60(4):450–5. PubMed PMID: 16940236.
33. Sakalidis VS, Geddes DT. Suck-Swallow-Breathe Dynamics in Breastfed Infants. J Hum Lact. 2016;32(2):201–11. quiz 393–5. PubMed PMID: 26319112.
34. Mathew OP, Bhatia J. Sucking and breathing patterns during breast- and bottle-feeding in term neonates. Effects of nutrient delivery and composition. Am J Dis Child. 1989;143(5):588–92. PubMed PMID: 2718995.
35. Lau C. Development of suck and swallow mechanisms in infants. Ann Nutr Metab. 2015;66(Suppl 5):7–14. PubMed PMID: 26226992. Pubmed Central PMCID: 4530609.
36. Lau C, Alagugurusamy R, Schanler RJ, Smith EO, Shulman RJ. Characterization of the developmental stages of sucking in preterm infants during bottle feeding. Acta Paediatr. 2000;89(7):846–52. PubMed PMID: 10943969.
37. Meier PP, Brown LP, Hurst NM, Spatz DL, Engstrom JL, Borucki LC, et al. Nipple shields for preterm infants: effect on milk transfer and duration of breastfeeding. J Hum Lact. 2000;16(2):106–14; quiz 29–31. PubMed PMID: 11153341.

38. McClellan H, Geddes D, Kent J, Garbin C, Mitoulas L, Hartmann P. Infants of mothers with persistent nipple pain exert strong sucking vacuums. Acta Paediatr. 2008;97(9):1205–9. PubMed PMID: 18489617.

39. Neifert M, Lawrence R, Seacat J. Nipple confusion: toward a formal definition. J Pediatr. 1995;126(6):S125–9. PubMed PMID: 7776072.

40. Mobbs EJ, Mobbs GA, Mobbs AE. Imprinting, latchment and displacement: a mini review of early instinctual behaviour in newborn infants influencing breastfeeding success. Acta Paediatr. 2016;105(1):24–30. PubMed PMID: 25919999. Pubmed Central PMCID: 5033030.

41. Mobbs AE. Human imprinting and breastfeeding. Breastfeed Rev. 1989;1(1):39–41.

42. Mobbs AE. Latchment before attachment. The first stage of emotional development: oral tactile imprinting. Sydney: G.T. Crarf Pty Ltd.; 2011.

43. Hurst NM. Recognizing and treating delayed or failed lactogenesis II. J Midwifery Womens Health. 2007;52(6):588–94. PubMed PMID: 17983996.

44. Genna CW, editor. Supporting sucking skills in breastfeeding infants. 3rd ed. Burlington: Jones & Bartlett Learning; 2017.

45. Messner AH, Lalakea ML, Aby J, Macmahon J, Bair E. Ankyloglossia: incidence and associated feeding difficulties. Arch Otolaryngol Head Neck Surg. 2000;126(1):36–9. PubMed PMID: 10628708.

46. O'Shea JE, Foster JP, O'Donnell CP, Breathnach D, Jacobs SE, Todd DA, et al. Frenotomy for tongue-tie in newborn infants. Cochrane Database Syst Rev. 2017;(3):CD011065. PubMed PMID: 28284020.

47. McClellan HL, Kent JC, Hepworth AR, Hartmann PE, Geddes DT. Persistent nipple pain in breastfeeding mothers associated with abnormal infant tongue movement. Int J Environ Res Public Health. 2015;12(9):10833–45. PubMed PMID: 26404342. Pubmed Central PMCID: 4586646.

48. Gardner H, Kent JC, Lai CT, Mitoulas LR, Cregan MD, Hartmann PE, et al. Milk ejection patterns: an intra- individual comparison of breastfeeding and pumping. BMC Pregnancy Childbirth. 2015;15:156. PubMed PMID: 26223256. Pubmed Central PMCID: 4520208.

49. Ramsay DT, Kent JC, Owens RA, Hartmann PE. Ultrasound imaging of milk ejection in the breast of lactating women. Pediatrics. 2004;113(2):361–7. PubMed PMID: 14754950.

50. Borr C, Hielscher-Fastabend M, Lucking A. Reliability and validity of cervical auscultation. Dysphagia. 2007;22(3):225–34. PubMed PMID: 17457548.

51. Leslie P, Drinnan MJ, Zammit-Maempel I, Coyle JL, Ford GA, Wilson JA. Cervical auscultation synchronized with images from endoscopy swallow evaluations. Dysphagia. 2007;22(4):290–8. PubMed PMID: 17554472.

52. Rankin MW, Jimenez EY, Caraco M, Collinson M, Lostetter L, DuPont TL. Validation of test weighing protocol to estimate enteral feeding volumes in preterm infants. J Pediatr. 2016;178:108–12. PubMed PMID: 27587072.

53. Haase B, Barreira J, Murphy PK, Mueller M, Rhodes J. The development of an accurate test weighing technique for preterm and high-risk hospitalized infants. Breastfeeding Med. 2009;4(3):151–6. PubMed PMID: 19739951.

54. Hurst NM, Meier PP, Engstrom JL, Myatt A. Mothers performing in-home measurement of milk intake during breastfeeding of their preterm infants: maternal reactions and feeding outcomes. J Hum Lact. 2004;20(2):178–87. PubMed PMID: 15117517.

55. Kent JC, Hepworth AR, Langton DB, Hartmann PE. Impact of measuring milk production by test weighing on breastfeeding confidence in mothers of term infants. Breastfeed Med. 2015;10(6):318–25. PubMed PMID: 26090790.

56. Feldman-Winter L, Barone L, Milcarek B, Hunter K, Meek J, Morton J, et al. Residency curriculum improves breastfeeding care. Pediatrics. 2010;126(2):289–97. PubMed PMID: 20603262.

57. Morton J, Hall JY, Pessl M. Five steps to improve bedside breastfeeding care. Nurs Womens Health. 2013;17(6):478–88. PubMed PMID: 24589048.

58. Meier PP, Patel AL, Hoban R, Engstrom JL. Which breast pump for which mother: an evidence-based approach to individualizing breast pump technology. J Perinatol. 2016;36(7):493–9. PubMed PMID: 26914013. Pubmed Central PMCID: 4920726.

59. Meier PP, Engstrom JL, Hurst NM, Ackerman B, Allen M, Motykowski JE, et al. A comparison of the efficiency, efficacy, comfort, and convenience of two hospital-grade electric breast pumps for mothers of very low birthweight infants. Breastfeed Med. 2008;3(3):141–50. PubMed PMID: 18778208.

60. Meier P, Hurst N, Rodriguez N, Ackerman B, Howard K, Allen M, et al. Comfort and effectiveness of the symphony breast pump for mothers of preterm infants: comparison of three suction patterns. Adv Exp Med Biol. 2004;554:321–3. PubMed PMID: 15384591.

61. Meier PP, Engstrom JL, Janes JE, Jegier BJ, Loera F. Breast pump suction patterns that mimic the human infant during breastfeeding: greater milk output in less time spent pumping for breast pump-dependent mothers with premature infants. J Perinatol. 2012;32(2):103–10. PubMed PMID: 21818062. Pubmed Central PMCID: 3212618.

62. Post ED, Stam G, Tromp E. Milk production after preterm, late preterm and term delivery; effects of different breast pump suction patterns. J Perinatol. 2016;36(1):47–51. PubMed PMID: 26540245.

63. Dennis CL. Theoretical underpinnings of breastfeeding confidence: a self-efficacy framework. J Hum Lact. 1999;15(3):195–201. PubMed PMID: 10578797.

64. de Jager E, Skouteris H, Broadbent J, Amir L, Mellor K. Psychosocial correlates of exclusive breastfeeding: a systematic review. Midwifery. 2013;29(5):506–18. PubMed PMID: 23099152.

65. Dennis CL. Identifying predictors of breastfeeding self-efficacy in the immediate postpartum period. Res Nurs Health. 2006;29(4):256–68. PubMed PMID: 16847899.

66. Mannion CA, Hobbs AJ, McDonald SW, Tough SC. Maternal perceptions of partner support during breastfeeding. Int Breastfeed J. 2013;8(1):4. PubMed PMID: 23651688. Pubmed Central PMCID: 3653816.

67. McQueen KA, Dennis CL, Stremler R, Norman CD. A pilot randomized controlled trial of a breastfeeding self-efficacy intervention with primiparous mothers. J Obstet Gynecol Neonatal Nurs. 2011;40(1):35–46. PubMed PMID: 21244493.

Chapter 4
Clinical Feeding-Swallowing Evaluation: Overview for the Healthcare Provider

Christina A. Rappazzo and Catherine L. Turk

Purpose of a Clinical Feeding-Swallowing Exam and Prerequisite Knowledge

The clinical feeding-swallowing evaluation is the most widely used method by the speech-language pathologist for assessing a child's ability to feed safely and efficiently. It is typically the first step taken in the overall assessment process and the most important as it often sets a plan in motion. The clinical swallow evaluation has various purposes and goals. Per the American-Speech-Language-Hearing Association (ASHA), the goals include (1) diagnosing or suspecting a feeding and/or swallowing impairment, (2) determining the phase of the swallow that may be involved in the disorder, (3) determining if the patient should be referred to an interdisciplinary team assessment or other medical specialist, (4) determining if an instrumental evaluation is warranted, and (5) developing a therapy/treatment program. The patient's age and history may influence the overall goal of the evaluation, but the overriding objective is to determine safety and efficiency of eating for all patients.

Though formal measures are currently available and discussed later, the assessment is most often a descriptive exam based on what is currently known regarding normal swallow physiology of infants and children, and general feeding development. With that in mind, prior to completing a clinical feeding-swallowing evaluation, the clinician must be well-versed in swallow physiology across the life span. This knowledge ranges from normal infant swallowing, including premature infants, to the young adult swallow, as is seen in adolescent patients. The clinician must

C. A. Rappazzo (✉) · C. L. Turk
Department of Speech, Language and Learning, Texas Children's Hospital, Houston, TX, USA
e-mail: carappaz@texaschildrens.org; clturk@texaschildrens.org

© Springer International Publishing AG, part of Springer Nature 2018
J. Ongkasuwan, E. H. Chiou (eds.), *Pediatric Dysphagia*,
https://doi.org/10.1007/978-3-319-97025-7_4

have a solid understanding of normal feeding development with special attention to changes during critical periods such as transitioning from reflexive suckling to volitional sucking, and transitioning from puree foods to chewable foods (mastication skills). Additionally, because feeding and swallowing is affected by multiple systems, extensive knowledge of neurologic, airway-respiratory, gastrointestinal, and genetic disorders is necessary. Though this background knowledge is not the emphasis of this chapter, it is critical and a prerequisite for any clinician completing the evaluation in order to differentiate between normal and delayed or impaired feeding-swallowing skills.

A cursory overview of feeding development will be provided. This section is not intended to be comprehensive, and the reader is invited to seek additional resources for more detailed information regarding feeding and swallowing development. In brief, infant suckling and swallowing skills begin in utero [1]. By 15–16 weeks of gestation, swallowing movements have been noted via ultrasound to emerge with a gradual increase in frequency noted [2]. This early swallowing behavior is critical for management of amniotic fluid and maturation of the gastrointestinal tract and lays the groundwork for later feeding [3]. Once the term infant is born, the infant relies on primitive reflexes such as rooting to help initiate feeding. An infant's initial sucking pattern is best described as "suckling" rather than "sucking." This suckling is more reflexive in nature and requires a simple anterior-posterior lingual motion [4]. At approximately 3–4 months, suckling transitions from a reflexive to a more volitional pattern, as some of the reflexes which support feeding dissipate. As the infant matures, the next major milestone in feeding is the introduction of spoon feedings (puree foods). This occurs at approximately 6 months and coincides with improved trunk control, growth of the oropharynx, and lowering of the laryngeal structures [5]. The tongue protrusion reflex also integrates at approximately this age which facilitates improved oral skills for spoon-feeding [6]. At this point, the infant is entering the "transitional feeder" stage of development where they are evolving from liquid-only to foods of increased texture gradually. The introduction of textured foods before the age of 10 months is recommended to avoid solid food refusal in the future [6]. At approximately 8–9 months, early dissolvables are introduced to facilitate the development of early chewing skills [7]. Initial chewing movement is up-down vertical jaw motion with the tongue suckling (mashing) on the solid [8]. As the infant matures, lateral lingual movements are noted to transfer the bolus to the molar table. The child then begins to increase the complexity and viscosity of the solid foods taken, and by 12–18 months, he or she receives the vast majority of calories from a toddler diet. Oral skills continue to refine until the age of 3 approximately [5].

With regard to swallowing, the swallow is often divided into the oral phase (oral preparatory and oral transit) and the pharyngeal phase. The oral phase involves latch and expression of liquid from the bottle, procurement of liquids or foods, and/or mastication of the solid. In the typical swallow, the bolus is formed and held in the groove or depression in the central portion of the tongue [9]. A seal is then formed by lingual-palatal contact to contain the bolus and prevent free spillage into the pharynx. Transfer of the bolus is initiated by elevation and anterior-posterior movement of the tongue tip with simultaneous release of the lingual-palatal seal. As the bolus is being propelled posteriorly, the soft palate begins to elevate to close off the nasopharyngeal area to prevent pharyngonasal backflow [10]. The pharyngeal phase is under voluntary and involuntary control [11]. Generally speaking, this phase begins with closure of the nasopharyngeal cavity by palatal elevation, anterior excursion of the hyoid, and initiation of tongue base propulsion [12]. The exact trigger point has some degree of variability in normals, but in infants most often at the level of the valleculae [7]. After the swallow is initiated, epiglottic inversion is viewed as the pressure of the tongue approximating the pharyngeal wall along with hyoid excursion enables the epiglottis to fully invert [13]. The posterior pharyngeal musculature contracts from a superior to inferior in conjunction with tongue base retraction which leads to the bolus coursing through the pharynx via the pressure generated by these actions [14]. Nearly simultaneously, the laryngeal-vestibule achieves closure. Closure of the airway is achieved by medial and forward movement of the arytenoids with eventual contact with the base of the epiglottis, epiglottic inversion, and adduction of the true and false vocal folds [15]. The precise and coordinated timing of these actions results in adequate airway protection and clearance of the bolus into the esophagus.

For the purposes of this chapter, we will first provide an overview of formal clinical measures of feeding-swallowing skills currently available and then discuss the six major components of a typical exam with an emphasis on the clinical saliency of each component:

1. Obtaining general medical history
2. Obtaining feeding-swallowing history
3. Completing oral mechanism exam and posture/positioning observations
4. Assessment of the oral phase of the swallow
5. Assessment of the pharyngeal phase of the swallow
6. Recommendations

Formal Assessment Measures

There are formal clinical feeding- swallowing assessments available for the pediatric population. These assessments were designed for patients ranging in age from birth (younger than 6 months) to adolescence with a variety of diagnoses. However, many focus on feeding refusal/behaviors with limited emphasis on oral-pharyngeal swallow skills. Additionally, many of these tests are population-specific and were designed for children with autism, cerebral palsy, or for breastfeeding. Furthermore, many of the tools are no longer commercially available. Of significance is that psychometric properties of these assessments are often not available or of poor quality. Heckathorn et al. and Pados et al. completed a comprehensive review of the available assessments and found that, in general, they lack information regarding validity and reliability [16, 17]. As such, both publications concluded that use of the currently available formal assessments should be administered "with caution" [16, 17].

Medical History

One of the first steps in completing a clinical feeding-swallowing evaluation is obtaining a thorough medical history. This background information allows the speech-language pathologist to formulate a hypothesis regarding risk of feeding delay and/or swallowing impairment, and develop a plan for the assessement. Additionally, the speech-language pathologist should be aware of all prescribed medications as they may impact swallowing. The following information in Table 4.1, though not exhaustive, should be obtained during a standard feeding-swallowing evaluation.

Table 4.1 Medical history and feeding-swallowing application

Prenatal/birth history	Clinical relevance
Is there a history of any prenatal or perinatal complications? 　Prematurity 　Low birth weight 　Intrauterine growth restriction (IUGR) 　Hypoxic ischemic event	Premature or term infants with comorbidities are at risk of feeding difficulties including oral-motor delays, delay in achieving full oral feedings, and poor growth [18–21]
Gastrointestinal history	**Clinical relevance**
Does the patient have a history of any motility disorders such as: 　Gastroesophageal reflux 　Gastroparesis 　Esophageal achalasia/dysmotility 　Chronic constipation	These diagnoses may result in feeding refusal, reduced esophageal motility, and discomfort with feeding which may contribute to poor weight gain [22–24]
Does the patient have a history of: 　Food intolerances 　Food allergies 　Eosinophilic gastrointestinal disorders 　Food protein-induced enterocolitis	These conditions may result in feeding refusal, oral aversion, coughing, poor oral-motor skills, regurgitation, and vomiting [25–31]
Does the patient have any history of structural anomalies: 　Congenital diaphragmatic hernia 　Esophageal strictures 　Trachea-esophageal fistula 　Esophageal atresia 　Omphalocele 　Short gut	These disorders have been associated with an array of feeding-swallowing difficulties including oral aversion/refusal, esophageal dysphagia, aspiration, and poor oral phase skills [32–36]
Respiratory and airway history	**Clinical relevance**
Does the patient have a history of or require: 　Chronic lung disease 　Bronchopulmonary dysplasia 　Noninvasive respiratory support (CPAP)	These disorders are associated with abnormal sucking patterns and tracheal aspiration [37, 38]
Does the patient have a history of respiratory infections such as: 　Bronchiolitis, bronchitis, or pneumonia	These diagnoses can be a sequela of chronic tracheal aspiration [39, 40]

Table 4.1 (continued)

Does the child have a history of airway disorders such as: Laryngomalacia Vocal fold immobility Subglottic stenosis Laryngeal cleft	Airway disorders can negatively affect breathing patterns resulting in poor feeding and reduced airway protection [41–45]
Neurologic history	**Clinical relevance**
Does the child have a history of: Epilepsy Cardiovascular accident/stroke Brain tumor Traumatic brain injury Traumatic spinal injury	These disorders can affect brainstem and cortical controls of swallowing resulting in various profiles of swallowing impairment including delayed swallow initiation, poor pharyngeal clearance, and tracheal aspiration [46–52]
Cardiac history	**Clinical relevance**
Does the child have a history of: Single ventricle PDA ASD/VSD Aortic arch abnormalities	Cardiac disorders can result in reduced oral-motor skills, poor endurance, delayed initiation of the pharyngeal swallow, reduced laryngeal-vestibular closure, and tracheal aspiration [43, 53–56]

Feeding and Swallowing History

The next consideration of the clinical evaluation is the completion of a feeding-swallowing history. This information allows the speech-language pathologist to better understand the infant or child's experience with feeding, identify fluctuations or regression in feeding skills, identify parent/caregiver concerns, and formulate a hypothesis regarding oral trials.

For young infants, critical information to obtain includes the timing of introduction of oral feeding, method of feeding (breast or bottle), volume prescribed per feed, volume consumed per feed, length of feeding, type of formula being provided, nipple flow rate, position of feeding, and interventions being utilized during feeding. Then, a descriptive summary of a typical feeding is obtained with emphasis on areas of concern. Common areas of inquiry are comprised of: infant latch, oral leakage/spillage, sucking rhythmicity, fluid expression, fatigue/endurance, and signs of potential pharyngeal swallow difficulties. This information allows the speech pathologist to systematically begin the process of formulating a differential diagnosis and predict where the breakdown of the feeding process occurs.

For children, the most critical information to obtain includes: timeline of introduction to puree and chewable foods, variety of foods consumed, current volume of each consistency consumed, drinking vessels utilized, modifications being implemented, and overall parental concerns regarding feeding-swallowing skills. Most importantly, the speech-language pathologist also inquires about any possible sign of pharyngeal phase dysfunction and/or tracheal aspiration such as coughing, choking, wet voice, wet respiration, or pharyngeal congestion.

Lastly, gathering information regarding any previous swallowing, gastrointestinal, or airway exams is important. The following studies provide valuable infomation regarding swallowing safety and integrity of the aerodigestive tract. They include: videofluoroscopic swallow studies (VFSS), Fiberoptic endoscopic evaluation of swallowing (FEES), upper gastrointestinal series exams, gastric emptying exams, pH-impedance testing, high-resolution manometry, or direct laryngoscopy and bronchoscopy (DL&B).

Oral Mechanism Exam and Positioning Considerations

Oral Mechanism

The oral mechanism exam is a detailed sensori-motor examination of the face, oral cavity and voice. The exam assesses the structures at rest, during non-feeding tasks and during feeding tasks as appropriate. For children who can not follow commands, this is completed via general observation during feeding rather than via direct tasks. The main purpose of this portion of the evaluation is to identify any structural defects or functional movement deficits that may interfere with successful feeding-swallowing. This is of importance because it provides insight into basic neurologic function that is critical for swallowing. Table 4.2 is a brief overview of the cranial nerves involved in swallowing and the clinical implications if affected.

Table 4.2 Cranial nerves and swallowing application

Cranial nerve	Sensory-motor function	Clinical relevance
Trigeminal (5)	Jaw muscles Facial sensation	Difficulty with mastication Decreased sensation of the lower face Decreased hyoid elevation
Facial (7)	Facial muscles Taste	Difficulty with labial seal/closure Residue in the buccal cavities Reduced taste anterior portion of tongue
Glossopharyngeal (9)	Pharyngeal sensation Posterior Tongue sensation Laryngeal elevation/ pharyngeal shortening Taste Gag reflex	Impaired sensation of the posterior tongue Impaired sensation of pharynx Delayed swallow initiation Decreased laryngeal elevation Absent gag
Vagus (10)	Palatal elevation Pharyngeal musculature Larynx	Pharyngo-nasal reflux Difficulty initiating swallow Difficulty with pharyngeal constriction Reduced vocal fold abduction/adduction Reduced UES opening Pharyngeal stasis
Hypoglossal (12)	Intrinsic and extrinsic tongue muscles	Difficulty forming bolus Difficulty with posterior containment Difficulty transferring bolus/oral stasis Difficulty retracting tongue base

Table 4.3 Oral reflexes [7]

Reflex	Age of integration
Rooting	3–6 months
Transverse tongue	6–9 months
Phasic bite	9–12 months
Gag	Persists

In infants, the intraoral structures are also examined as are the oral reflexes. From a structural standpoint, facial symmetry is assessed; labial integrity and the presence/absence of sucking pads are noted. As sucking requires intact palate structure/function, palatal shape/height and general integrity is assessed. The jaw is also examined to ensure micrognathia and/or retrognathia is not present. Also, lingual frenulum is then evaluated for any evidence of ankyloglossia. Vocal quality is informally assessed via quality of the cry or spontaneous vocalizations. Baseline vitals such as respiratory and heart rate are noted. The oral reflexes listed in Table 4.3 are assessed as they are most pertinent to feeding-swallowing.

Positioning

It is well-documented that positioning as well as neuromuscular control can influence one's swallowing ability [57]. Therefore, when performing a clinical feeding-swallowing evaluation, the patient's overall gross motor function should be kept in mind. Optimal positioning depends on the patient's age, medical history, and postural control. We will briefly discuss infants, neurotypical children, and children with neuromuscular impairment.

With regard to term infants, they are typically held in a semi-upright position with adult-provided head/neck and trunk support, whereas premature infants or those with a history of airway or pulmonary compromise may require additional positional considerations. For instance, side-lying positioning has been shown to help maintain physiologic stability [58]. Additional postural supports include: hands to midline, swaddling, and bracing of the feet. By contrast, a more upright position may be the best option for an infant with cleft palate to reduce pharyngo-nasal backflow.

The neurotypical toddler or child is placed in a high chair or chair for the clinical swallow. With this in mind, optimal positioning for feeding includes: neutral head position with balance between flexion and extension, symmetrical shoulder-girdle stability, pelvic stability, and hips, knees, and ankles each at 90 degrees with appropriate foot support [59]. This is critical because an unstable pelvis and trunk may result in poor head and neck positioning impairing the individual's ability to control oral-pharyngeal patterns for a safe swallow [57].

Positioning the infant or child with neuromuscular compromise becomes crucial as the potential effects of impaired motor control can negatively impact the safety of the swallow. A study by Benfer et al. compared clinical swallowing evaluation results in children with cerebral palsy with gross motor assessments and found that the more impaired levels on the Gross Motor Function Classification System (GMFCS) correlated with increased number of clinical markers of oropharyngeal dysphagia [60]. In general, patients with abnormal tone often exhibit a poor base of stability that affects mobility of oral-motor structures. Poor head position (neck hyperextension) has been associated with compromised airway protection in two ways: (1) creating a more "open" airway and (2) increasing the rate of bolus transit to the pharynx via gravity assist. These variables, taken in concert with known postural and swallowing deficits, create an added demand in an already compromised system resulting in increased aspiration risk. Additionally, individuals with changes in alignment of the cervical spine such as in lordosis may experience swallowing difficulties as these changes can result in: narrowing of the pharyngeal space, reduction of the pharyngeal squeeze, and reduction of laryngeal elevation [61]. A wide variety of anomalies such as kyphosis or torticollis may be associated with malformation of craniovertebral junction (CVJ) resulting in compression of cervico-medullary junction [62].

Assessment of the Oral Phase of the Swallow

Term Infant (Bottle-Feeding)

A typical swallowing exam begins with assessment of the infant's non-nutritive skills. Rooting response and non-nutritive sucking should be present in healthy, term infants. The rooting response occurs when an infant turns toward the stimulus and displays sucking motion with his/her mouth when the cheek or lip is touched [63]. In addition, non-nutritive sucking of a newborn is elicited by placing a pacifier or gloved finger gently inside the infant's mouth to the mid-tongue area. The infant should close his mouth around the pacifier/finger and initiate suckling motion. The rate should be two sucks per second with a mature sucking burst [64]. Information gathered regarding the non-nutritive suck includes: rhythmicity, number of sucking bursts and pauses, and relative strength of the suck [65]. In addition, observation of tongue cupping can be noted. The presence of a non-nutritive suck is an indicator for readiness to bottle-feeding; however, it is not necessarily predictive of successful nutritive feeding [65, 66].

Regarding nutritive sucking, there are two primary components of mature sucking mechanics that should be evaluated: expression and suction [67, 68]. Expression refers to positive pressure generated as the tongue compresses the nipple against the hard palate [64, 68, 69]. Suction refers to the negative intraoral pressure that is created by closure of the nasopharyngeal port with lips sealed around the bottle and lowering of the jaw, thus creating a vacuum [70]. These coordinated actions result in the extraction of the liquid out of the bottle. One suck per swallow is the ideal pattern of sucking expression with normal variance up to three sucks per swallow.

Sucking bursts of 10–30 suck-swallow sequences are viewed with brief ventilation pauses of 1–2 seconds between bursts [7]. A healthy term infant should be able to latch onto the nipple with ease and initiate a coordinated, rhythmical sucking pattern and complete a feeding within 20-30 minutes.

Premature Infant (Bottle-Feeding)

With medical and technological advances, the survival rate for the extremely premature and medically complex infant is increasing [71]. Premature infants may also have concomitant comorbidities involving the cardiac, neurologic, or respiratory systems that additionally impact their ability to feed/swallow effectively. These infants have an increased risk of oropharyngeal dysphagia and coordination difficulties. Because nutrition and oral intake is essential for brain and development, early assessment of feeding-swallowing is warranted [72].

A preterm infant is any infant born before 37 weeks of gestation. Depending on individual readiness, bottle-feeding/breastfeeding typically begins around 32–34 weeks of gestation [73]. Factors influencing the infant's readiness to feed include, but are not limited to: gestational age, neurologic maturity, medical stability, physiologic stability with care and handling, behavioral and motor regulation, and appropriate infant feeding cues [74]. Some of the feeding cues specific to the infant include the presence of non-nutritive suck and rooting response, the ability to maintain calm and quiet state, the presence of appropriate motor tone with hands at midline toward mouth, and the ability to maintain respiratory and heart rate at optimal levels [75]. Once the infant is deemed "ready," the feeding-swallowing evaluation is initiated and consists of assessing latch, spillage, tongue position, sucking burst length, suck-swallow ratio, rhythmicity, and most importantly the coordination of the suck-swallow-breathe triad. The main goal is for the infant to maintain physiologic stability during bottle attempts and demonstrate no signs of distress. If deficits are noted, then potential critical interventions include flow rate of the nipple, position of the infant, postural support, position of the bottle, and pacing. These are utilized dependent on clinical findings. In healthy preterm infants ("feeders and growers"), if deficits are noted, they may be a reflection of immaturity rather than a true oral-pharyngeal dysphagia. This is especially true if the infant is assessed prior to reaching term gestation. Please see Table 4.4 for summary of oral phase deficits.

Child

When assessing the child, the liquid and foods presented are largely dependent on the feeding history and age. The swallow exam is performed with the child seated in a high chair, typical chair, specialty chair, or wheelchair depending on his/her trunk/neck stability. The clinical swallow exam attempts to mimic a typical meal

Table 4.4 Oral phase deficits for bottle-feeding

Possible deficits	Clinical relevance
Oral phase	
Absent rooting	Developmental immaturity (<32 weeks) neurologic compromise
Weak/absent suction	Developmental immaturity (<36 weeks) Structural palate deficit Neurologic compromise
Anterior spillage	Excessive flow rate Reduced labial seal
Reduced tongue cupping	Inefficient expression
Excessive jaw excursion	Inefficient expression
Increased suck-swallow ratio	Inefficient expression Prolonged feeding
Poor coordination of suck-swallow-breathe	Risk of apnea Risk of bradycardia Risk of tracheal aspiration
Decreased length of sucking bursts	Respiratory compromise Limited endurance
Pharyngo-nasal regurgitation	Structural defect of the palate Palatal weakness or incoordination
Pulling off the nipple	Respiratory compromise Airway protection Poor endurance Gastrointestinal disturbances
Arching/discomfort/crying	Gastrointestinal disturbances
Extended feeding times	Inefficient sucking Poor weight gain

if clinically appropriate, especially for children consuming all nutrition orally. If the child has minimal or reduced oral intake, then the assessment begins at the current level and gradually introduces new liquid/food items in a patient-directed manner. In oral feeders, the caregiver brings in feeding supplies and foods to be provided during the evaluation. The child's preferred food or drink is presented first with gradual progression to more challenging foods or liquids. Liquids may be provided using cups brought from home. Clinical observation of the oral preparatory phase and oral transit of swallowing includes: labial seal/closure, anterior spillage, formation/control of bolus, mastication skills, efficiency of transfer to the pharynx, and the presence of oral residue. If oral phase deficits are noted, then possible interventions are introduced during the evaluation. These interventions may be changes in positioning, posture, flavors, type of drinking vessel used, bite sizes, cyclic swallows, allowing "dry swallows" between bites, placement of chewable foods on molars, and/or blending of foods. Interventions such as thickened liquids are typically not recommended based on clinical evaluation alone. Please see Table 4.5 for possible oral phase deficits in children (non-bottle-fed).

A summary of possible deficits and their significance includes the following.

Table 4.5 Oral phase deficits in children

Possible deficits	Clinical relevance
Oral phase	
Reduced lip closure	Oral spillage Reduced bolus procurement Inefficient transport
Anterior spillage	Fast flow rate of liquid Labial weakness
Reduced bolus control	Reduced/weak tongue movement/elevation
Tongue thrust	Oral spillage Inefficient transport
Tongue retraction	Inefficient bolus formation Inefficient bolus transport
Reduced oral transport	Inefficient bolus formation and transfer
Pocketing of foods or liquids	Decreased oral sensation/hyposensitivity Reduced buccal tension
Immature/reduced chewing	Reduced jaw movements/stability Reduced tongue lateralization Risk of choking/gagging/swallowing whole
Pharyngo-nasal regurgitation	Structural defect of palate Reduced palatal closure/incoordination
Expelling	Texture hypersensitivity Flavor hypersensitivity Immature chewing
Refusal	Gastrointestinal disturbances Airway protection
Gagging	Flavor hypersensitivity Texture hypersensitivity Gastrointestinal disturbances Immature chewing
Prolonged mealtimes	Reduced oromotor functioning Sub-optimal nutrition Poor weight gain

Assessment of the Pharyngeal Phase of the Swallow

One of the major purposes of the clinical evaluation is to determine the safety of oral feeding. More specifically, it is to determine whether the patient displays clinical signs suspicious for pharyngeal dysphagia and/or aspiration. As pharyngeal phase dysphagia can only be properly diagnosed instrumentally, the speech-language pathologist attempts to identify markers concerning for aspiration or pharyngeal dysphagia such as: cough, choking, chest congestion, gagging, desaturations/apneas, throat clearing, wet voice quality, wet respirations (wet/noisy breathing), increased respiratory effort, and audible swallows. It should be noted, however, that to date, there is a paucity of data to support that all these signs, in fact, predict pharyngeal dysphagia/tracheal aspiration in pediatrics.

One specific study attempted to determine which of the above clinical markers were predictive of tracheal aspiration, laryngeal penetration, or pharyngeal residue on a Videofluoroscopic Swallow Study (VFSS). Weir et al. did a retrospective study of 150 children comparing signs concerning for aspiration observed during a clinical feeding-swallowing evaluation to the documented results of the VFSS. In the study, the statistically significant clinical markers associated with tracheal aspiration of thin liquids on the VFSS were: wet voice, wet breathing, and cough. In addition, cough was associated with post-swallow residues on thin liquids. Of note, there were no clinical markers associated with aspiration, penetration, or post-swallow residues for purees [76].

Although Weir identified signs predictive of aspiration of thin liquid, another study noted minimal predictive value of the clinical evaluation in identifying patients that were aspirating. In a study by Duncan et al., 40% of the children (<2 years of age), who were reported to have "normal" clinical feeding-swallowing evaluations, demonstrated tracheal aspiration on their VFSS. Even when adjusted for comorbidities, no single symptom (including but not limited to choking, coughing, noisy breathing, congestion, slow feeding, respiratory distress, and recurrent pneumonia) predicted aspiration on the VFSS [77]. The difficulty of identifying aspiration clinically likely stems from the fact that many children experience "silent" aspiration. "Silent aspiration," as viewed on the VFSS, occurs when contrast falls below the vocal folds and there is no cough response to the event. In a study done by Arvedson, J et al., aspiration was "silent" in 94% of neurologically-impaired children [78]. Furthermore, another study documented significant rates of "silent" tracheal aspiration in populations with laryngeal clefts, laryngomalacia, and vocal fold paralysis with the highest rate in infants < 6 months of age (95%) [79]. As such, the clinical feeding-swallowing evaluation is not without its deficiencies. Therefore the clinician must base their decision on clinical observations along with risk factors inherent in the child's medical and developmental history which may include a referral for an imaging examination.

Though we highlighted limitations with regard to the clinical evaluation's ability to detect tracheal aspiration, the evaluation still has merit as it provides information regarding oral phase skills and developmental feeding levels that can aid in diet selection, therapeutic recommendations, and improve the overall management of the dysphagia and/or feeding delay. Lastly, the exam may assist the clinician in preparing/planning for an instrumental examination, if warranted.

Recommendations

The final portion of the clinical feeding-swallowing evaluation is to provide the caregiver with suggestions to aid in successful feeding/swallowing. Though a wide range of possible recommendations exist, most center on providing appropriate utensils/drinking vessels, ensuring optimal positioning, and assisting in selecting foods commensurate with oromotor skills. In addition, a therapeutic plan for addressing any oral-sensory or oral phase deficits appreciated during the exam, such as aversion or immature mastication, is provided. Of note, decisions regarding significant diet modifications (i.e., use of thickened liquids) are often reserved for after the completion of an instrumental swallow evaluation to ensure appropriateness.

Summary and Future Needs

In summary, the clinical feeding-swallowing examination provides the speech-language pathologist with an initial framework or profile of the child's feeding and swallowing abilities. It provides baseline information from which recommendations and modifications may be derived. Because current formal assessment tools used to evaluate feeding-swallowing lack sufficient psychometric testing data or are often population-specific, most often the evaluation is an informal, descriptive exam. The clinician obtains information on medical and feeding history, evaluates oral mechanism functioning, and assesses oral phase abilities through direct observation. During the assessment, the clinician attempts to glean information regarding pharyngeal phase skills and swallowing safety cautiously, as currently there are only a few validated clinical markers predictive of tracheal aspiration documented in pediatrics and these results have yet to be duplicated [76, 77, 79]. With this in mind, instrumental swallow exams are often a suggested complement to the clinical evaluation as both have distinct, but inherent value in the overall management of patients with feeding and swallowing difficulties.

Future needs in the area of pediatric dysphagia and clinical swallow assessment are numerous. However, most importantly, they include additional research on clinical markers predictive of tracheal aspiration across consistencies and ages, and the development of valid and reliable formal test measures.

References

1. Miller JL, Sonies BC, Macedonia C. Emergence of oropharyngeal, laryngeal and swallowing activity in the developing fetal upper aerodigestive tract: an ultrasound evaluation. Early Hum Dev. 2003;71(1):61–87. www.elsevier.com/locate/earlhumdev. Accessed 17 July 2017
2. de Vries JIP, Visser GHA, Prechtl HFR. The emergence of fetal behaviour. II. Quantitative aspects. Early Hum Dev. 1985;12:99. https://doi.org/10.1016/0378-3782(85)90174-4.
3. Ross M, Nijland M. Fetal swallowing: relation to amniotic fluid regulation. Clin Obstet Gynecol. 1997;40(2):352–65. https://doi.org/10.1097/GRF.0b013e31821859c3.
4. Lau C. Development of infant oral feeding skills: what do we know?. https://doi.org/10.3945/ajcn.115.109603.
5. Delaney AL, Arvedson JC. Development of swallowing and feeding: prenatal through first year of life. Dev Disabil Res Rev. 2008;14(2):105–17. https://doi.org/10.1002/ddrr.16.

6. Illingworth RS, Lister J. The critical or sensitive period, with special reference to certain feeding problems in infants and children. J Pediatr. 1964;65(6):839–48. https://doi.org/10.1016/S0022-3476(64)80006-8.

7. Arvedson JC, Brodsky L. Pediatric swallowing and feeding: assessment and management. Albany: Singular Thomson Learning; 2002.

8. Morris S. The normal acquisition of oral feeding skills: implications for assessment and treatment. Central Islip: Therapeutic Media; 1982.

9. Logemann JA. Critical factors in the oral control needed for chewing and swallowing. J Texture Stud. 2014;45(3):173–9.

10. Molfenter SM, Steele CM. Temporal variability in the deglutition literature. Dysphagia. 2012;27(2):162–77.

11. Jean A. Brain stem control of swallowing: neuronal network and cellular mechanisms. Physiol Rev. 2001;81(2):929–69.

12. Molfenter SM, Leigh C, Steele CM. Event sequence variability in healthy swallowing: building on previous findings. Dysphagia. 2014;29(2):234–42.

13. Logeman J. Evaluation and treatment of swallowig disorders. 2nd ed. Austin: Pro-Ed; 1998.

14. Martin-Harris B, Jones B. The videofluorographic swallowing study. Phys Med Rehabil Clin N Am. 2008;19(4):769–85.

15. Van Daele DJ, McCulloch TM, Palmer PM, Langmore SE. Timing of glottic closure during swallowing: a combined electromyographic and endoscopic analysis. Ann Otol Rhinol Laryngo. 2016;114(6):478–87.

16. Heckathorn DE, Speyer R, Taylor J, Cordier R. Systematic review: non-instrumental swallowing and feeding assessments in pediatrics. Dysphagia. 2016;31(1):1–23. https://doi.org/10.1007/s00455-015-9667-5.

17. Pados BF, Park J, Estrem H, Awotwi A. Assessment tools for evaluation of oral feeding in infants younger than 6 months. Adv Neonatal Care. 2016;16(2):143–50. https://doi.org/10.1097/ANC.0000000000000255.

18. Jadcherla SR, Wang M, Vijayapal AS, Leuthner SR. Impact of prematurity and co-morbidities on feeding milestones in neonates: a retrospective study. J Perinatol. 2010;30(3):201–8. https://doi.org/10.1038/jp.2009.149.

19. Törölä H, Lehtihalmes M, Yliherva A, Olsén P. Feeding skill milestones of preterm infants born with extremely low birth weight (ELBW). Infant Behav Dev. 2012;35(2):187–94. https://doi.org/10.1016/j.infbeh.2012.01.005.

20. Wrotniak BH, Stettler N, Medoff-Cooper B. The relationship between birth weight and feeding maturation in preterm infants. Acta Paediatr Int J Paediatr. 2009;98(2):286–90. https://doi.org/10.1111/j.1651-2227.2008.01111.x.

21. Krüger E, Kritzinger A, Pottas L. Breastfeeding and swallowing in a neonate with mild hypoxic-ischaemic encephalopathy. South African J Commun Disord = Die Suid-Afrikaanse Tydskr vir Kommun. 2017;64(1):e1–7. http://www.ncbi.nlm.nih.gov/pubmed/28582997. Accessed 26 July 2017

22. Fishbein M, Branham C, Fraker C, Walbert L, Cox S, Scarborough D. The incidence of oropharyngeal dysphagia in infants with GERD-like symptoms. J Parenter Enter Nutr. 2013;37(5):667. https://doi.org/10.1177/0148607112460683.

23. Ferris L, Rommel N, Doeltgen S, et al. Pressure-flow analysis for the assessment of pediatric oropharyngeal dysphagia. J Pediatr. 2016;177:279. https://doi.org/10.1016/j.jpeds.2016.06.032.

24. Smits M, van Lennep M, Vrijlandt R, et al. Pediatric achalasia in the Netherlands: incidence, clinical course, and quality of life. J Pediatr. 2016;169:110–115.e3. https://doi.org/10.1016/j.jpeds.2015.10.057.

25. Meyer R, Rommel N, Van Oudenhove L, Fleming C, Dziubak R, Shah N. Feeding difficulties in children with food protein-induced gastrointestinal allergies. J Gastroenterol Hepatol. 2014;29(10):1764–9. https://doi.org/10.1111/jgh.12593.

26. Mukkada VA, Haas A, Maune NC, et al. Feeding dysfunction in children with eosinophilic gastrointestinal diseases. Pediatrics. 2010;126(3):e672–7. https://doi.org/10.1542/peds.2009-2227.

27. Furuta GT, Maune NC, Haas A. Feeding difficulties in children with eosinophilic esophagitis. Perspect Swallowing Swallowing Disord. 2010;19(3):59–63.
28. Yamada Y, Kato M, Toki F, et al. Eosinophilic gastrointestinal disorder in an infant with feeding dysfunction. Int Arch Allergy Immunol. 2012;158(SUPPL. 1):83–6. https://doi.org/10.1159/000337797.
29. Wu YP, Franciosi JP, Rothenberg ME, Hommel KA. Behavioral feeding problems and parenting stress in eosinophilic gastrointestinal disorders in children. Pediatr Allergy Immunol. 2012;23(8):730–5. https://doi.org/10.1111/j.1399-3038.2012.01340.x.
30. Maslin K, Dean T, Arshad SH, Venter C. Fussy eating and feeding difficulties in infants and toddlers consuming a cows' milk exclusion diet. Pediatr Allergy Immunol. 2015;26(6):503–8. https://doi.org/10.1111/pai.12427.
31. Herbert LJ, Mehta P, Sharma H. Mealtime behavior among parents and their young children with food allergy. Ann Allergy Asthma Immunol. 2017;118(3):345–50. https://doi.org/10.1016/j.anai.2016.12.002.
32. Rayyan M, Allegaert K, Omari T, Rommel N. Dysphagia in children with esophageal atresia: current diagnostic options. Eur J Pediatr Surg. 2015;25(4):326–32. https://doi.org/10.1055/s-0035-1559818.
33. Gottrand M, Michaud L, Sfeir R, Gottrand F. Motility, digestive and nutritional problems in esophageal atresia. Paediatr Respir Rev. 2016;19(2016):28–33. https://doi.org/10.1016/j.prrv.2015.11.005.
34. Rommel N, Rayyan M, Scheerens C, Omari T. The potential benefits of applying recent advances in esophageal motility testing in patients with esophageal atresia. Front Pediatr. 2017;5:1–7. https://doi.org/10.3389/fped.2017.00137.
35. Rudra S, Adibe OO, Malcolm WF, Smith PB, Cotten CM, Greenberg RG. Gastrostomy tube placement in infants with congenital diaphragmatic hernia: frequency, predictors, and growth outcomes. Early Hum Dev. 2016;103(2016):97–100. https://doi.org/10.1016/j.earlhumdev.2016.08.003.
36. Mahoney L, Rosen R. Feeding problems and their underlying mechanisms in the esophageal atresia–tracheoesophageal fistula patient. Front Pediatr. 2017;5(May):127. https://doi.org/10.3389/fped.2017.00127.
37. Gewolb IH, Bosma JF, Taciak VL, Vice FL. Abnormal developmental patterns of suck and swallow rhythms during feeding in preterm infants with bronchopulmonary dysplasia. Dev Med Child Neurol. 2001;43(7):454–9. http://www.ncbi.nlm.nih.gov/pubmed/11463175. Accessed 26 July 2017
38. Ferrara L, Bidiwala A, Sher I, et al. Effect of nasal continuous positive airway pressure on the pharyngeal swallow in neonates. J Perinatol. 2017;37(4):398–403. https://doi.org/10.1038/jp.2016.229.
39. de Benedictis FM, Carnielli VP, de Benedictis D. Aspiration lung disease. Pediatr Clin N Am. 2009;56(1):173–90. https://doi.org/10.1016/j.pcl.2008.10.013.
40. Owayed AF, Campbell DM, Wang EE. Underlying causes of recurrent pneumonia in children. Arch Pediatr Adolesc Med. 2000;154(2):190–4. https://doi.org/10.1001/archpedi.154.2.190.
41. Simons JP, Greenberg LL, Mehta DK, Fabio A, Maguire RC, Mandell DL. Laryngomalacia and swallowing function in children. Laryngoscope. 2016;126(2):478–84. https://doi.org/10.1002/lary.25440.
42. Chun RH, Wittkopf M, Sulman C, Arvedson J. Transient swallowing dysfunction in typically developing children following supraglottoplasty for laryngomalacia. Int J Pediatr Otorhinolaryngol. 2014;78(11):1883–5. https://doi.org/10.1016/j.ijporl.2014.08.017.
43. Sachdeva R, Hussain E, Moss MM, et al. Vocal cord dysfunction and feeding difficulties after pediatric cardiovascular surgery. J Pediatr. 2007;151(3):312. https://doi.org/10.1016/j.jpeds.2007.03.014.
44. Thottam PJ, Georg M, Chi D, Mehta DK. Outcomes and predictors of surgical management in type 1 laryngeal cleft swallowing dysfunction. Laryngoscope. 2016;126(12):2838–43. https://doi.org/10.1002/lary.26069.

45. Svystun O, Johannsen W, Persad R, Turner JM, Majaesic C, El-Hakim H. Dysphagia in healthy children: characteristics and management of a consecutive cohort at a tertiary centre. Int J Pediatr Otorhinolaryngol. 2017;99:54–9. https://doi.org/10.1016/j.ijporl.2017.05.024.
46. Buckley RT, Morgan T, Saneto RP, Barber J, Ellenbogen RG, Ojemann JG. Dysphagia after pediatric functional hemispherectomy. J Neurosurg Pediatr. 2014;13(1):95–100. https://doi.org/10.3171/2013.10.PEDS13182.
47. Newman LA, Boop FA, Sanford RA, Thompson JW, Temple CK, Duntsch CD. Postoperative swallowing function after posterior fossa tumor resection in pediatric patients. Childs Nerv Syst. 2006;22(10):1296–300. https://doi.org/10.1007/s00381-006-0065-z.
48. Afsharkhar L, Khalessi N, Karimi P. Intraventricular hemorrhage in term neonates: sources, severity and outcome. Iran J Child Neurol. 2015;9(3):34–9.
49. Valenzano TJ, Waito AA, Steele CM. A review of dysphagia presentation and intervention following traumatic spinal injury: an understudied population. Dysphagia. 2016;31(5):598–609. https://doi.org/10.1007/s00455-016-9728-4.
50. Morgan AT, Mageandran SD, Mei C. Incidence and clinical presentation of dysarthria and dysphagia in the acute setting following paediatric traumatic brain injury. Child Care Health Dev. 2010;36(1):44–53. https://doi.org/10.1111/j.1365-2214.2009.00961.x.
51. Morgan AT. Dysphagia in childhood traumatic brain injury: a reflection on the evidence and its implications for practice. Dev Neurorehabil. 2010;13(3):192–203. https://doi.org/10.3109/17518420903289535.
52. Stephanie K, Huckabee Maggie-Lee D. Dysphagia following stroke. 2nd ed. San Diego, CA: Singulair; 2016.
53. Jadcherla S, Vijayapal A, Leuthner S. Feeding abilities in neonates with congenital heart disease: a retrospective study. https://doi.org/10.1038/jp.2008.136.
54. McGrattan KE, McGhee H, DeToma A, et al. Dysphagia in infants with single ventricle anatomy following stage 1 palliation: physiologic correlates and response to treatment. Congenit Heart Dis. 2017;12(3):382–8. https://doi.org/10.1111/chd.12456.
55. Skinner ML, Halstead LA, Rubinstein CS, Atz AM, Andrews D, Bradley SM. Laryngopharyngeal dysfunction after the Norwood procedure. J Thorac Cardiovasc Surg. 2005;130(5):1293–301. https://doi.org/10.1016/j.jtcvs.2005.07.013.
56. Averin K, Uzark K, Beekman Iii RH, Willging JP, Pratt J, Manning PB. Postoperative assessment of laryngopharyngeal dysfunction in neonates after Norwood operation. Ann Thorac Surg. 2012;94:1257–61. https://doi.org/10.1016/j.athoracsur.2012.01.009.
57. Larnert G, Ekberg O. Positioning improves the oral and pharyngeal swallowing function in children with cerebral palsy. Acta Paediatr. 1995;84(6):689–92. https://doi.org/10.1111/j.1651-2227.1995.tb13730.x.
58. Clark L, Kennedy G, Pring T. Improving bottle feeding in preterm infants: investigating the elevated side-lying position. Infant (3). 2007;3(4):154–8. http://www.infantgrapevine.co.uk/pdf/inf_016_ife.pdf.
59. Alexander R. Oral-motor treatment for infants and young children with cerebral palsy. Semin Speech Lang. 1987;8(1):87–100.
60. Benfer KA, Weir KA, Bell KL, Ware RS, Davies PSW, Boyd RN. Clinical signs suggestive of pharyngeal dysphagia in preschool children with cerebral palsy. Res Dev Disabil. 2015;38:192–201. https://doi.org/10.1016/j.ridd.2014.12.021.
61. Tian W, Yu J. The role of C2-C7 and O-C2 angle in the development of dysphagia after cervical spine surgery. Dysphagia. 2013;28(2):131–8. https://doi.org/10.1007/s00455-012-9421-1.
62. Menezes AH. Craniovertebral junction database analysis: incidence, classification, presentation, and treatment algorithms. Childs Nerv Syst. 2008;24(10):1101–8. https://doi.org/10.1007/s00381-008-0605-9.
63. Sheppard JJ, Mysak ED. Ontogeny of infantile oral reflexes and emerging chewing. Child Dev. 1984;55(3):831–43. https://doi.org/10.2307/1130134.
64. Wolff PH. The serial organization of sucking in the young infant. Pediatrics. 1968;42(6):943–56. https://doi.org/10.1017/S1431927603445509.

65. Lau C, Kusnierczyk I. Quantitative evaluation of infant's nonnutritive and nutritive sucking. Dysphagia. 2001;16(1):58–67. https://doi.org/10.1007/s004550000043.
66. Pinelli J, Symington AJ. Non-nutritive sucking for promoting physiologic stability and nutrition in preterm infants. In: Pinelli J, editor. Cochrane database of systematic reviews. Chichester: John Wiley & Sons, Ltd; 2005. https://doi.org/10.1002/14651858.CD001071.pub2.
67. Eishima K. The analysis of sucking behaviour in newborn infants. Early Hum Dev. 1991;27(3):163–73. https://doi.org/10.1016/0378-3782(91)90192-6.
68. Colley JRT, Creamer B. Sucking and swallowing in infantes. Br Med J. 1958;2:422–3. https://doi.org/10.1136/bmj.2.5093.422.
69. Sameroff AJ. The components of sucking in the human newborn. J Exp Child Psychol. 1968;6(4):607–23. https://doi.org/10.1016/0022-0965(68)90106-9.
70. Lau C. Development of suck and swallow mechanisms in infants. Ann Nutr Metab. 2015;66:7–14. https://doi.org/10.1159/000381361.
71. Perrin JM, Anderson LE, Van Cleave J. The rise in chronic conditions among infants, children, and youth can be met with continued health system innovations. Health Aff. 2014;33(12):2099–105. https://doi.org/10.1377/hlthaff.2014.0832.
72. Knudsen EI. Sensitive periods in the development of the brain and behavior. J Cogn Neurosci. 2004;16(8):1412–25. https://doi.org/10.1162/0898929042304796.
73. Bu'Lock F, Woolridge MW, Baum JD. Development of co-ordination of sucking, swallowing and breathing: ultrasound study of term and preterm infants. Dev Med Child Neurol. 1990;32(8):669–78. https://doi.org/10.1111/j.1469-8749.1990.tb08427.x.
74. Pickler RH. A model of feeding readiness for preterm infants. Neonatal Intensive Care. 2004;17(4):31–6. http://www.ncbi.nlm.nih.gov/pubmed/16429606. Accessed 26 July 2017
75. Thoyre SM, Shaker CS, Pridham KF. The early feeding skills assessment for preterm infants. Neonatal Netw. 2005;24(3):7–16. https://doi.org/10.1891/0730-0832.24.3.7.
76. Weir K, McMahon S, Barry L, Masters IB, Chang AB. Clinical signs and symptoms of oropharyngeal aspiration and dysphagia in children. Eur Respir J. 2009;33(3):604–11. https://doi.org/10.1183/09031936.00090308.
77. Duncan DR, Mitchell PD, Larson K, Rosen RL. Presenting signs and symptoms do not predict aspiration risk in children. J Pediatrics. 2018.
78. Arvedson J, Rogers B, Buck G, Smart P, Msall M. Silent aspiration prominent in children with dysphagia. Int J Pediatr Otorhinolaryngol. 1994;28(2–3):173–81. https://doi.org/10.1016/0165-5876(94)90009-4.
79. Velayutham P, Irace AL, Kawai K, Dodrill P, Perez J, Londahl M, Mundy L, Dombrowski ND, Rahbar R Silent aspiration: Who is at risk? Laryngoscope.

Chapter 5
The Videofluoroscopic Swallow Study: Indoduction, Limitations, and Challenges

Christina A. Rappazzo and Catherine L. Turk

General Introduction

Assessing dysphagia in the pediatric population can be a challenge even for the most skilled speech-language pathologist. Clinical markers of tracheal aspiration are difficult to delineate in pediatrics as some of the hallmark signs present in the adult population such as cough may not be present in the pediatric population [1, 2]. The literature identifying validated clinical indicators of tracheal aspiration across consistencies in pediatrics is limited at the present time [2, 3]. Yet we do have evidence that "silent" tracheal aspiration occurs to a significant degree in various pediatric populations such as those with neurologic impairment, airway disorders, and congenital heart anomalies. [4–7]. Due to these current limitations, instrumental tools such as the videofluoroscopic swallow study (also referred to as the Modified Barium Swallow Study) play an important role in the assessment and management of pediatric dysphagia.

The videofluoroscopic swallow study (VFSS) is radiographic exam of swallowing completed by a radiologist and a speech-language pathologist. This collaboration allows for the most comprehensive and accurate assessment to be completed. The VFSS has evolved since the early prototype by Dr. Martin Donner, a radiologist [8, 9]. An early version of the exam utilized cineradiography; however, it evolved to the exam it is today due to the contributions of speech-language pathologists most notably Dr. Jerilyn Logemann [10]. Though other instrumental exams are available and have a valid and important role in the assessment of dysphagia, the VFSS is still one of the

C. A. Rappazzo (✉) · C. L. Turk
Department of Speech, Language and Learning,
Texas Children's Hospital, Houston, TX, USA
e-mail: carappaz@texaschildrens.org; clturk@texaschildrens.org

© Springer International Publishing AG, part of Springer Nature 2018
J. Ongkasuwan, E. H. Chiou (eds.), *Pediatric Dysphagia*,
https://doi.org/10.1007/978-3-319-97025-7_5

few methods to visualize the oral-pharyngeal phases of the swallow in their entirety with minimal discomfort to the patient. The general purpose of the exam is to detail oral-pharyngeal swallow physiology, identify structural differences of the oropharynx, document airway protection assess effectiveness of treatment strategies as indicated and assist with diet recommendations. The exam also allows the clinician an opportunity to possibly capture events of tracheal aspiration but is by no means a "pass/fail" exam or an exam focused solely on the presence or absence of tracheal aspiration.

Indications, Contraindications, and General Limitations of the VFSS

The American Speech-Language-Hearing Association (ASHA) and the American College of Radiology (ACR) have both developed practice parameters and recommendations regarding key indicators for when to consider a videofluoroscopic swallow study [11, 12]. Indicators may stem from risk factors in the patient's medical history to clinical signs and symptoms present during completion of a clinical swallow evaluation. For the purposes of this chapter, we have categorized risk factors into three categories based on ASHA's guidelines. They include: clear need for instrumental evaluation, possible need for instrumental evaluation, and no need for instrumental evaluation.

Clear indicators for a VFSS include signs of swallowing dysfunction noted during clinical evaluation, differential diagnosis required for medical team, nutritional or pulmonary compromise due to suspected oral-pharyngeal dysphagia, swallow rehabilitation program development, identification of compensations or postural changes that may ease the swallow dysfunction, and known structural differences of the oral-pharyngeal cavity that may result in dysphagia. An exam may be considered for the following reasons: the child has impaired cognition and/or communication which does not allow for a thorough clinical examination, pre-surgical baseline when known procedure may negatively impact the swallow, and diagnosis present that is associated with a high risk for dysphagia such as neurologic impairments.

Contraindications for completion of a videofluoroscopic swallow study may include a variety of conditions and/or situations. First, all patients must be medically stable to tolerate the procedure and the risks inherent in the procedure. If the child is too ill or the risk of possible aspiration would result in injury, then the exam would be contraindicated at that time. Also, if the patient's level of consciousness is such that they cannot maintain an alert state for eating due to either medical acuity or cognitive dysfunction, then an exam would be contraindicated as well. Additionally, the child must have had an opportunity for feeding/swallowing practice for a reasonable amount of time prior to completing an exam in order for the exam to be valid. This is especially important in the infant population where developmental processes and skills are evolving at a rapid rate or in children who have had limited practice with oral intake in their lifetime. In addition, premature infants are not typically considered appropriate for videofluoroscopic swallow studies until they reach term to allow for maturation. Lastly, it is important to consider whether the exam is going to alter the plan of care presently or in the future. If regardless of the results, the plan of care would not be altered, then it would not be beneficial to complete an exam.

As with all medical procedures, a VFSS has its own set of limitations. The primary limitation is the radiation exposure inherent in the exam. This places restrictions on the number of trials and consistencies a clinician can present during the exam. Therefore, this makes testing for respiratory fatigue, as often utilized during infant exams, a challenge. Additionally, this limits the number of times an exam can be repeated to avoid excessive radiation exposure. Lastly, breastfeeding cannot be assessed as the test requires the administration of barium sulfate.

Overall, a videofluoroscopic swallow study should be considered when a threshold of risk has been reached based on either medical history or direct observation via clinical evaluation. As much of the aspiration in pediatric dysphagia is "silent," advancing to instrumental evaluation based solely on the classic presentation of cough rather than the entire clinical picture needs to be questioned [4, 5, 7].

Radiation Safety Considerations, Exam Settings and Length

Speech-language pathologists and radiologists are well-versed in the ALARA principle. The concept expressed in the ALARA principal, as low as reasonably achievable, and the application has evolved over time but now applies to all medical imaging procedures [13]. The aim is to manage "the radiation does to the patient to be commensurate with the medical purpose" [14]. With this philosophy in place, radiation time and dosage during a VFSS is always kept to a minimum by the speech-language pathologist and radiologist while still capturing the needed diagnostic and therapeutic information.

The pulse rate utilized during a VFSS had varied. A rate of 30 pulses per second is recommended for the accurate assessment of oral-pharyngeal swallow physiology as the pharyngeal swallow often lasts less than 0.5 s [15]. Utilizing pulse rates less than 30 has been identified in the adult literature as resulting in differences in judging various aspects of swallowing impairment and in the treatment recommendations [16]. Though we currently have no published data in pediatrics regarding whether reduction in rates results in different treatment recommendations, we do have some evidence by Cohen that laryngeal penetration could potentially be missed if rate is reduced [17]. This pulse rate is especially important during the assessment of liquids. It has been suggested that rate for solid foods can be reduced to 15 pulses per second in an attempt to reduce radiation exposure without jeopardizing the quality of the exam. This is generally considered an acceptable "middle ground" for solid food for exams especially in children who have completed multiple exams.

The duration of the videofluoroscopic swallow study should be kept as short as possible without jeopardizing the validity of the exam. In adult literature, when using a standardized approach, exams averaged 2.98 minutes with the inclusion of intervention strategies [18]. Per Arvedson, most infant swallow studies can be completed in 60–90 seconds [19]. In an effort to minimize radiation exposure, yet assess for fatigue during bottle-feeding, the radiologist will often turn the fluoroscope on and off at various intervals. This allows for a more representative sample of feeding while still maintaining radiation exposure time to a minimum. In older children, exam lengths have been documented to range from 2 to 3 minutes [20]. In a study by Henderson, average radiation time was 1.58 min [15]. Exams exceeding these lengths are discouraged and would be considered an exception rather than the standard.

Basics in Performing the Exam

It is difficult to know if a child is "ready" for a VFSS especially when the child is receiving primary nutrition via gastrostomy tube. The typical guidelines include medical stability, ability to maintain alertness, and experiences with "small amounts" of food or liquid. Ideally, the VFSS should not be the very first feeding for the patient in order for the exam to be representative.

A variety of liquids and foods are presented to the patient based on age, developmental level and oral experiences. All liquids and food contain barium for visualization. Liquid viscosity levels include thin, nectar, and honey-thick liquid as developed by the National Dysphagia Diet [21]. The infant and child's standard feeding utensils such as bottles and cups are utilized during the exam to promote a more natural form of eating. Modifications are then provided based on performance.

Positioning of the patient is critical for an accurate assessment of swallowing abilities. Positioning varies depending on the age of the child and medical history of the child. For young infants, typically, the exam is completed with the infant in a sidelying semi-upright position. For infants with known unilateral vocal fold involvement, the infant is placed with the non-paralyzed side down [22]. For older infants (>3 months) or infants with cleft palate, a more upright position may be more appropriate. For children, the VFSS is conducted with the patient in an upright, seated position with adequate head and trunk support [22]. For patients with cerebral palsy or other neurologic conditions, the use of supportive seating is of utmost importance as trunk and head instability can negatively impact swallowing abilities. In general, a neutral head position and neck-trunk elongation with hips, knees, and ankles each at 90 degrees is the optimal position. For populations that must remain in their wheelchair or bed, a C-arm can be used. A C-arm is an imaging scanning intensifier that is mobile and functions much like the standard videofluoroscopic equipment.

Terminology of Modified Liquids and Foods

As mentioned briefly in the previous section, liquids and foods are currently being classified by categories developed by the National Dysphagia Diet (NDD) [21]. The NDD established by the Academy of Nutrition and Dietetics (formerly American Dietetic Association) was created by a task force of dietitians, speech-language pathologists, and food scientists in 2002 [21]. The NDD is the most commonly used system in North America. Its aim was to establish standard terminology when referring to altered foods and liquids for consistent practice patterns and standardization in dysphagia management. The task force utilized an instrumental texture analyzer that leads to the development of anchor foods to represent points along a continuum of textures/foods. Terms were developed for both liquid viscosities and solid food textures. Please see Table 5.1 for terminology for food levels and liquids as defined by the NDD include [23].

Table 5.1 Terminology utilized for modified liquids/foods

Liquid viscosities	
Thin liquid	1–50 centipoise
Nectar-like	51–350 centipoise
Honey-like	351–1750 centipoise
Spoon-thick	>1750 centipoise
Foods	
Level 1 Puree	Cohesive, pudding-like
Level 2 Mechanical altered	Cohesive, moist semisolid foods
Level 3 Advance	Soft solids
Regular	All foods

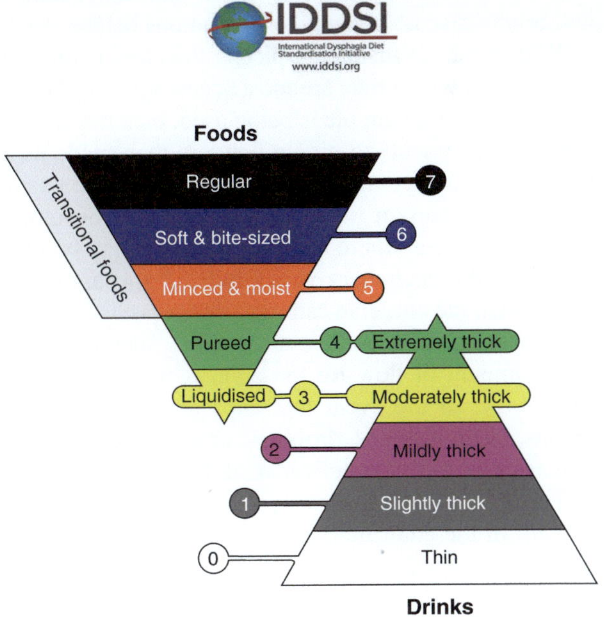

Fig. 5.1 The International Dysphagia Diet Standardisation Initiative 2016. (c) The International Dysphagia Diet Standardisation Initiative 2016 @http://iddsi.org/resources/framework [24]

Though the NDD is currently the most prevalent system, the International Dysphagia Diet Standardisation Initiative (IDDSI) is gaining consideration and endorsements by both the American Speech-Language-Hearing Association and the Academy of Nutrition and Dietetics. The initiative came to completion in 2015 and has developed new terminology for both liquids and solid foods, and new testing methodology [24]. The systems framework consists of a diet of eight levels (0–7). The liquid levels range from thin liquid to extremely thick liquids, and foods range from liquidized to regular. Please see Fig. 5.1 for the terminology utilized by IDDSI.

The importance of understanding the terminology from both systems cannot be overemphasized as they are standards used daily in dysphagia management.

Order, Manner, and Volume Presentation of Liquid and Food

There are significant benefits to standardizing the protocol for administration of food and liquid during the videofluoroscopic swallow study. This goal has been successfully accomplished in the adult population with many suggested protocols available [25–27]. Though currently in development for bottle-fed patients, protocols have not been established in pediatrics [28]. Due to the paucity of standardized methods, the clinician must consider multiple factors including: diagnosis, age, developmental level, oral-motor skills, and feeding experiences in order to carefully design and execute the exam.With this in mind, it is fair to state that the manner, order, and volume of the food and liquid presented during a pediatric videofluoroscopic swallow study may vary more than adult exams. Due to these limitations, we will briefly discuss general considerations below.

With regard to manner, typically the child is presented the liquid consistency in the vessel in which they are most accustomed to. For instance, in the infant population, if a slow flow nipple is being used, then the clinician typically begins with that nipple. Adjustments to nipple flow are then made as appropriate based on performance. In toddlers and older children, again the customary vessel is used. This is especially important in children with global developmental delays and/or neurologic impairment where a specialized cup may be the preferred method. If during the exam, the customary vessel utilized appears not to be supportive of safe oral intake, then the clinician can trial other vessels including sippy cups, open cups, cut-out cups, squeeze bottles, and straws. Identifying vessels that deliver the "just right" amount of flow for the child is the goal in order to promote best swallow physiology. In the event that cups are not supportive of safe swallowing, then spoons, medicine cups, droppers, or syringes can be utilized. This allows the clinician an opportunity to deliver small boluses first to gauge airway protection.

The order in which consistencies are presented requires thoughtful consideration as well. In the adult literature, though not mandated, beginning with thin liquid is often the accepted standard [25, 27, 29]. Though this is often the case in pediatrics as well, there may be variation in the order of presentation due to multiple factors. One thought is to begin with the consistency that the patient consumes best as this will allow the child to become acclimated and comfortable with the exam. Another consideration is the reason for the exam or the nature of the suspected dysphagia. For example, if the patient has a history of difficulty with thin liquids the exam would begin with thin liquid to ensure that the consistency of concern is assessed. Lastly, patient compliance is unpredictable in pediatrics. In these situations, the clinician has to use his/her judgment to obtain the most important information and may reorder the consistencies based on the patient's acceptance rather than his/her initial plan.

Lastly, with respect to volume (sip size), the presentation is also influenced by many factors. In adult literature, typically boluses are presented in a structured and calculated volume often beginning with 5 ml and increasing in a graduated method [25, 27]. This is a bottom-up approach [30]. Using this approach in pediatrics, the clinician begins with small boluses presented via spoon or a calculated amount in a small cup, and then increases incrementally based on performance. This approach is likely to be of benefit with patients recovering from any neurologic insult, patients with unknown swallowing abilities, and patients with limited feeding/swallowing experiences. However, If the patient is currently consuming all nutrition-hydration orally, then the volume presented is similar to what the child is currently accustomed to drinking. For instance, if the child takes liquids via straw or drinks from an open cup, then the clinician often begins at that level. This is a "top-down" approach as described by Gropher and Crary [30], where the clinician begins with more typical bolus sizes first and then provides smaller, more calculated volumes as needed. If during those trials, the child displays difficulty managing the bolus and/ or airway contamination is noted, the clinician modifies and controls volume to determine if the dysphagia is volume-dependent.

Neurology of Swallowing and Phases of Swallowing

For purposes of this chapter, a brief review of the neurology of swallowing and the phases of swallowing will be provided. This review is not considered comprehensive but merely an overview to highlight key information and general constructs.

Swallowing is a complex sensorimotor activity involving activation of sensory afferent and motor efferent pathways at different levels [31]. It involves the coordinated contraction of more than 20 pairs of muscles in the oropharynx, larynx, and esophagus [32]. It has subcortical and cortical controls. The subcortical controls are believed to be located in the medulla oblongata and can be divided into two major regions: the dorsal region and the ventral region [33]. The dorsal region contains the neural tractus solitarius or NTS. The NTS is the primary sensory nucleus for the facial, glossopharyngeal, and vagus nerves [34]. These neurons are considered "programming" interneurons and provide critical information to motor neurons for the swallow [35]. The ventral region contains the nucleus ambiguous (NA). The NA is the primary motor nucleus for the glossopharyngeal nerve and vagal nerve. Therefore, these NA neurons send out commands that control the muscles of the pharynx, larynx, and esophagus [26]. The cortical controls of the swallow play an important role as well. Per Lang, swallowing is a neurologic response that can be influenced cortically rather than isolated to the brain stem level [31]. Research shows that cortical control is responsible for initiation of the volitional swallow and "priming" of the pharyngeal swallow [36]. Its primary role is believed to center around modulation and regulation of the swallow based on the feeding circumstance such as bolus size and viscosity. The centers responsible for this include the sensorimotor and premotor regions located in the frontal lobe [36].

For ease of discussion and analysis, dysphagia specialists have delineated three phases of swallowing [37]. However, it is important to note that these phases are interdependent and influence one another greatly. The phases are briefly summarized below.

Oral Preparatory/Oral Transit

The oral phase is under volitional neural control and involves latch and expression of liquid from the bottle, procurement of liquids or foods, and/or mastication of the solid. Timing of this phase varies depending on the type of food consumed and patient's oromotor functioning. However, liquids are held in the oral cavity for less than 2 s in typical pediatric patients [22]. In the "normal" swallow, the bolus is formed and held in the groove or depression in the central portion of the tongue [38]. The extent of the depression is based on the volume of the liquid or food. A seal is then formed by lingual-palatal contact to contain the bolus and prevent free spillage into the pharynx. Transfer of the bolus is initiated by elevation and posterior movement of the tongue tip with simultaneous release of the lingual-palatal seal. This transfer typically takes approximately 1 s [39]. As the bolus is being propelled posteriorly, the soft palate begins to elevate to close off the nasopharyngeal area to prevent pharyngonasal backflow [40].

Pharyngeal Phase The pharyngeal phase is under both voluntary and involuntary neural control [33]. Examples of involuntary swallowing acts include swallowing of secretions in sleep. Though recent investigations have noted subtle variability in healthy adults with regard to specific sequences, generally speaking, this phase begins with closure of the nasopharyngeal cavity by palatal elevation, anterior excursion of the hyoid bone, and initiation of tongue base propulsion/retraction [41]. The exact trigger point, or pharyngeal swallow initiation, has some degree of variability in normals [42]. In infants, most often the pharyngeal swallow is initiated at the level of the valleculae [19]. However, findings in young healthy adults have noted that the swallow can be produced inferior to the valleculae [43–45]. Additionally, bolus characteristics such as volume and texture influence timing as does the swallowing task [38]. For instance, a "cued" swallow is typically initiated in a more timely swallow than a non-cued swallow [42]. After the swallow is initiated, epiglottic inversion is then viewed as the pressure of the tongue approximating the pharyngeal wall along with hyoid excursion enable the epiglottis to fully invert in older infants/toddlers and adults [39]. However, in young infants, complete epiglottic inversion is not noted due to normal airway differences as the laryngeal is positioned high which acts an added measure of airway protection. Next, the posterior pharyngeal musculature contracts from a superior to inferior in conjunction with tongue base retraction which leads to the bolus coursing through the pharynx via the pressure generated by these actions [37]. Nearly simultaneously, the laryngeal vestibule achieves closure. Closure of the airway is achieved by medial and forward movement of the arytenoids with eventual contact with the base of the epiglottis, epiglottic inversion, and adduction of the true and false vocal folds [46]. The precise and coordinated timing of these actions results in adequate airway protection.

Cervical Esophageal Phase During this phase, the upper esophageal sphincter (UES) fully relaxes via vagal-mediated control, thus allowing entrance of the bolus into the esophagus [47]. Successful entrance is accomplished via an interaction of sphincter relaxation and opening of the segment by anterior and superior hyolaryngeal elevation and pharyngeal shortening [48]. Simultaneously, positive pressure produced by the upper digestive tract, primarily the tongue base, drives the bolus through the open UES. Relaxation of the UES lasts between 0.32 and 0.5 s, depending on bolus volume/size [49]. See Fig. 5.2 below for the illustration of the sequence of normal swallowing.

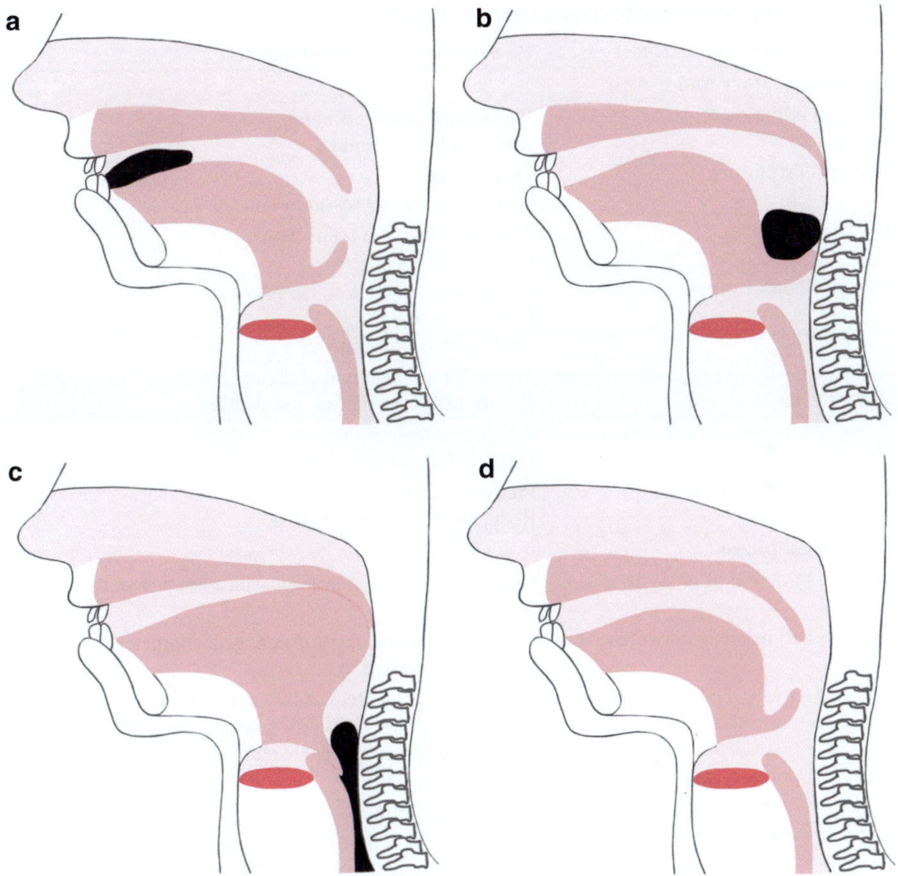

Fig. 5.2 Normal swallowing sequence

Analysis and Interpretation of the Oral-Pharyngeal Swallow

With thorough understanding of normal swallowing, the clinician can then advance to analyzing swallowing dysfunction. Below, in Table 5.2, is a summary of swallowing deficits commonly depicted on a videofluoroscopic study and their subsequent consequence. Deficits are organized by phase of the swallow with emphasis on children >12 months of age (non-bottle). Additionally, in Fig. 5.3 please see the radiographic images of pharyngeal swallow impairments.

Table 5.2 Possible deficits for children (non-bottle fed)

Swallow physiology deficits	Possible consequences of deficits
Oral preparatory and transit	
Delay in initiation of oral preparatory	Pocketing/packing of bolus Inefficient eating/intake
Reduced lip closure	Oral spillage Reduced anterior pressure point
Reduced chewing	Transferring of the bolus whole Gagging or choking
Reduced bolus formation/control	Premature spillage into the pharynx Piecemeal deglutition Oral residue after transfer
Reduced posterior oral containment/lingual-velar seal	Premature spillage into pharyngeal recesses Increased risk for aspiration before the swallow
Reduced oral transfer efficiency	Piecemeal deglutition Inefficient feeding/oral intake
Reduced palatal elevation	Pharyngonasal backflow Reduced pressure/bolus drive
Pharyngeal phase	
Delayed initiation of pharyngeal swallow	Increased risk of penetration/aspiration before the swallow
Absent pharyngeal swallow response	No opening of the upper esophageal sphincter Tracheal aspiration
Reduced elevation of hyolaryngeal complex	Delayed or incomplete of laryngeal closure Risk of penetration/aspiration during the swallow Reduced upper esophageal sphincter opening
Reduced epiglottic inversion	Pharyngeal residue Laryngeal penetration
Reduced tongue base retraction	Vallecular and tongue base residue Risk of penetration/aspiration after the swallow on residue Reduced pressure/bolus drive
Reduced constriction/stripping	Residue in pharyngeal recesses Risk of penetration/tracheal aspiration after the swallow on residue Reduced pressure/bolus drive
Reduced glottic closure	Tracheal aspiration during the swallow Reduce cough efficiency
Upper 1/3 cervico-esophageal phase	
Achalasia	Aspiration before the swallow
Reduced opening of pharyngeal-esophageal segment	Residue in the pyriform sinuses Laryngeal penetration after the swallow Tracheal aspiration after the swallow
Cricopharyngeal bar	Reduced clearance into esophagus Retrograde flow to the hypopharynx

Oral phase analysis for infants/bottle-fed patients are as follows in Table 5.3.

Table 5.3 Deficits for infants (bottle fed)

Swallow physiology deficits	Possible consequences of deficits
Oral phase	
Reduced latch	Inefficient feeding Inadequate intake Poor expression
Reduced nipple compression/suction	Inefficient feeding Extends length of feeding Poor expression of fluid
Reduced length of sucking burst	Extends length of feeding
Reduced rhythmicity of suck	Impacts coordination Risk of aspiration
Reduced labial seal	Anterior spillage
Excessive jaw excursion	Reduced expression Anterior spillage Air ingestion/aerophagia
Reduced bolus control/formation	Premature spillage into the pharynx Oral residue
Reduced posterior oral containment/lingual-velar seal	Premature spillage into pharyngeal recesses Increased risk for aspiration before the swallow
Reduced palatal elevation	Impacts suction (negative intraoral pressure) Pharyngonasal backflow Reduced pressure/bolus drive

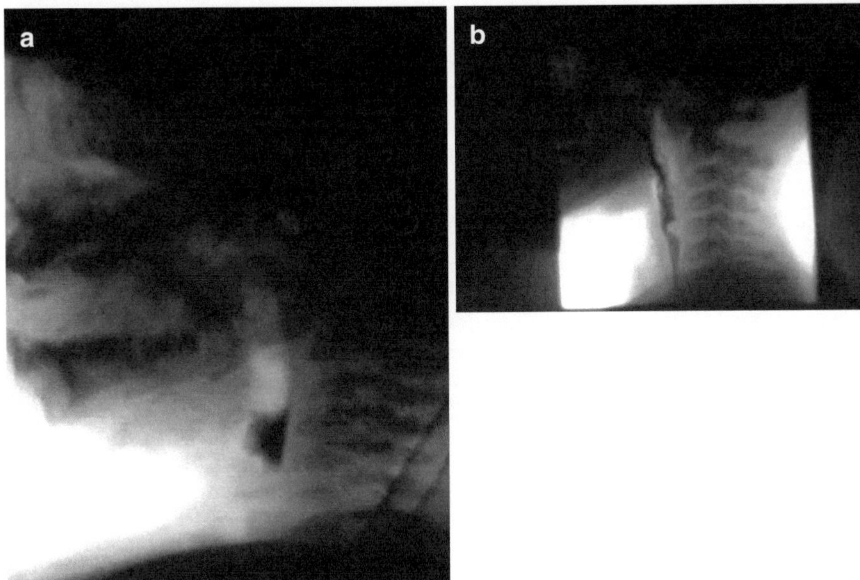

Fig. 5.3 Radiographic image of (**a**) oral residue on the lingual surface and pharyngeal residue in pyriform sinuses after the swallow (**b**) cricopharyngeal bar in the pharyngo-esophageal segment

Airway Protection

As noted in the section above, during a videofluoroscopic swallow study, the clinician's main role is to describe oral-pharyngeal swallow physiology and pathophysiology, if present. When physiology is normal, it leads to adequate airway protection. However, in patients with oral-pharyngeal dysphagia, airway protection may be compromised. This compromise may lead to airway contamination with liquid or food entering the airway. A lapse in airway protection has been described by the presence or absence of laryngeal penetration and/or tracheal aspiration. If they occur during an exam, these two events are documented and described in detail by the speech-language pathologist.

Laryngeal penetration is defined as food or liquid entering the vestibule or entrance of the airway to any level but not falling below the superior surface of the true vocal folds [29, 50]. When laryngeal penetration occurs, special consideration should be given to the depth and the clearance of the penetrated material. The depth of the laryngeal penetration can vary [51]. Clinicians often use the terms "flash," or "high" to describe penetration that enters only the upper portion of the laryngeal vestibule and does not contact the superior surface of the true vocal folds. When this occurs, the natural clearing mechanism for "high" penetration is the upward and forward movement of the larynx that results in the "squeezing" action of the larynx [52]. Several studies in the adult literature have documented "high" laryngeal penetration that clears as a normal phenomenon with incidence rates in normal at 9.9% [52]. In pediatrics, the incidence (frequency) of penetration in typically developing infants/children is unknown; however, there is some data to support that isolated penetration in non-dysphagic children is a normal finding as well [53].

On the other hand, "deep" laryngeal penetration is defined as liquid or food that contacts the true vocal folds but does not go beneath them [50, 54]. This level or depth of penetration has not been documented to occur in normal subjects in the available literature [52]. Furthermore, in infants, "deep" penetration as defined by contrast that enters the lower 1/3 of the laryngeal vestibule is associated with subsequent tracheal aspiration on videofluoroscopic swallow studies [54]. Additionally, pediatric patients who exhibited laryngeal penetration early in their videofluoroscopic exams then went on to demonstrate tracheal aspiration further in the study [1]. Lastly, the patient's ability to clear the laryngeal penetration is of importance. If an individual does not clear the penetration, then there is risk of tracheal aspiration as the penetrated material can subsequently fall into the airway post-swallow. Please see Figs. 5.4, and 5.5 for images of penetration.

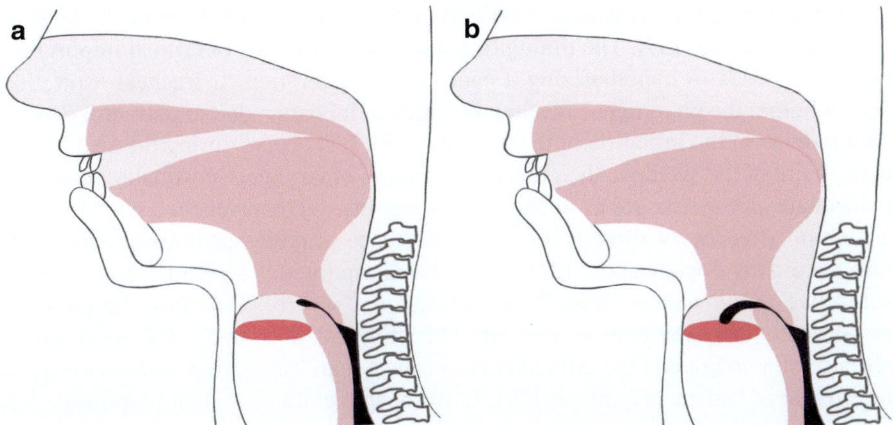

Fig. 5.4 Sketching of laryngeal penetration: (**a**) Shallow penetration which enters the laryngeal vestibule but does not contact the true vocal folds. (**b**) Deep penetration which enters the vestibule and contacts the superior surface of the true vocal folds but does not go beneath them

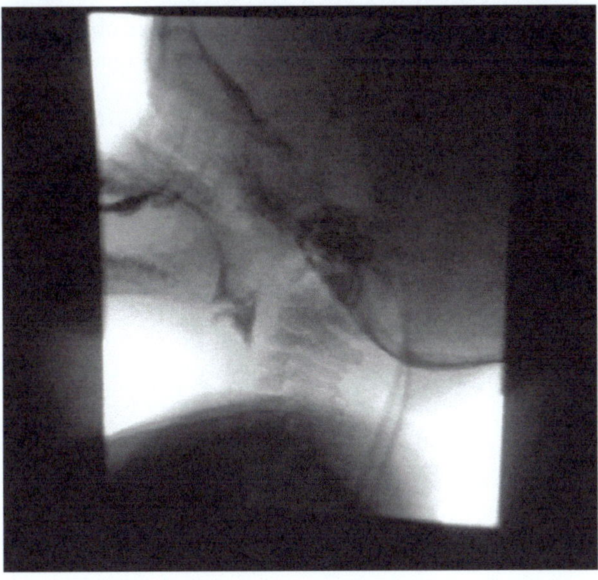

Fig. 5.5 Radiographic image of laryngeal penetration

Tracheal aspiration is defined as liquid or food that has fallen below the level of the true vocal folds [55]. The timing of the aspiration event is of critical importance because it leads to hypothesizing a cause of the aspiration. If tracheal aspiration occurs before the pharyngeal swallow is initiated, it is often due to poor oral control and/or delay in the initiation of the swallow [39]. If it occurs during the swallow or at the point of the swallow, then it is due to timing of laryngeal-vestibular closure or inadequate airway closure as in patients with glottic incompetence. Lastly, tracheal aspiration after the swallow is due to the presence of pharyngeal residue that falls into the airway post-swallow [22]. The volume aspirated is typically reported with subjective terms such a "trace," "moderate," or "severe." Detailing the patient's response to the aspiration is critical. The clinician documents the presence or absence of a cough and the effectiveness of the cough. Aspiration with no cough is referred to as "silent" aspiration [39]. In dysphagic children "silent" aspiration has been noted to predominate in both patients with neurologic impairment and those without [4, 5, 56]. "Silent" aspiration is especially prominent in infants < 6 months of age [7]. Of note, in infants the cough reflex has been hypothesized to have a developmental overlay with normal infants developing their protective cough after the third month of life [57]. Please see the illustration of tracheal aspiration in Fig. 5.6 below and radiographic image in Fig. 5.7.

Though clinicians often report their airway protection findings descriptively, scales have been developed to provide more objective and consistent reporting. The 8-point penetration-aspiration scale was designed to increase uniformity in reporting

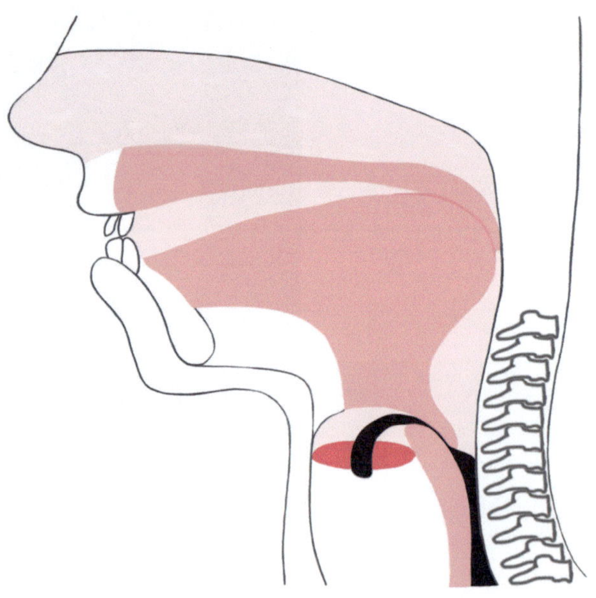

Fig. 5.6 Illustrative image of tracheal aspiration

penetration and aspiration but is not a dysphagia severity scale [50]. Reliability has been established. It is an 8-point scale that reports on (1) the depth of entrance into the airway, (2) the presence or absence of the cough, and (3) the clearance of the airway. It is well recognized in the adult population and is gaining more use in the pediatric population with some emerging supportive data [58]. Please see Table 5.4 below.

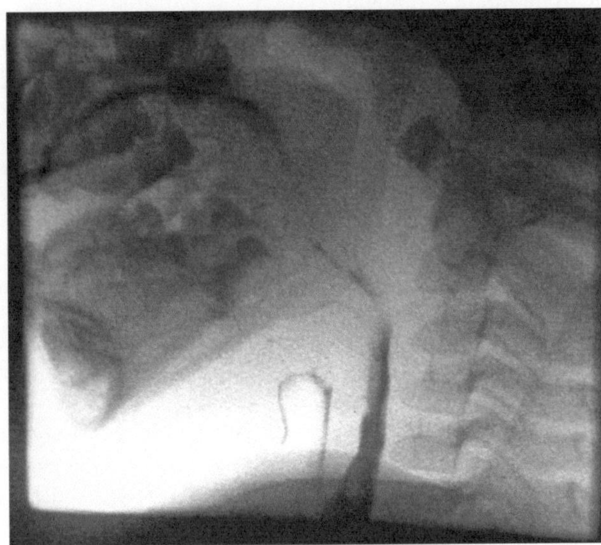

Fig. 5.7 Radiographic image of tracheal aspiration

Table 5.4 8-point penetration-aspiration scale

Score	Description	Category
1	Material does not enter airway	
2	Material enters supraglottic space but then is ejected from the airway	Penetration
3	Material enters supraglottic space and is not ejected from the airway	
4	Material contacts the vocal folds but is then ejected from the airway	
5	Material contacts the vocal fold but is not ejected from the airway	
6	Material passes the glottis but no subglottic residue is visible	Aspiration
7	Material passes the glottis; visible subglottic residue is present despite patient response	
8	Material passes the glottis; visible subglottic residue is present; no patient response	

Intervention Options

The VFSS is not only a diagnostic exam but also an interventional exam. This is as important in pediatrics as it is in the adult population. When the speech-language pathologist identifies an interruption in swallow physiology, their responsibility is to implement strategies to improve swallowing function. Intervention options are based on age and cognitive abilities. The aim of the intervention is twofold. The first is to maintain as much oral intake as possible, and the second is to create a plan to help alleviate the dysphagia and improve swallowing function by targeting the pathophysiology of the swallow. Table 5.5 provides a summary of interventions that may be implemented during the exam. Of note, many of the interventions listed in the school-age population have only been researched in adult populations.

Table 5.5 Intervention summary

	Interventions	Rationale
Infants	Positioning sidelying	Regulates respiratory function Slow flow of feeds
	Postural support	Provides postural stability which can improve coordination
	Nipple flow rate changes	Slow flow promotes coordination and improved oral control
	Pacing	Ventilation breaks and maintains coordination of SSB triad
	[a]Thickening	May slow the bolus and facilitate forming a more cohesive bolus
Toddlers	Reduced sip/bite size	Improves oral control
	Sip-swallow-pause	Regulates rate of intake
	Altering liquids-solids	Clears oral-pharyngeal residuals
	Dry swallow	Clears oral-pharyngeal residuals
	Chink down/tuck	Widens the valleculae for improved airway protection
	[a]Thickening liquids	Slows the bolus and facilitates forming a more cohesive bolus
School age and adolescent	Volume regulation	Improves oral control of bolus
	Chin tuck/down	Compensates for delayed swallow response Improves contact of tongue base and posterior pharyngeal wall Increases duration of laryngeal vestibule closure
	Supraglottic swallow	Improves airway closure at the level of the glottis
	Supra-supraglottic swallow	Improves airway closure at the level of the glottis and above at the level of the arytenoids
	3-second swallow prep	Increase central volitional control for swallowing
	Alternating liquids-solids	Clears oral-pharyngeal residue
	Head turn	Redirect bolus away from "closed" side Reduces pharyngeal residue on "closed" side Facilitates UES opening
	Effortful swallow	Improves base of tongue retraction Extends the duration of hyolaryngeal excursion
	Thickened liquids	Slows the bolus and facilitates forming a more cohesive bolus

[a]To be used as a last resort when all other interventions have failed. Use of thickened liquids in the infant population requires careful consideration before implementation.

Summary and Future Needs

In summary, the VFSS is one important tool in the assessment of infants and children with swallowing disorders. It is a complementary exam to both the clinical feeding-swallow evaluation and other instrumental swallow exams. It provides the speech-language pathologist critical information regarding swallow physiology and airway protection in order to develop a safe and efficient feeding-swallowing plan. Lastly, the VFSS guides the treating speech-language pathologist with the necessary information to devise a comprehensive therapy plan for rehabilitation/habilitation as appropriate.

The field of pediatric dysphagia is an emerging field of science relative to other medical sciences with many more questions than answers. Future needs are plentiful, but one priority is standardizing the administration and interpretation of the VFSS for pediatrics as is available for adults [26]. As detailed in the sections above, currently it is a descriptive exam with heterogenous methods of administration and interpretation. A standardized approach would allow all speech-language pathologist to assess in a manner that is consistent and reliable to one another, thus improving the quality of care for patients with dysphagia.

References

1. Newman L. Videofluoroscopy in infant and pediatric populations. Perspectives on Swallowing and Swallowing Disorders. 2007;16(1):11–5. https://doi.org/10.1044/sasd16.1.11.
2. Benfer KA, Weir KA, Bell KL, Ware RS, Davies PSW, Boyd RN. Clinical signs suggestive of pharyngeal dysphagia in preschool children with cerebral palsy. Res Dev Disabil. 2015;38:192–201. https://doi.org/10.1016/j.ridd.2014.12.021.
3. Weir K, McMahon S, Barry L, Masters IB, Chang AB. Clinical signs and symptoms of oropharyngeal aspiration and dysphagia in children. Eur Respir J. 2009;33(3):604–11. https://doi.org/10.1183/09031936.00090308.
4. Weir KA, McMahon S, Taylor S, Chang AB. Oropharyngeal aspiration and silent aspiration in children. Chest. 2011;140(3):589–97. https://doi.org/10.1378/chest.10-1618.
5. Arvedson J, Rogers B, Buck G, Smart P, Msall M. Silent aspiration prominent in children with dysphagia. Int J Pediatr Otorhinolaryngol. 1994;28(2–3):173–81. https://doi.org/10.1016/0165-5876(94)90009-4.
6. Duncan DR, Mitchell PD, Larson K, Rosen RL. Presenting signs and symptoms do not predict aspiration risk in children. J Pediatr. 2018:1–6.
7. Velayutham P, Irace AL, Kawai K, Dodrill P, Perez J, Londahl M, Mundy L, Dombrowski ND, Rahbar R. Silent aspiration: Who is at risk? Laryngoscope. 2017:1–6.
8. Donner M. Martin Donner. J Am Coll Radiol. 2013;10(5):386. https://doi.org/10.1016/j.jacr.2013.01.020.
9. Donner M, Silbiger M. Cinefluorographic analysis of pharyngeal swallowing in neuromuscular disorders. Am J Med Sci. 1966;5:600–16.
10. Miller RM, Groher ME. Speech-language pathology and dysphagia: a brief historical perspective. Dysphagia. 1993;8(3):180–4.
11. American College of Radiology. Practice guideline modified barium swallow / 1; 2014:8.
12. American Speech-Language-Hearing Association. Clinical indicators for instrumental assessment of dysphagia. Rockville, MD; 1997.
13. Strauss KJ, Kaste SC. ALARA in pediatric interventional and fluoroscopic imaging: striving to keep radiation doses as low as possible during fluoroscopy of pediatric patients-a white

paper executive summary. J Am Coll Radiol. 2006;3(9):686–8. https://doi.org/10.1016/j.jacr.2006.04.008.

14. Miller DL, Schauer D. The Alara principle in medical imaging. AAPM Newsl. 2015;40(1):38–40.

15. Henderson M, Miles A, Holgate V, Peryman S, Allen J. Application and verification of quantitative objective videofluoroscopic swallowing measures in a pediatric population with dysphagia. J Pediatr. 2016;178:200–5. https://doi.org/10.1016/j.jpeds.2016.07.050.

16. Bonilha HS, Blair J, Carnes B, et al. Preliminary investigation of the effect of pulse rate on judgments of swallowing impairment and treatment recommendations. Dysphagia. 2013;28(4):528–38. https://doi.org/10.1007/s00455-013-9463-z.

17. Cohen MD. Can we use pulsed fluoroscopy to decrease the radiation dose during video fluoroscopic feeding studies in children? Clin Radiol. 2009;64(1):70–3. https://doi.org/10.1016/j.crad.2008.07.011.

18. Bonilha HS, Humphries K, Blair J, et al. Radiation exposure time during MBSS: influence of swallowing impairment severity, medical diagnosis, clinician experience, and standardized protocol use. Dysphagia. 2013;28(1):77–85. https://doi.org/10.1007/s00455-012-9415-z.

19. Arvedson JC, Brodsky L. Pediatric swallowing and feeding: assessment and management. Albany: Singular Thomson Learning; 2002.

20. Weir KA, McMahon SM, Long G, et al. Radiation doses to children during modified barium swallow studies. Pediatr Radiol. 2007;37(3):283–90. https://doi.org/10.1007/s00247-006-0397-6.

21. McCullough G, Pelletier C, Steele C. National dysphagia diet: what to swallow? ASHA Leader. 2003;8:16.

22. Arvedson JC, Lefton-Greif MA. Pediatric videofluoroscopic swallow studies. 1st ed: Elsevier; 1998.

23. National Dysphagia Diet Task Force, American Dietetic Association. National dysphagia diet: standardization for optimal care. American Dietetic Association; 2002. https://books.google.com/books?id=MZ5mSbGPOE4C&pgis=1.

24. Cichero JAY, Lam P, Steele CM, et al. Development of international terminology and definitions for texture-modified foods and thickened fluids used in dysphagia management: the IDDSI framework. Dysphagia. 2017;32(2):293–314. https://doi.org/10.1007/s00455-016-9758-y.

25. Martin-Harris B, Brodsky MB, Michel Y, et al. MBS measurement tool for swallow impairment-MBSimp: establishing a standard. Dysphagia. 2008;23(4):392–405. https://doi.org/10.1007/s00455-008-9185-9.

26. Stephanie K, Huckabee Maggie-Lee D. Dysphagia following stroke. 2nd ed: Singulair; 2016.

27. Jaffer NM, Ng E, Wing F, et al. Fluoroscopic evaluation of oropharyngeal dysphagia: anatomic, technical, and common etiologic factors. 2015; https://doi.org/10.2214/AJR.13.12374.

28. Lefton-Greif MA, McGrattan KE, Carson KA, Pinto JM, Wright JM, Martin-Harris B. First steps towards development of an instrument for the reproducible quantification of oropharyngeal swallow physiology in bottle-fed children. Dysphagia. 2018;33(1):76–82.

29. Logemann J. Manual for the videofluorographic study of swallowing. 2nd ed. Austin: ProEd; 1993.

30. Groher M, Crary M. Dysphagia: Clinical Management in Adults and Children. 2nd ed: Elsevier; 2016.

31. Lang IM. Brain stem control of the phases of swallowing. https://doi.org/10.1007/s00455-009-9211-6.

32. Lefton-Greif MA. Pediatric dysphagia. Phys Med Rehabil Clin NA. 2008;19:837–51. https://doi.org/10.1016/j.pmr.2008.05.007.

33. Jean A. Brain stem control of swallowing: neuronal network and cellular mechanisms. Physiol Rev. 2001;81(2):929–69. https://doi.org/10.1002/cne.902830207.

34. Jean A, Jean A. Control of the central swallowing program by inputs from the peripheral receptors. A review J Auton Nerv Syst. 1984;10:225–33. http://ac.els-cdn.com.ezproxyhost.library.

tmc.edu/0165183884900171/1-s2.0-0165183884900171-main.pdf?_tid=f30dc53e-5c06-11e7-9607-00000aacb35e&acdnat=1498657237_3dfe91ad005330e768f82c6a93788d25. Accessed 28 Jun 2017

35. Amri M, Car A, Roman C. Experimental brain research axonal branching of medullary swallowing neurons projecting on the trigeminal and hypoglossal motor nuclei: demonstration by electrophysiological and fluorescent double labeling techniques. Exp Brain Res. 1990;81:384–90. https://link-springer-com.ezproxyhost.library.tmc.edu/content/pdf/10.1007%2FBF00228130.pdf. Accessed 28 Jun 2017

36. Sasegbon A, Hamdy S. The anatomy and physiology of normal and abnormal swallowing in oropharyngeal dysphagia. Neurogastroenterol Motil. May 2017;29:e13100. https://doi.org/10.1111/nmo.13100.

37. Martin-Harris B, Jones B. The videofluorographic swallowing study. Otorinolaringologia. 2009;59(1):19–29. https://doi.org/10.1016/j.pmr.2008.06.004.

38. Logemann JA, Ralph B-S, Sundin J. Critical factors in the oral control needed for chewing and swallowing. https://doi.org/10.1111/jtxs.12053.

39. Logemann J. Evaluation and treatment of swallowing disorders. 2nd ed. Austin: Pro-Ed; 1998.

40. Arvedson JC, Lefton-Greif MA. Pediatric videofluoroscopic swallow studies: a professional manual with caregiver guidelines. San Antonio: Communication Skill Builders; 1998.

41. Molfenter SM, Leigh C, Steele CM. Event sequence variability in healthy swallowing: building on previous findings. Dysphagia. 2014;29(2):234–42. https://doi.org/10.1007/s00455-013-9501-x.

42. Molfenter SM, Steele CM. Temporal variability in the deglutition literature. Dysphagia. 2012;27(2):162–77. https://doi.org/10.1007/s11103-011-9767-z.Plastid.

43. Daniels SK, Foundas AL. Swallowing physiology of sequential straw drinking. Dysphagia. 2001;16(3):176–82. https://doi.org/10.1007/s00455-001-0061-0.

44. Nagy A, Leigh C, Hori SF, et al. Timing differences between cued and noncued swallows in healthy young adults. https://doi.org/10.1007/s00455-013-9456-y.

45. Martin-Harris B, Brodsky MB, Michel Y, Lee F-S, Walters B. Delayed initiation of the pharyngeal swallow: normal variability in adult swallows. J Speech Lang Hear Res. 2007;50(3):585–94. https://doi.org/10.1044/1092-4388(2007/041).

46. Van Daele DJ, McCulloch TM, Palmer PM, Langmore SE. Timing of glottic closure during swallowing: a combined electromyographic and endoscopic analysis. Ann Otol Rhinol Laryngol. 2005;114(6):478–87. https://doi.org/10.1177/000348940511400610.

47. Lang IM, Shaker R. An overview of the upper esophageal sphincter. Curr Gastroenterol Rep. 2000;2(3):185–90. https://link-springer-com.ezproxyhost.library.tmc.edu/content/pdf/10.1007%2Fs11894-000-0059-z.pdf. Accessed 21 Jun 2017

48. McConnel FMS, Cerenko D, Jackson RT, TNJ G. Timing of major events of pharyngeal swallowing. Arch Otolaryngol – Head Neck Surg. 1988;114:1413–8.

49. Mittal R. Motor function of the pharynx, esophagus, and its sphincters – PubMed – NCBI. San Diego: Morgan & Claypool Life Sciences; 2011. https://www-ncbi-nlm-nih-gov.ezproxyhost.library.tmc.edu/pubmed/21634068. Accessed 21 Jun 2017.

50. Rosenbek JC, Robbins JA, Roecker EB, Coyle JL, Wood JL. A Penetration-Aspiration Scale. Dysphagia. 1996;11:93. https://doi.org/10.1007/BF00417897.

51. Rosenbek JC, Robbins JA, Roecker PDEB, Coyle JL, Wood JL. Dysphagia. 1996;98:93–8. https://doi.org/10.1007/BF00417897.

52. Daggett A, Logemann J, Rademaker A, Pauloski B. Laryngeal penetration during deglutition in normal subjects of various ages. https://doi.org/10.1007/s00455-006-9051-6.

53. Delzell PB, Kraus RA, Gaisie G, Lerner GE. Laryngeal penetration: a predictor of aspiration in infants? Pediatr Radiol. 1999;29(10):762–5. https://doi.org/10.1007/s002470050690.

54. Friedman B, Frazier JB. Deep laryngeal penetration as a predictor of aspiration. Dysphagia. 2000;15(3):153–8. https://doi.org/10.1007/s004550010018.

55. Arvedson JC. Assessment of pediatric dysphagia and feeding disorders: clinical and instrumental approaches. Dev Disabil Res Rev. 2008;14(2):118–27. https://doi.org/10.1002/ddrr.17.

56. Lefton-Greif MA, Carroll JL, Loughlin GM. Long-term follow-up of oropharyngeal dysphagia in children without apparent risk factors. Pediatr Pulmonol. 2006;41(11):1040–8. https://doi.org/10.1002/ppul.20488.
57. Thach BT. Maturation of cough and other reflexes that protect the fetal and neonatal airway. Pulm Pharmacol Ther. 2007;20(4):365–70. https://doi.org/10.1016/j.pupt.2006.11.011.
58. Holman SD, Campbell-Malone R, Ding P, et al. Development, reliability, and validation of an infant mammalian penetration-aspiration scale. Dysphagia. 2013;28(2):178–87. https://doi.org/10.1007/s00455-012-9427-8.

Chapter 6
Who Should Pass the Endoscope During a Fiberoptic Evaluation of Swallowing Procedure

Jay Paul Willging

Introduction

Susan Langmore, PhD, developed fiberoptic endoscopic evaluation of swallowing (FEES) in 1988 while working with adult patients at the Veterans Administration Hospital in Ann Arbor, Michigan. The pediatric application of FEES began in 1993 at Cincinnati Children's Hospital Medical Center, with Claire Miller, PhD, and J. Paul Willging, MD. Today, the safety of FEES is well established in both adults and children, as is its ability to accurately assess the patient's ability to protect the airway during swallowing.

Visualization of laryngeal and hypopharyngeal structures allows an assessment of the influence of abnormal anatomy on swallowing safety. Similarly, the influence of abnormal neurologic function (sensory or motor) can be demonstrated on FEES. Based on the assessment of swallowing safety, compensation techniques can be recommended to improve the patient's swallowing efficiency and safety.

There is controversy over who should be conducting the FEES examination. Should a physician be involved with the procedure or is it appropriate for a speech-language pathologist (SLP) to conduct the examination independently? I feel the answer hinges on the specifics of the situation.

J. P. Willging
Department of Otolaryngology, Cincinnati Children's Hospital Medical Center,
University of Cincinnati, Cincinnati, OH, USA
e-mail: paul.willging@cchmc.org

© Springer International Publishing AG, part of Springer Nature 2018
J. Ongkasuwan, E. H. Chiou (eds.), *Pediatric Dysphagia*,
https://doi.org/10.1007/978-3-319-97025-7_6

The FEES Procedure

The FEES examination can be broken down into several discrete steps.

1. An initial history is taken to define the problem the patient is experiencing. This allows a plan to be developed on how to execute the FEES procedure: what food items and textures are appropriate, what order should specific liquids and solids be offered, and what bolus sizes should be offered. A sample feeding may be observed.
2. The patient is prepared for the examination. The test is explained to the patient and family. Topical anesthetic agents may be used in select situations. Assignments are made for people to assist during the evaluation.
3. Endoscope passage is undertaken, with an assessment of the relevant structures of the upper aerodigestive tract made as the endoscope passes them. The endoscope is advanced such that the tip of the endoscope is in the oropharynx, providing complete visualization of the larynx and hypopharyngeal structures.
4. Evaluation of swallowing safety. The patient is offered foods and liquids appropriate for their developmental age and medical condition. Their ability to protect the airway is assessed. Their ability to clear all material from the hypopharynx is determined. A qualitative assessment of hypopharyngeal sensation is made based on the patient's ability to manage secretions and prevent their accumulation in the hypopharynx.
5. The examination is reviewed and a treatment plan is generated. If the study is conducted jointly by a physician and a SLP, both should review the examination and come to consensus on what the findings are and what the treatment strategy should be for the patient.
6. The findings and recommendations are discussed with the family.
7. A report of the findings and recommendations is generated and placed in the medical record.

Both the SLP and the physician can perform all the steps of the FEES examination.

Training

Speech pathologists are trained in dysphagia. It is estimated by the American Speech-Language-Hearing Association (ASHA) that 45% of a SLP's time working with adults, and 16% of the time working with children, is related to swallowing and feeding disorders [1]. Their professional training provides the foundation for the assessment and treatment of dysphagia associated with medical problems encountered in these patients. ASHA provides recognition to SLP who meet stringent requirements of the Specialty Board on Swallowing and Swallowing Disorders. After completing a clinical tract that takes 3–5 years to complete, the individual is able to apply to sit for the board examination. The training criteria are extensive and include clinical exposure to patients with swallowing and swallowing disorders; continuing education in the area of dysphagia; education and mentorship that include research and presentation of projects at local, state, or regional conferences; demonstration of leadership and engagement in local or national groups focusing on dysphagia; and scholarship or research in the area of dysphagia. Individual SLP who complete the program and pass the certification examination are designated as Board Recognized in Swallowing and Swallowing Disorders and may use the initials "BRS-S" following their name [2].

Physicians receive a broad education in medical school to prepare them for practice and seek further specialty or subspecialty training in residency and fellowship programs. Dysphagia is a clinical area shared by multiple medical/surgical disciplines: otolaryngology, gastroenterology, pulmonary medicine, physical medicine and rehabilitation, neurology, and pediatrics. Essentially all otolaryngologists have training and expertise in dysphagia. Practice interests may enhance or limit the percentage of time a practitioner spends in this area of concentration. Those with a special interest in dysphagia perform many of the evaluation studies and surgical procedures to improve/correct problems related to dysphagia.

Both SLP and physicians have the training opportunities available to be competent in the field of dysphagia and the instrumental examinations that evaluate swallowing function and safety.

Etiology of Dysphagia

The etiology of dysphagia can vary widely based on the age of the patient. Adults in general have had normal swallowing function until a specific event occurred leading to their dysphagia. Common problems leading to dysphagia include neurologic events such as stroke or progressive degenerative neurologic disorders (dementia), progression of benign or malignant intracranial neoplasms, postoperative conditions following neurosurgical procedures, and surgical ablation of head and neck tumors. Long-term sequela of radiation treatments to the head and neck area or chest can lead to significant dysphagia due to the increasing fibrosis of surrounding tissues and subsequent deterioration of swallowing function.

The etiology of dysphagia in children is much more varied. Many children with feeding problems have never orally fed. They may have significant developmental delays affecting the maturation of normal oral-motor skills. There may be neurologic problems affecting the acquisition of normal feeding skills. Seizure disorders, Chiari malformations, increased intracranial pressures, or structural abnormalities of the corpus callosum or brain stem may prevent the acquisition of normal feeding skills. Genetic disorders may interfere with normal swallowing function. Chromosomal duplications or deletions, mitochondrial DNA abnormalities, and many syndromes have dysphagia commonly associated with their diagnosis. Cardiorespiratory problems can affect swallowing in multiple ways. Tachypnea associated with some cyanotic congenital heart defects can interfere with the ability to coordinate a suck-swallow-breathe sequence, as can severe bronchopulmonary dysphasia and laryngomalacia. Structural anomalies can preclude normal swallowing function as there may not be a separation of the airway and the esophagus. Laryngeal clefts, tracheoesophageal fistula, and esophageal atresia create a condition where safe swallowing is not possible. Eighty percent of pediatric patients have a behavioral component complicating their dysphagia problems. Many of these children exhibit signs of oral aversion, hypersensitivity, or hyposensitivity issues. Addressing an underlying structural issue will not always eradicate the secondary behavioral issues without continued therapy. There are also specific metabolic issues such as cystinuria that induce severe swallowing problems.

Clinical Experience

Clinicians involved with the evaluation and treatment of patients with dysphagia need to be experienced with the patient population they will be dealing with. Otolaryngologists receive training in conditions affecting the head and neck region of adults and children. The clinical experience of SLPs is more varied, as it depends on the mentors selected after their initial training. The Speech-Language Pathology Clinical Fellowship Year (CFY) is the transition period between being a student enrolled in training and being an independent provider of speech-language pathology services. The CFY involves a mentored professional experience after completion of the academic course work and the clinical practicum. The CFY can focus any area of speech-language pathology. It requires a minimum of 1260 h over a minimum of 36 weeks. Eighty percent of this time must be in direct clinical work [3]. Additional mentorship is required in the field of dysphagia if the original training was inadequate to satisfy ASHA's code of ethics, which states that "individuals shall engage in the provision of the profession that are within the scope of their competence, consistent with their level of education, training and experience."[4] ASHA's practice policy documents include knowledge and skills statements that can be used to guide members and institutions in developing competency assessment programs.

Physicians have the ability to diagnose and treat. Additionally, they may prescribe medications to facilitate the cooperation of patients undergoing diagnostic evaluations. In the hospital setting, physicians are limited in their scope of practice to that which the Hospital Board gives them privileges to perform. The physician's delineation of privileges is based on their educational experiences and their demonstrated competence in the specialty area.

Speech-language pathologists work to prevent, assess, diagnose, and treat speech, language, social communication, and cognitive-communication and swallowing disorders in children and adults. Their scope of practice may be limited by the State Board that issues their license and controls their activities.

Controversy

Controversy exists around the area of who should pass the endoscope during FEES examinations. In some states, the passage of flexible endoscopes is considered outside the scope of practice of SLP practicing their state. Other states require a physician to be available during the procedure. Other states allow the SLP to be an independent provider of endoscopy services as it relates to the evaluation of voice and swallowing problems. The SLP is not able to diagnose an abnormality found on endoscopy. They are required to refer the patient to a physician for further evaluation, diagnosis, and treatment.

Who "can" pass an endoscope during a FEES examination is not the same question as who "should" pass an endoscope during a FEES examination. Where there are state limitations on scope of practice involving flexible endoscopes, the SLP cannot pass the scope, and a physician must perform the instrumental aspect of the examination. In states where a scope passage is within the scope of practice of a SLP, the SLP should be able to perform FEES as long as they have the requisite training as determined by ASHA for independent scope passage and interpretation of a FEES examination [5].

The model we have developed at Cincinnati Children's Hospital Medical Center, and continue to use at this point, is a collaborative clinic model with a physician and SLP jointly performing the examinations in children. The patient population that we serve has a high percentage of patients with structural abnormalities of the upper aerodigestive tract. The otolaryngologist is present at the time of the examination to assess specifically the structural elements of the upper aerodigestive tract. Many of these patients are tracheotomy dependent, with a goal of treatment to achieve decannulation. The patients require an assessment of their ability to protect their airway but also to judge the adequacy of the upper airway to support respiration without a tracheotomy tube in place: vocal fold function, arytenoid prolapse, irritation of the laryngeal structures from gastroesophageal reflux, retrognathia and glossoptosis, nasopharyngeal or oropharyngeal stenosis, choanal atresia or stenosis, and adenotonsillar hypertrophy.

Many patients with subglottic stenosis have abnormal swallowing function. A determination needs to be made as to whether an airway reconstruction should be performed or delayed till swallowing function improves. A severe laryngeal stenosis may present with no sign of aspiration preoperatively, as no significant communication exists from the hypopharynx through the larynx to the trachea. Once the airway is reconstructed, however, a possibility exists where life-threatening aspiration and pulmonary complications could develop from aspiration of oral secretions and food/drink. Only a physician can make these determinations.

Having a physician present at the time of the FEES minimizes the need to have the child repeat flexible endoscopic examinations in the office setting. If a SLP independently performs the FEES procedure, these patients will often need a second procedure to complete the assessment. We have combined pediatric voice and FEES evaluations specifically to minimize the number of procedures patients need to undergo. We have a physician present to participate in both the voice evaluation with one SLP and to facilitate the FEES examination with another SLP.

The variety of diagnoses associated with pediatric dysphagia also supports having a physician present for an initial FEES examination in pediatric patients. Many of these children need an assessment of the structural aspects of the upper aerodigestive tract to ensure no further evaluations are required.

Follow-up FEES evaluations can certainly be done in the pediatric population by SLP independently. The initial evaluation has determined the presence or absence of other diagnoses that would affect swallowing function. FEES examinations in the adult population can certainly be done independent of physician involvement.

The team approach to FEES has many advantages. While not essential, it minimizes repeat endoscopic evaluations by the physician. It maximizes the clinical findings of the evaluation and provides an opportunity for the family to explore the medical and functional aspects of their child's dysphagia problem. Who passes the endoscope is not as important as the expertise held by the person passing the endoscope. Maximizing the information obtained from a FEES evaluation is essential, and to obtain this, one should include an assessment of the likely etiologies associated with child's problem and consciously make a decision as to who should be present for a given examination.

Bibliography

1. http://www.asha.org/.
2. http://www.swallowingdisorders.org/?page=apply.
3. http://www.asha.org/Certification/Certification-Standards-for-SLP%2D%2DClinical-Fellowship/.
4. http://www.asha.org/Code-of-Ethics/.
5. http://www.asha.org/News/2016/New-SLP-Scope-of-Practice-Now-Available/.

Chapter 7
Fiberoptic Endoscopic Evaluation of Swallowing: Assessing Dysphagia in the Breastfeeding Patient

James W. Schroeder Jr, Susan Willette, and Laura Hinkes Molinaro

The etiology of feeding and swallowing disorders in the pediatric population is multifactorial. Therefore, the workup and treatment of children with these problems is complex and requires a multidisciplinary approach. Feeding and swallowing disorders are relatively common in early infancy and in some instances may be markers for conditions that do not become apparent until later in life [1]. Feeding and swallowing disorders can include difficulties with efficient intake for adequate growth and nutrition as well as an inability to maintain functional airway protection when swallowing. Classifying complex pediatric feeding problems can be complicated by the comorbidities that can be associated with an infant's medical and developmental history. The most frequently described categories of feeding problems have been listed by Burklow et al. [2]; see Table 7.1. The incidence of feeding disorders is reported to be 25–45% of typically developing children and up to 80% of children with developmental disabilities [3]. According to Reynolds et al. [4], health-care professionals have been influenced by the World Health Organization/United Nations Children's Fund Baby-Friendly Hospital Initiative to more actively promote breastfeeding as the exclusive option for parents to provide nutrition to their infant. Feeding and swallowing difficulties can complicate a mother's ability to exclusively breastfeed and should be considered when the breastfeeding process is not progressing smoothly. Evaluating breastfeeding physiology creates new challenges for the health-care providers who must

J. W. Schroeder Jr (✉)
Pediatric Otolaryngology, Ann and Robert H. Lurie Children's Hospital of Chicago,
Department of Otolaryngology Head and Neck Surgery, Northwestern University,
Chicago, IL, USA
e-mail: jschroeder@luriechildrens.org

S. Willette · L. H. Molinaro
Speech and Language Pathology, Ann and Robert H. Lurie Children's Hospital of Chicago,
Chicago, IL, USA
e-mail: swillette@luriechildrens.org; lhinkes@luriechildrens.org

© Springer International Publishing AG, part of Springer Nature 2018
J. Ongkasuwan, E. H. Chiou (eds.), *Pediatric Dysphagia*,
https://doi.org/10.1007/978-3-319-97025-7_7

Table 7.1 Categories for identifying complex pediatric feeding disorders

Diagnostic category	
Behavioral	Resulting from psychosocial difficulties
Neurologic	Associated with CNS insult or musculoskeletal disorders
Structural	Anatomic abnormalities of the structures associated with feeding
Cardiorespiratory	Associated with diseases/symptoms that compromise the cardiovascular and respiratory systems
Metabolic	Associated with metabolic diseases/symptoms that interfere with normal feeding patterns
Normal	

Adapted from Burklow et al. [2]

develop diagnostic and treatment paradigms to address specifically swallowing concerns. Early and effective evaluation of feeding difficulties in healthy full-term infants should be considered as a part of the effort to sustain breastfeeding in the early stages of infant feeding [5].

Clinical Assessment of Feeding

Speech-language pathologists have extensive knowledge of anatomy and physiology of the aerodigestive tract for swallowing, including the oral, pharyngeal, and cervical esophageal anatomic regions. Speech-language pathologists are trained to understand how underlying medical and behavioral etiologies of swallowing and feeding disorders impact functional performance. Because of the complexities of assessing infants with swallowing and feeding disorders, speech-language pathologists and other professionals work as a team with families, caregivers, and patients (ASHA position paper).

When addressing an infant who is having difficulty with breastfeeding, a thorough clinical feeding evaluation should be performed by a pediatric speech-language pathologist. This consists of a review of the infant's medical, developmental, and feeding history, an examination of the oral structures, and a feeding observation that includes evaluation of both the non-nutritive sucking (NNS) pattern and the nutritive sucking (NS) pattern during breast- or bottle-feeding [1]. Breastfeeding evaluation tools such as the LATCH or Bristol Breastfeeding Assessment Tool outline a specific focus on the integrity of the infant's latch, the adequacy of milk transfer, and the position of the baby during breastfeeding [6]. However, these breastfeeding assessment tools do not integrate an evaluation of the infant's ability to manage variation in milk flow, suck-swallow-breathe (SSB) coordination, or evidence of dysphagia/aspiration concerns [7]. A clinical feeding observation provides for the opportunity to assess the quality of the feeding and apply compensatory strategies when appropriate. These may include slower nipple flow rates for bottle-feeding, use of nipple shields for breastfeeding, use of external pacing to improve suck-swallow-breathe coordination for both breast- and bottle-feeding, and position changes for both breast- and bottle-feedings. The goal of the treating speech pathologist should be to determine a safe and effective feeding plan based on the patient's reaction to various compensatory strategies and to decide when further evaluation is warranted.

Suck-Swallow-Breathe Coordination and Physiologic Stability for Breast- vs Bottle-Feeding

Inherent to the evaluation of an infant's feeding is the fundamental understanding of suck-swallow-breathe (SSB) coordination for both breast- and bottle-feeding. The frequency of sucking, compared to the rate of breaths taken and the length of the infant's pause for breathing, is arranged in a series of bursts. With each swallow, breathing is interrupted affecting the infant's ventilation, oxygen saturation, and heart rate. For example, if the infant is swallowing frequently, the breathing rate will likely be lower. The integrity of the infant's SSB pattern can be influenced by underlying cardiorespiratory issues, the infant's age/development, state regulation and level of alertness during feeding, nipple flow, and rate of milk flow during breastfeeding [8].

Several studies have evaluated the difference in SSB coordination, the mechanics of sucking, and oxygen saturation for breastfeeding infants compared to bottle-feeding infants. There are clear differences between the two that have clinical implications. Goldfield et al. found that oxygen saturation was higher in breastfeeding infants, suggesting that breastfeeding infants are better able to regulate the frequency of sucking and breathing pauses to allow for less interruption of breathing with swallowing [9]. This study also concluded that differences in bottle systems and nipple flow rates may impact an infant's SSB coordination. Moral et al. evaluated breastfeeding and bottle-feeding in healthy full-term infants at 21–28 days of life and at 3–5 months of age and found that babies that are exclusively breastfed show different NS patterns than those babies that are exclusively bottle-fed [10]. Sakalidis et al. hypothesized that SSB coordination may change as the infant ages. This study found that infants became more efficient breastfeeders within the first 4 months by transferring the same volume of milk in a shorter amount of time, by increasing the length of suck bursts, and by decreasing the time spent pausing. The authors also described breastfeeding infants as being able to adapt weaker vacuum levels during sucking to maintain both cardiorespiratory stability and SSB coordination [11].

Indications for Instrumental Evaluation

A feeding observation and clinical feeding assessment can provide valid information regarding the oral phase of swallowing, including the integrity of the infant's sucking pattern, the infant's efficiency to extract liquids in a timely manner, and the infant's ability to manage the bolus from the oral cavity into the pharynx. If an infant is observed to have clinical indications of aspiration, they may require further evaluation of the pharyngeal and esophageal phases of the swallow via a videofluoroscopic swallow study (VFSS) or fiberoptic endoscopic evaluation of swallowing (FEES). Clinical indications of aspiration may include a direct cough during feeding, wet vocal quality, noisy breathing or wet upper airway congestion, changes in oxygen saturation or heart rate, weight loss or poor weight gain, frequent respiratory infections, and disengagement of the feeding [11].

Instrumental Evaluation of Swallowing

Videofluoroscopic Swallow Study

The videofluoroscopic swallow study allows for dynamic imaging of the oral, pharyngeal, and upper esophageal phases of swallowing [12]. This exam is most often performed in the medical imaging suite with both a radiologist and speech-language pathologist jointly administering the exam. It involves a lateral fluoroscopic view of the patient and includes a moving image of the patient swallowing various consistencies of liquid contrast material, typically barium. Both the relevant anatomic structures and the swallow physiology can be evaluated, and the clinician is able to identify if aspiration occurs before, during, or after the swallow is completed. This test does allow for the implementation of various compensatory strategies in real time to determine the safest feeding plan for the child. Several disadvantages to using fluoroscopy have been described, including the infant's exposure to radiation, use of barium for feeding, cost, and inability to assess swallow physiology for breastfeeding [4]. VFSS does allow for view of the oral phase of feeding and identification of aspiration during the swallow and allows for evaluation of the upper esophagus during and after the swallow.

Fiberoptic Endoscopic Evaluation of Swallowing

Fiberoptic endoscopic evaluation of swallowing (FEES) is another instrumental evaluation of swallowing that is available to assess both the relevant anatomic structures and the swallow physiology for patients with identified feeding difficulty. The exam is ideally performed with a team of clinicians that consists of an otolaryngologist, a nurse, and a speech-language pathologist. Typically, for the FEES exam, the infant is held by the parent in a cradled position; the endoscope, coated with lidocaine gel, is passed through one naris and into the nasopharynx and positioned so that the oropharynx, hypopharynx, and larynx are in full view. The scope remains in place as the child is presented with food and begins to eat. Anatomic structures are observed, and swallow physiology is evaluated to identify laryngeal penetration or direct aspiration with feeding. Both Reynolds et al. [4] and Langmore [13] describe studies that have demonstrated the safety, efficacy, sensitivity, and specificity of FEES in its ability to detect laryngeal penetration and direct aspiration in both adults and pediatric patients when compared to VFSS. In contrast to VFSS, FEES allows for swallow evaluation without the exposure to radiation; patients are allowed to use formula or breast milk instead of barium; it allows for evaluation of secretion management and pharyngeal/laryngeal sensation; visualization of the vocal folds is possible; the exam can be repeated more frequently to asses improvement in swallow function; and finally, it allows for evaluation of swallowing during breastfeeding [11].

Application of FEES for Breastfeeding Infants

Because there is a clear difference in how infants coordinate their SSB pattern when bottle-feeding as compared to when they are breastfeeding, it is difficult to apply the results of a VFSS performed using bottle-feeding to an infant that is primarily breastfed. In addition, respiratory difficulties such as stridor and laryngomalacia can impact SSB coordination and can contribute to breastfeeding difficulties and/or early cessation of breastfeeding [8]. The application of FEES for breastfeeding infants allows for safe evaluation of SSB coordination, swallow physiology, and the influence of airway anomalies on swallowing safety. The multidisciplinary team can utilize the results of this exam for early intervention to help maintain safe and effective breastfeeding when possible.

Multidisciplinary Approach to FEES Procedure

FEES Process

The process for performing FEES to evaluate breastfeeding is described in Willette et al. [14]. FEES for breastfeeding is conducted utilizing a multidisciplinary team approach which includes a pediatric nurse, a pediatric otolaryngologist, and one or two pediatric speech-language pathologists (SLP). Before the exam begins, the nurse and the SLP discuss the patient's medical and feeding histories with the parents/caregivers, the parents' goals of the exam, and how the procedure is conducted. A pulse oximeter is placed on the patient's foot to monitor the patient's physiologic stability (heart rate, respiratory rate, and oxygen saturation) throughout the exam. The SLP completes an oral mechanism exam and the otolaryngologist performs a head and neck exam prior to placement of the endoscope. Four percent lidocaine gel is applied to the distal end of the 2.7 mm pediatric flexible endoscope to achieve topical anesthesia of the nasal mucosa during the exam, the nurse stabilizes the patient's head, and the endoscope is inserted into one of the patient's nostrils. An endoscopic evaluation of the patient's anatomical structures (nasal cavity, nasophar-ynx, oropharynx, hypopharynx, and larynx) is performed, and this is followed by an evaluation of the patient's ability to safely manage secretions. Standard grocery store green food coloring is swabbed inside the patient's mouth with a toothette, and the patient is placed into mother's preferred breastfeeding position to initiate breast-feeding. For all patients, the SLP and RN should work with the parent to achieve the most typical and optimal feeding position while maintaining neutral head and neck alignment. A video of the endoscopic exam is recorded, and the results of the exam are reviewed as a team.

In the event that aspiration is identified during breastfeeding, various compensatory strategies may be evaluated. These include changing the breastfeeding position to promote better bolus control, external pacing by breaking the baby's latch to allow for breathing breaks, or offering breast milk through a slow flow bottle nipple. If aspiration continues with use of these compensatory strategies, then thickened liquids may be assessed via bottle drinking. Different consistencies of thickened liquids, various nipple flow rates, changes in feeding position, and/or external pacing during bottle-feeding may be trialed until a safe feeding plan is determined.

After the exam is completed, the otolaryngologist and SLP interpret the information obtained about the anatomical structures and the influence of swallow physiology on breathing, airway protection during feeding, and the patient's overall feeding difficulties. Should the infant require further evaluation or support to establish a safe and effective feeding plan, the family may be referred for lactation, nutrition, gastroenterology, feeding therapy/speech services, and occupational or physical therapy services.

Willette et al. [14] evaluated the safety and efficacy of using FEES to evaluate swallow physiology for breastfeeding. The authors demonstrated that FEES is a safe, a well-tolerated, and an easy-to-perform option for instrumental evaluation of swallowing for infants that are primarily breastfed. FEES can provide meaningful information to direct the medical plan of care for patients with feeding difficulty including airway management, feeding recommendations, and referrals for various supports including nutrition services, gastroenterology consultation, and occupational or physical therapy services. This diagnostic tool allows for a comprehensive investigation of the (upper) airway and provides objective data that aids in the development of a customized feeding plan to optimize the patient's safety with continued breastfeeding.

References

1. Arvedson J. Swallowing and feeding in infants and young children. GI Motility Online. 2006.
2. Burklow K, Phelps A, Schultz J, McConnell K, Rudolph C. Classifying complex pediatric feeding disorders. J Pediatr Gastroenterol Nutr. 1998;27(2):143–7.
3. Linscheid TR, Budd KS, Rasnake LK. Pediatric feeding problems. In: Roberts MC, editor. Handbook of pediatric psychology. New York: Guilford Press; 2003.
4. Reynolds J, Carrol S, Sturdivant C. Fiberoptic endoscopic evaluation of swallowing: a multidisciplinary alternative for assessment of infants with dysphagia in the neonatal intensive care unit. Adv Neonatal Care. 2016;16(1):37–43.
5. Walker N. Management of selected early breastfeeding problems seen in clinical practice. Birth. 1989;16:148–58.

6. Schlomer JA, Kemmerer J, Twiss JJ. Evaluating the association of two breastfeeding assessment tools with breastfeeding problems and breastfeeding satisfaction. J Hum Lact. 1999;15:35–9.
7. Riordan J, Gill-Hopple K, Angeron J. Indicators of effective breastfeeding and estimates of breast milk intake. J Hum Lact. 2005;21(4):406–12.
8. Glass RP, Wolf LS. Incoordination of sucking, swallowing, and breathing as an etiology for breastfeeding difficulty. J Hum Lact. 1994;10(3):185–9.
9. Goldfield EC. Coordination of sucking, swallowing and breathing and oxygen saturation during early infant breast-feeding and bottle-feeding. Pediatr Res. 2006;60:450–5.
10. Moral A, et al. Mechanics of sucking: comparison between bottle feeding and breastfeeding. BMC Pediatr. 2010;10(6):1–8.
11. Sakalidis VS, et al. Longitudinal changes in suck-swallow-breathe, oxygen saturation, and heart rate patterns in term breastfeeding infants. J Hum Lact. 2013;29(2):236–45.
12. Arvedson JC. Assessment of pediatric dysphagia and feeding disorders: clinical and instrumental approaches. Dev Disabil Res Rev. 2008;14:118–27.
13. Langmore S. History of fiberoptic endoscopic evaluation of swallowing for evaluation and management of pharyngeal dysphagia: changes over the years. Dysphagia. 2017;32:27–38.
14. Willette S, et al. Fiberoptic examination of swallowing in the breastfeeding infant. Laryngoscope. 2016;126(7):1681–6.

Chapter 8
Use of Bronchoscopy and Bronchoalveolar Lavage in the Evaluation of Chronic Pulmonary Aspiration

Shailendra Das

Chronic pulmonary aspiration in children presents a challenging problem to medical providers, causing significant morbidity in affected patients. Chronic respiratory signs and symptoms include chronic cough, wheezing, and recurrent pneumonia and can sometimes lead to bronchiectasis (abnormal dilation of the bronchi, usually irreversible, resulting from recurrent infection and inflammation leading to destruction of the elastic and muscle tissue of the airways) [1]. Although many diagnostic tests exist to aid in recognizing the presence of aspiration, there is currently no true gold standard. Direct visualization of the airways with flexible bronchoscopy can help detect (with some exceptions) anatomic abnormalities, such as tracheoesophageal fistula, or airway inflammation causing endobronchial damage. Bronchoalveolar lavage (BAL) is often coupled with flexible bronchoscopy, to allow for sampling of the airways. BAL fluid can detect the presence of acute infection or provide more evidence of chronic aspiration with several biomarkers. This chapter focuses on the utility of the flexible bronchoscopy and bronchoalveolar lavage in chronic pulmonary aspiration.

Essentials of Flexible Bronchoscopy

A full detailed summary of flexible bronchoscopy is beyond the scope of this chapter. Both flexible and rigid bronchoscopes are used for diagnostic and therapeutic purposes, and each has its own advantages depending on the situation. Flexible scopes can be passed further down into the fourth- and fifth-generation airways and provide better maneuvering into these airways. Flexible bronchoscopes 2.8 mm or

S. Das
Department of Pediatrics, Texas Children's Hospital (Baylor College of Medicine),
Houston, TX, USA
e-mail: sxdas@texaschildrens.org

© Springer International Publishing AG, part of Springer Nature 2018
J. Ongkasuwan, E. H. Chiou (eds.), *Pediatric Dysphagia*,
https://doi.org/10.1007/978-3-319-97025-7_8

Table 8.1 Indications for flexible bronchoscopy

Recurrent aspiration
Persistent wet cough
Recurrent/persistent pneumonia
Persistent abnormal CXR/chest CT
Foreign body aspiration
Hemoptysis/pulmonary hemorrhage
Persistent wheezing
Tracheostomy evaluation
Stridor
Respiratory symptoms in an immunocompromised host

greater (outer diameter) also have a small suction channel, which serves multiple purposes: (1) it provides a channel through which secretions/mucus can be aspirated; (2) fluids may be delivered to the airways; and (3) small flexible instruments, such as biopsy forceps or cytology brush, may be passed. The channel in pediatric flexible bronchoscopes, however, is usually small (1.2 or 2.0 mm in diameter). General indications for flexible bronchoscopy are listed in Table 8.1. Flexible bronchoscopy is *not* usually the modality of choice for removal of foreign body. Rigid bronchoscopy allows for more control of the airway and involves larger forceps and other tools ideal for foreign body extraction.

Diagnostic flexible bronchoscopy is often coupled with bronchoalveolar lavage. Bronchoalveolar lavage (BAL) involves instillation of saline through the suction port, with return of some of the sample to be collected and sent for studies. The scope is introduced into the lower airway, and wedged in a subsegment, to allow sufficient return of fluid. Being wedged ensures a better alveolar and airway sample and also prevents saline spilling into other bronchi. The laboratory studies include cell count, cytology, microbial cultures, special stains, and polymerase chain reaction (PCR) testing. There are special assays as well, which will be discussed later when evaluating biomarkers for aspiration.

Flexible Bronchoscopy in the Evaluation of Pulmonary Aspiration

As mentioned earlier, flexible bronchoscopy can be a useful tool in delineating the airway anatomy, looking for abnormalities, and evaluating airway inflammation/edema. A follicular or nodular pattern ("cobblestoning") of the airways can be indicative of inflammation and/or lymphoid hyperplasia (Fig. 8.1), although no direct correlation between cobblestoning and inflammation is noted [2, 3]. Other findings may include tracheoesophageal fistula, laryngomalacia, and tracheomalacia. One limitation to the usefulness of flexible bronchoscopy is the evaluation for laryngeal cleft, which must be performed using direct laryngoscopy and palpation of the interarytenoid groove [4].

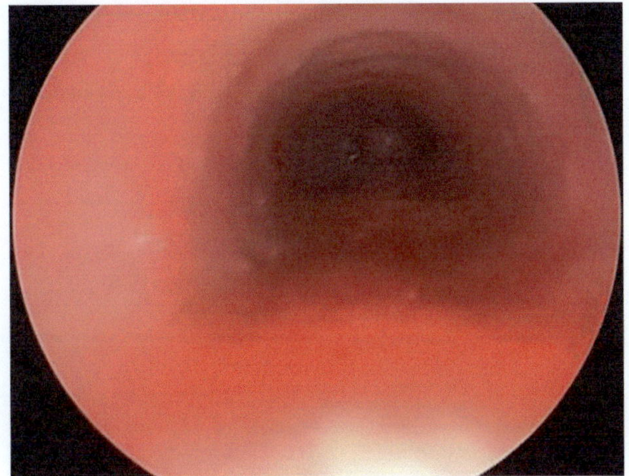

Fig. 8.1 Chronic endobronchial inflammation in a patient with recurrent aspiration. Although nonspecific, this follicular pattern, also known as "cobblestoning," can be representative of chronic pulmonary aspiration

Obtaining a BAL sample is important in the evaluation of patients that are suspected to aspirate. In many cases, chronic pulmonary aspiration is a set up for mucus stasis and endobronchial bacterial growth. Thus, obtaining cultures can be helpful to direct antimicrobial therapy. Several biomarkers found in lavage fluid have been studied to suggest aspiration (most commonly used being the lipid-laden macrophage); however none of them have been shown to have consistently good specificity. The remainder of this chapter examines the various biomarkers and their value in evaluating for aspiration.

Lipid-Laden Macrophages

The lipid-laden macrophage is the first described and most commonly used biomarker for aspiration of food contents in BAL fluid. Lipid stains red on Oil Red O stain when engulfed by alveolar macrophages. First reported in the 1980s, the lipid-laden macrophage index (LLMI) originally presented with promising results, with a sensitivity of 100% and specificity of 57%. An LLMI is based on a scoring of 100 macrophages. Intracellular lipid levels within macrophages are graded with a score of 0 to 4, where 0 = not opacified and 4 = complete opacification. The index is determined by adding the total grades of 100 cells, allowing for a maximum of 400 for each individual specimen [5–8] (Fig. 8.2).

Unfortunately, more recent studies have refuted the utility of this test as a gold standard for aspiration, for several reasons. First, the presence of lipid does not distinguish aspiration from above related to dysphagia versus from below related to gastroesophageal reflux (GER). Even with regard to GER, there is poor correlation between GER and the LLMI. Second, LLMs, though sensitive, are not specific for aspiration and can be seen in a wide variety of pulmonary disorders as an indicator of airway

Fig. 8.2 Modified
lipid-laden macrophage
index. (Reprinted from [8],
with permission from
Elsevier)

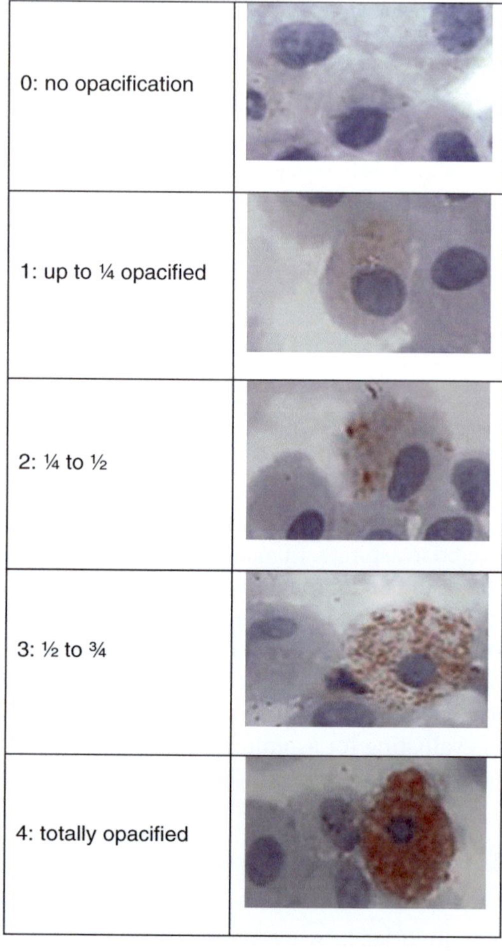

inflammation. Indeed, the lipid-laden macrophage index correlates well with airway neutrophils, reflecting parenchymal inflammation. A study by Reilly et al. demonstrated the presence of lipid-laden macrophages in comparable quantities in six different airway disease states: asthma, cystic fibrosis, immunocompromised patients, aspiration, airway malacia, and recurrent pneumonia; immunocompromised patients demonstrated the highest LLMI in BAL fluid, and perhaps more importantly, there was wide variability within each disease [5]. This leads to a third problem with the lipid-laden macrophage index: there are no clear cutoff values. Several small studies have been done, with variable results for cutoff values [9]. A more recent study published in 2007 suggested a higher cutoff value of >165, leading to a specificity of 78% [10]. As shown, although the presence the lipid-laden macrophages can be a good screening tool for aspiration, even with a higher cutoff value, the LLMI does distinguish from other types of chronic lung diseases.

Pepsin

Pepsin is formed by the cleavage of its inactive form pepsinogen, which is secreted by the gastric chief cells, to the active form in acidic pH. Pepsin is cytotoxic to bronchial epithelial cells. Previous studies have demonstrated the role of pepsin as a biomarker of gastroesophageal reflux-related pulmonary aspiration. Farrell et al. evaluated GER-related aspiration in 56 children undergoing anesthesia as part of the workup for GER [11]. The study group was compared to patients with proven aspiration (positive control) with milk suctioned from endotracheal tube and negative controls. The study demonstrated that patients with proven aspiration had significantly higher pepsin compared to negative controls. Furthermore, out of the patients in the study group, those with proximal (but not distal) GER, and those with chronic cough, were noted to have significantly elevated pepsin levels. Most studies evaluating pepsin as a biomarker do not compare it to a gold standard and assume its validity as a marker, limiting its use. Another problem is that pepsin is only detectable in BAL fluid for a short period of time following aspiration, which limits the ability for its utility in many clinical settings [12]. Furthermore, pepsin does not account for aspiration from "above" (i.e., swallow dysfunction), only GER-related aspiration.

BAL Cytology

Aspiration of food metabolites and/or acid stimulates a proinflammatory reaction in the airways. Neutrophil recruitment may be mediated by proinflammatory cytokines released by lung parenchymal cells. Analysis of bronchoalveolar lavage fluid does frequently demonstrate neutrophilia in the setting of aspiration, and higher percentage of neutrophils in BAL has been shown to be directly correlated with higher LLMI [13]. Unfortunately, these results have not been consistently seen; in one study, patients without gastroesophageal reflux were shown to have a statistically significantly higher percentage of BAL neutrophils than those with GER (albeit small clinical difference) [14]. In addition, similar to LLMI, BAL neutrophilia is also seen in a wide variety of disease processes as a marker of airway inflammation [15]. Moreover, neutrophilia can be a result of a secondary bacterial process (i.e., protracted bacterial bronchitis), and not a direct sequela of aspiration.

Future Directions

Currently, the diagnosis of aspiration is made on the cumulative basis of clinical and supportive studies: imaging, endoscopic findings, and biomarkers (such as lipid-laden macrophages). Other tests in lavage fluid have been/are being considered. Inflammatory markers such as C-reactive protein, various cytokines, and endothelin-1 have not been systematically evaluated with regard to aspiration.

One novel tool has been use of 16S RNA pyrosequencing of the microbial communities of the oral, gastric, and bronchoalveolar tracts. This has helped to determine similarities/differences among the communities and possibly identify patients that are chronically aspirating [16, 17]. In the future it is conceivable that a specific species may be identifiable in those patients known to aspirate [18].

Summary

Flexible bronchoscopy and bronchoalveolar lavage aid in the diagnostic workup of chronic pulmonary aspiration. Endoscopic visualization can detect inflammation of the airways. Several biomarkers exist; unfortunately, none that are used have significant enough specificity to be considered as gold standard. The evolution of utilizing bronchoscopy and lavage will involve discovery of a novel biomarker that can be used for diagnostic purposes.

References

1. Euler AR, Byrne WJ, Ament ME, Fonkalsrud EW, Strobel CT, Siegel SC, et al. Recurrent pulmonary disease in children: a complication of gastroesophageal reflux. Pediatrics. 1979;63(1):47–51.
2. Dave MH, Gerber A, Bailey M, Gysin C, Hoeve H, Hammer J, et al. Prevalence and characteristics of tracheal cobblestoning in children. Pediatr Pulmonol. 2015;50(1):995–9.
3. Duval M, Meier J, Asfour F, Jackson D, Grimmer JF, Muntz HR, Park AH. Association between follicular tracheitis and gastroesophageal reflux. Int J Pediatr Otorhinolaryngol. 2016;82:8–11.
4. Rahbar R, Rouillon I, Roger G, Lin A, Nuss RC, Denoyelle F, et al. The presentation and management of laryngeal cleft: a 10-year experience. Arch Otolaryngol Head Neck Surg. 2006;132(12):1335–41.
5. Reilly BK, Katz ES, Misono AS, Khatwa U, Didas A, Huang L, et al. Utilization of lipid-laden macrophage index in evaluation of aerodigestive disorders. Laryngoscope. 2011;121(5):1055–9.
6. Corwin RW, Irwin RS. The lipid-laden alveolar macrophage as a marker of aspiration in parenchymal lung disease. Am Rev Respir Dis. 1985;132(3):576–81.
7. Colombo JL, Hallberg TK. Recurrent aspiration in children: lipid-laden alveolar macrophage quantitation. Pediatr Pulmonol. 1987;3(2):86–9.
8. Gibeon D, Zhu J, Sogbesan A, Banya W, Rossios C, Saito J, et al. Lipid-laden bronchoalveolar macrophages in asthma and chronic cough. Respir Med. 2014;108(1):71–7. Figure 8.2, Modified lipid laden macrophage index; p. 73
9. Boesch RP, Daines C, Willging JP, Kaul A, Cohen AP, Wood RE, Amin RS. Advances in the diagnosis and management of chronic pulmonary aspiration in children. Eur Respir J. 2006;28(4):847–61.
10. Furuya ME, Moreno-Cordova V, Ramirez-Figueroa JL, Vargas MH, Ramon-Garcia G, Ramirez-San Juan DH. Cutoff value of lipid-laden alveolar macrophages for diagnosing aspiration in infants and children. Pediatr Pulmonol. 2007;42(5):452–7.

11. Farrell S, McMaster C, Gibson D, Shields MD, McCallion WA. Pepsin in bronchoalveolar lavage fluid: a specific and sensitive method of diagnosing gastro-oesophageal reflux-related pulmonary aspiration. J Pediatr Surg. 2006;41(2):289–93.
12. Jaoude PA, Knight PR, Ohtake P, El-Solh AA. Biomarkers in the diagnosis of aspiration syndromes. Expert Rev Mol Diagn. 2010;10(3):309–19.
13. Sacco O, Silvestri M, Sabatini F, Sale R, Moscato G, Pignatti P, et al. IL-8 and airway neutrophilia in children with gastroesophageal reflux and asthma-like symptoms. Respir Med. 2006;100(2):307–15.
14. Chang AB, Cox NC, Purcell J, Marchant JM, Lewindon PJ, Cleghorn GJ, et al. Airway cellularity, lipid laden macrophages and microbiology of gastric juice and airways in children with reflux oesophagitis. Respir Res. 2005;6:72.
15. Yawn RJ, Fazili M, Provo-Bell G, Wootten CT. The utility of bronchoalveolar lavage findings in the diagnosis of eosinophilic esophagitis in children. Int J Pediatr Otorhinolaryngol. 2015;79(11):1834–7.
16. Bassis CM, Erb-Downward JR, Dickson RP, Freeman CM, Schmidt TM, Young VB, et al. Analysis of the upper respiratory tract microbiotas as the source of the lung and gastric microbiotas in healthy individuals. MBio. 2015;6(2):e00037.
17. Rosen R, Hu L, Amirault J, Khatwa U, Ward DV, Onderdonk A. 16S community profiling identifies proton pump inhibitor related differences in gastric, lung, and oropharyngeal microflora. J Pediatr. 2015;166(4):917–23.
18. Vece TJ, Magee A, Runge JK, Rubio-Gonzales M, Chiou EH, Ongkasuwan J, Cope J, Hollister EB, Versalovic J, Luna RA. The microbiome of the aerodigestive tract as a tool in the diagnosis of aspiration in children. Poster presented at: American Thoracic Society 2015 International Conference; 2015 May 15–20; Denver, CO.

Chapter 9
Diagnosis and Treatment of Pediatric Dysphagia: Radiography

William Stoudemire, Lynn Ansley Fordham, and Timothy J. Vece

Abbreviations

Chest CT	Computed tomography of the chest
Chest MR	Magnetic radiography of the chest
VFSS	Videofluoroscopic swallowing study

Introduction: Overview of Imaging Studies for Dysphagia and Aspiration

The diagnosis of aspiration using radiologic and other imaging studies can be difficult for a number of reasons, including a lack of consensus on which studies should be used. Evidence of recurrent aspiration can be seen on several radiographic studies; however, there are varying degrees of sensitivity, partially because aspiration does not always occur with every swallow. Some studies are used specifically for the diagnosis of aspiration, while others do not show direct evidence of aspiration but reveal sequelae of it including pneumonia and chronic lung disease. Imaging studies that can directly show evidence of aspiration, and therefore diagnose aspiration, include videofluoroscopic swallowing study (VFSS), radionuclide salivagram, and gastroesophageal scintigraphy. VFSS has the added advantage of being sufficient to

W. Stoudemire (✉) · T. J. Vece
Department of Pediatrics, University of North Carolina at Chapel Hill,
Chapel Hill, NC, USA
e-mail: William_stoudemire@med.unc.edu; tjvece@email.unc.edu

L. A. Fordham
Department of Radiology, North Carolina Children's Hospital,
Chapel Hill, NC, USA
e-mail: fdh@med.unc.edu

© Springer International Publishing AG, part of Springer Nature 2018
J. Ongkasuwan, E. H. Chiou (eds.), *Pediatric Dysphagia*,
https://doi.org/10.1007/978-3-319-97025-7_9

"

diagnosis dysphagia and other swallowing disorders without direct aspiration. Barium esophagrams also can diagnose aspiration, though only in the presence of H-type fistulas or severe gastroesophageal reflux. Other imaging studies that are not utilized to directly diagnose aspiration but can show signs of aspiration include chest radiograph, computed tomography of the chest (chest CT), lung ultrasound, and magnetic radiography of the chest (chest MR). These imaging studies can assess the degree of lung injury associated with chronic aspiration, which cannot be shown with a VFSS. Key findings of aspiration on these imaging studies will be addressed in this chapter except for VFSS which is covered in a previous chapter.

Part I: Chest Radiography

Chest radiographs are the most commonly used imaging study in the evaluation of respiratory symptoms and are typically the first radiographic study obtained in patients with respiratory difficulty. As signs of aspiration on chest radiographs are neither sensitive nor specific, they should not be used for the primary purpose of diagnosing or ruling out aspiration [1]. However, there are several abnormalities seen on chest radiograph that are suggestive of aspiration and should prompt the clinician to perform further diagnostic workup to evaluate for aspiration. Knowing the key findings of aspiration on chest radiograph is therefore useful, regardless of the initial indication for the study. Chest radiographs can also be useful in determining degree of lung injury from chronic aspiration, though will not detect early lung damage from aspiration.

Acute aspiration events are difficult to distinguish radiographically from infectious pneumonia. Indeed, radiographic evidence of acute aspiration pneumonia is typically defined as a new infiltrate consistent with bacterial pneumonia in patients at risk for aspiration [2]. Clinical suspicion, based on the risk of aspiration, including a witnessed aspiration event, previous history of aspiration, timing of the event, and presence of other infectious symptoms, is critically important in determining whether a new infiltrate on chest radiograph is an aspiration pneumonia and/or more common infectious pneumonia. Location of an acute pneumonia, described below, may increase the likelihood that pneumonia is secondary to aspiration, though this is non-specific finding for aspiration pneumonia.

Abnormalities seen on chest radiographs in chronic aspiration reflect tissue damage and inflammation that results from chronic entrance of saliva (salivary aspiration), ingested materials (solids or liquids), or stomach contents (gastric aspiration) into the airways and lungs. Inflammation of small airways can result in airway obstruction, with evidence of hyperinflation seen on radiographs, such as flattening of the diaphragms, increased number of ribs visible over the lung fields, and increased retrosternal space on a lateral film. Larger airway inflammation from aspirated contents results most often in peribronchial thickening. Segmental or subsegmental infiltrates can also be found, which results from inflammation and remodeling of lung tissue where aspiration occurs [1] (Fig. 9.1). Localized infiltrates are the

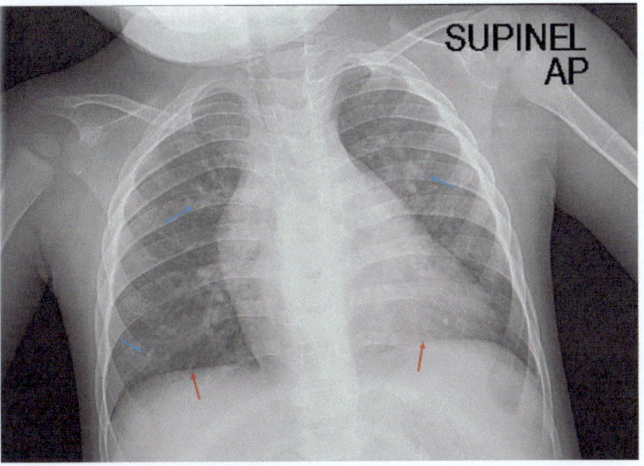

Fig. 9.1 Chest radiograph of an 18-month-old male with chronic aspiration and obstructive sleep apnea. Radiograph shows diffuse patchy infiltrates (red arrows) and flattening of the diaphragms (blue arrows)

most common abnormality seen on chest radiograph in patients with aspiration, followed by diffuse infiltrates, bronchial wall thickening, and hyperinflation [3]. These findings are often subtle, and are not specific to aspiration, but should raise clinical suspicion of aspiration in at risk patients. Unfortunately, chronic findings on chest x-ray are not seen in mild or early lung damage from aspiration and are only evident with significant aspiration over time. Severe or long-standing aspiration can eventually lead to bronchiectasis seen on chest x-ray, though this is a late finding and also not specific for aspiration [1].

The anatomic pattern of chest radiograph abnormalities can also be suggestive of aspiration. In older children and adolescents, the most common areas of chest radiograph findings are the superior and posterior segments of the lower lobes. This pattern is likely because this is the pathway of least resistance for aspirated content while upright. Infants are more likely to show abnormalities from aspiration in the dependent areas, such as the upper lobes and posterior segments of the lower lobes, since the majority of their time is spent supine [1, 3, 4]. These patterns, however, can vary between patients, and location of abnormalities on chest radiograph can be seen in many different anatomic patterns.

Part II: Computed Tomography of the Chest

Computed tomography of the chest (chest CT) offers high-resolution images that can reveal evidence of chronic aspiration into the lungs. As findings on chest CT are not diagnostic, but suggestive, aspiration chest CTs should not be used with the intent to diagnose aspiration. However, chest CTs are often obtained when the underlying respiratory diagnosis is unclear and may show signs of early airway and parenchymal damage suggestive of chronic aspiration in the appropriate clinical setting. Chest CTs can also reveal the extent of lung damage caused by chronic aspiration and have a higher sensitivity for early and less severe changes than chest radiographs.

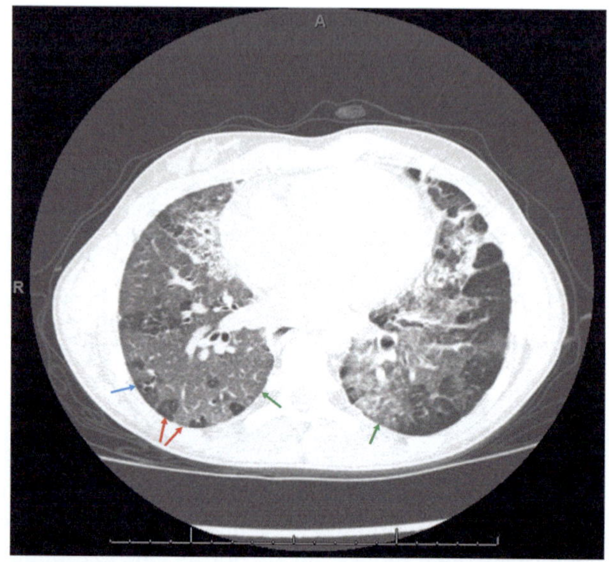

Fig. 9.2 Chest CT of a 15-year-old female with trisomy 21 and an occult H-type tracheoesophageal fistula. Images show mosaic attenuation (red arrows), ground-glass opacities (green arrows), and bronchiectasis (blue arrows)

Abnormalities seen on chest CT reflect damage to the airways and surrounding parenchyma. Airway inflammation from aspirated oral or gastric secretions can be seen as bronchial wall thickening, which is typically the earliest radiographic finding of chronic aspiration on chest CT. Small airway inflammation from aspiration can also result in air trapping, which is shown on chest CT as mosaic attenuation with areas of darker lung parenchyma next to lighter areas (Fig. 9.2) can be seen on chest CT. Severe, long-standing aspiration can eventually lead to traction bronchiectasis, which results from chronic inflammation and fibrosis of lung parenchyma and resultant stretching of the airways from decreased lung compliance. Pulmonary fibrosis also manifests as septal thickening and areas of ground-glass opacities. Since damage results from insult from the airway, centrilobular opacities can also be seen [1, 5]. Honeycombing, which are small (0.3–1 cm) cystic spaces generally in the periphery with well-defined thickened walls, can also be seen with fibrosis from chronic aspiration [6, 7]. This pattern is similar to idiopathic pulmonary fibrosis, and in fact, chronic aspiration is a known mimic of idiopathic pulmonary fibrosis in adults. Location of chest CT abnormalities is similar to those seen on chest radiographs, as described above.

Part III: Other Imaging Studies

Nuclear Medicine Studies Used in the Diagnosis of Aspiration

Besides VFSS, which is covered in the previous chapter, other imaging studies can be used for the diagnosis of aspiration. The primary imaging modalities available are radionuclide salivagram and gastroesophageal scintigraphy. Both studies involve administration of technetium-99m and subsequent imaging of the chest to determine if the nucleotide has been aspirated into the airway.

With gastroesophageal scintigraphy, frequently called a "milk scan," a technetium-99m containing liquid is administered to a patient for ingestion, and imaging is performed to detect for aspiration. The radiolabeled solution is mixed with a set volume of milk or other liquid, depending on child's typical diet. After fasting, the patient actively drinks the solution over a short period of time (approximately 10 min) [8] (Fig. 9.3). This may also be done via nasogastric or gastrostomy tube if necessary. A gamma camera is then used to take sequential images of the lung fields. Any radionuclide signal in the lung fields is considered a positive test for aspiration. Timing of aspiration after swallowing is noted as well, which can be clinically useful information.

A radionuclide salivagram is performed by slowly infusing a small amount of solution containing technetium-99m or another radiolabeled molecule into the mouth of a

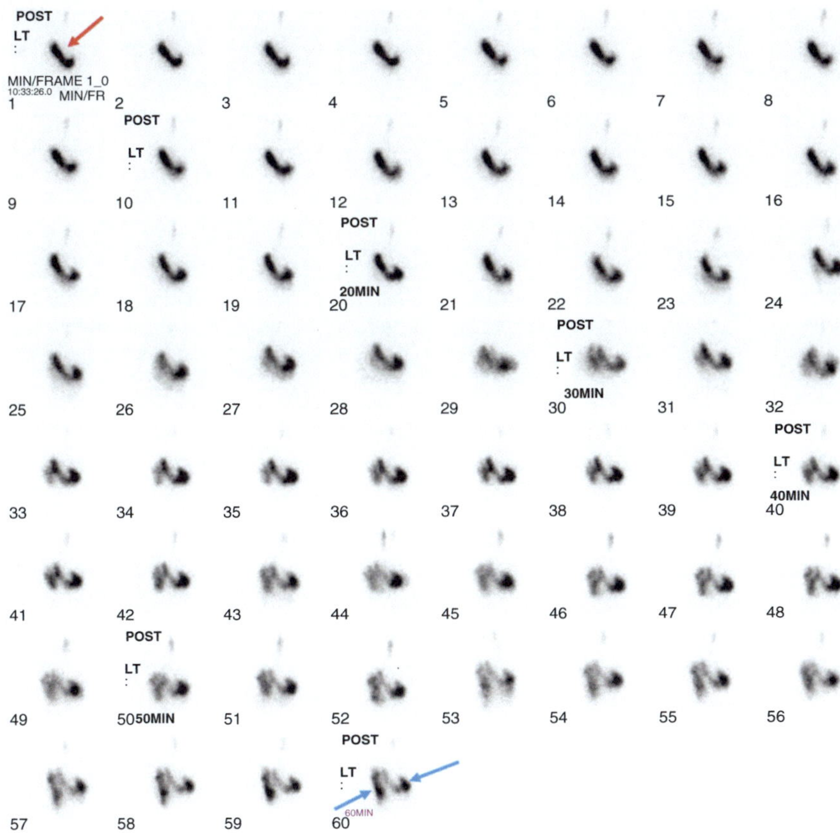

Fig. 9.3 A gastroesophageal scintigraphy scan positive for aspiration. Images are shown each minute over a 60 min time period. Initial signal is seen in the stomach (red arrow). Positive signal in the respiratory tract and lungs at the end of 60 min indicates aspiration (blue arrows). (Image courtesy of Jorge Oldan, M.D.)

patient, typically over an hour. Volumes used are smaller than those used with gastroesophageal scintigraphy. Images of the chest are then obtained with scintigraphy cameras (Figs. 9.4 and 9.5). As with gastroesophageal scintigraphy, any radionuclide signal seen in the lung fields is interpreted as a positive test, indicating anterograde aspiration of saliva into the lungs [8]. Salivagrams are used to detect aspiration of swallowing small amounts, including oral secretions and possible gastric secretions from gastroesophageal reflux that can become mixed with oral secretions.

Radionuclide salivagrams and gastroesophageal scintigraphy are similar tests but may be used preferentially for certain patient types and indications. Salivagrams may be more useful for patients that do not feed by mouth but are at high risk for aspiration of oral secretions (salivary aspiration) such as patients with significant neurodevelopmental disorders [9]. Gastroesophageal scintigraphy may be more useful in detecting aspiration in patients who feed by mouth but have symptoms concerning for dysphagia with swallowing but have had normal VFSS studies. Gastroesophageal aspiration may also be better detected with gastroesophageal scintigraphy than radionuclide salivagrams. However, children with dysphagia may

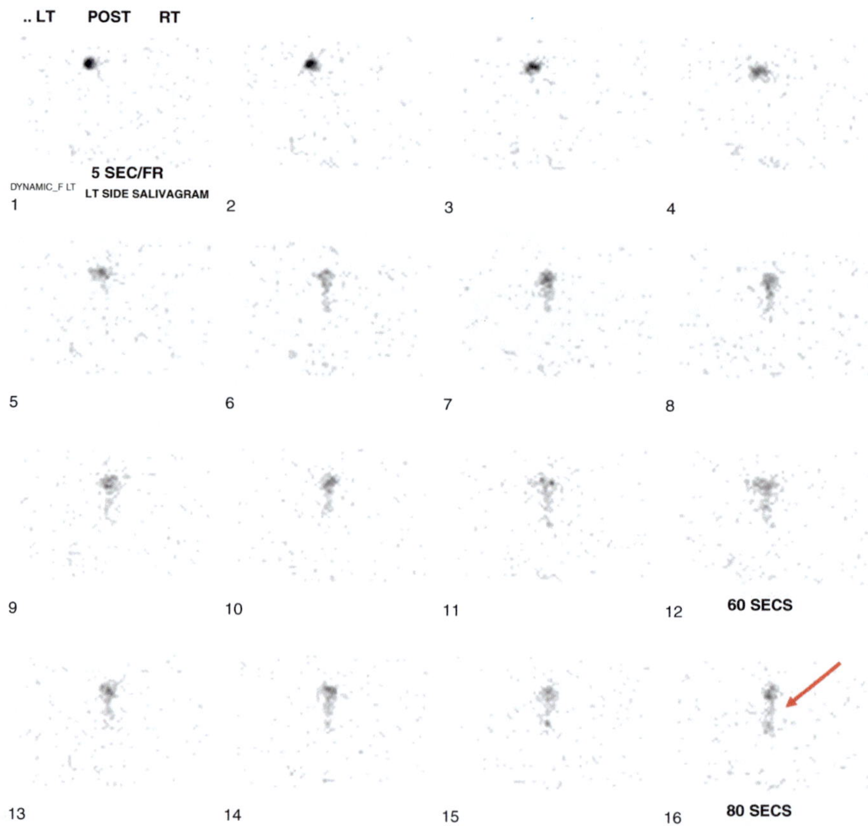

Fig. 9.4 A negative radionuclide salivagram showing signal only in the gastrointestinal tract (red arrow) and none in the respiratory tract. (Image courtesy of Jorge Oldan, M.D.)

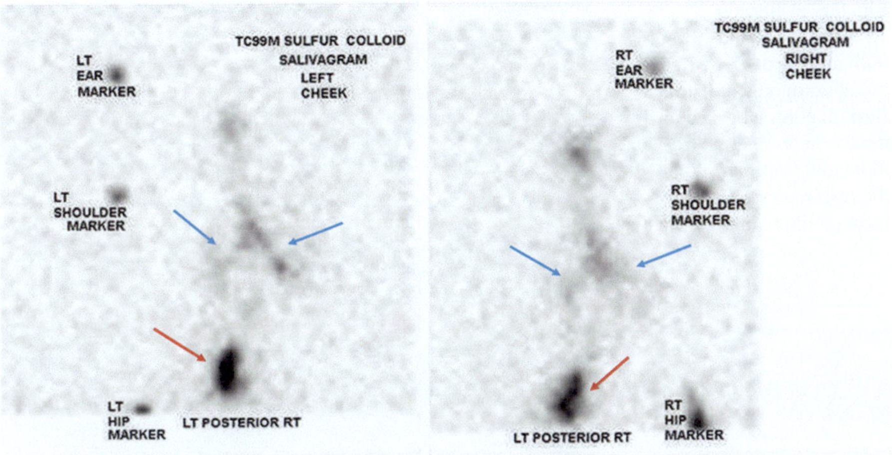

Fig. 9.5 A positive radionuclide salivagram showing signal in the respiratory tract (blue arrows) in addition to signal in the stomach (red arrow). (Image courtesy of Jorge Oldan, M.D.)

also not be able to swallow large volumes, resulting in a lower likelihood of developing increased pressure on the lower esophageal sphincter leading to reflux and a false negative for aspiration for both tests [8]. Overall sensitivity for aspiration is low for both salivagrams and gastroesophageal scintigraphy.

Other Imaging Studies

Barium esophagram is an imaging study in which a contrast agent is swallowed or placed into the esophagus and stomach and is sometimes used to diagnose reflux aspiration, tracheoesophageal fistula, or bronchoesophageal fistula. If there is significant gastroesophageal reflux of contrast that occurs during the study, aspiration of contrast into the lungs can be seen with fluoroscopy (Fig. 9.6). Anatomic abnormalities, such as tracheoesophageal fistulas leading to aspiration into the lungs, may also be seen on a barium esophagram. Small H-type fistulas can be missed by esophagram; therefore a negative test does not rule out a fistula. Laryngeal clefts are also occasionally seen on barium esophagram; however it is not the diagnostic modality of choice, as VFSS and/or endoscopic visualization is more sensitive. Barium esophagram should not routinely be used as a diagnostic test for aspiration in the absence of suspicion for communicating anatomic defects.

Magnetic resonance imaging of the chest (chest MR) is an imaging modality that has been used for a limited number of indications of respiratory pathology in children. Despite the potential benefits including lack of radiation exposure, there are significant limitations to chest MR due to deflection of the signal by air in the lungs. Chest MR is able to visualize soft tissue of the chest well, including the mediastinum and pleura. Visualization of small airway disease, as is most commonly seen with chronic aspiration is limited, however, and inferior to chest CT. New tech-

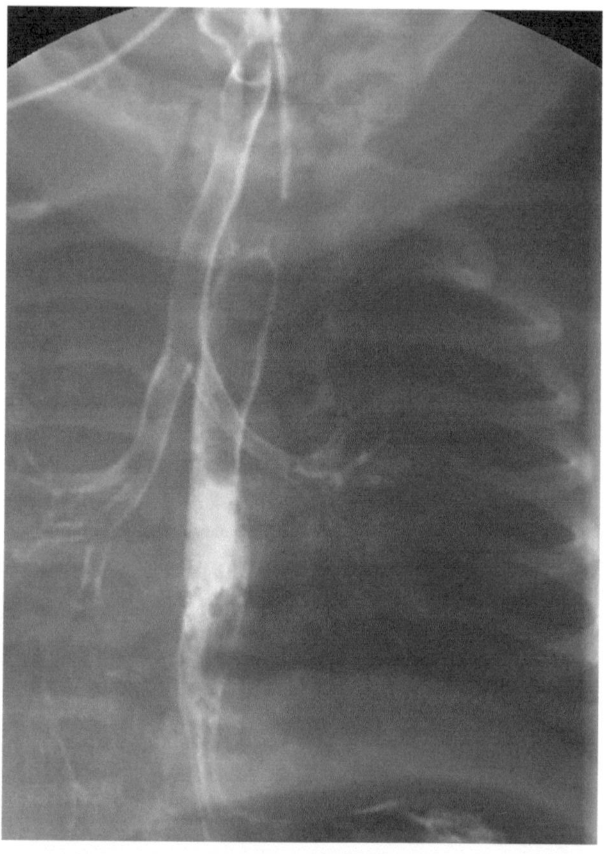

Fig. 9.6 A barium swallow study of a patient with an H-type tracheoesophageal fistula. Barium contrast is seen in the tracheobronchial tree, indicating aspiration into the respiratory tract through the fistula

niques such as using hyperpolarized gas and Fourier decompensation are being developed to improve the utility of chest MR and may be useful in imaging for children with aspiration in the future [10].

Lung ultrasound is being used increasingly to evaluate lung pathology given its low cost, lack of radiation exposure, and widespread availability. While lung ultrasound has been studied in the diagnosis of pneumonia and may be useful for diagnosis of acute aspiration pneumonia, no studies have looked at the use of lung ultrasound for chronic aspiration [11]. Given poor ability of lung ultrasound to visualize small airway disease, it is unlikely that lung ultrasound will have a significant role in diagnosis of chronic aspiration.

Sensitivity and Specificity of Imaging Studies in Aspiration

Several studies have sought to determine the sensitivity and specificity of different imaging studies for diagnosis of chronic aspiration in adults and children (Table 9.1). There has overall been poor agreement between different imaging studies, which

Table 9.1 Summary of radiographic tests for aspiration

	Findings of aspiration	Advantages	Disadvantages
Used directly to diagnose aspiration			
VFSS	Pooling of liquid, penetration of liquid into the airway	Detailed evaluation of swallowing, able to test multiple consistencies Highest overall sensitivity for aspiration	Unable to perform in a child who does not feed orally Relatively high radiation exposure
Gastroesophageal scintigraphy	Contrast detected in the airway or lungs	Low radiation exposure	Low sensitivity
Radionuclide salivagram	Contrast detected in the airway or lungs	Can be performed in patients who do not feed orally	Longer time required for imaging Low sensitivity
Barium esophagram	Contrast penetration into the airway or lungs	Can assess esophageal abnormalities	Only detects aspiration from severe reflux and major anatomic defects
Incidental findings for aspiration			
Chest radiograph	Hyperaeration, subsegmental or segmental infiltrates, peribronchial thickening, bronchiectasis (late stage)	Relatively low radiation exposure Widely available Low cost	Cannot detect early lung damage Low sensitivity and specificity for aspiration
Chest CT	Bronchial wall thickening, air trapping, bronchiectasis, ground-glass opacities, honeycombing, centrilobular opacities	Able to detect early lung damage Can assess degree of lung damage	High radiation exposure Not specific for aspiration

points to the difficulty in establishing a gold standard for a diagnosis of aspiration. This discrepancy is likely due to a number of reasons, including the intermittent nature of aspiration and different types of aspiration (aspiration from swallowing dysfunction, gastroesophageal reflux aspiration, and salivary aspiration), which may be best evaluated by different tests. VFSS has been shown to have the highest sensitivity when compared to other tests of aspiration, with a reported sensitivity of 100% and a specificity of 63% in adults, though given that there is no clear gold standard test and sensitivity may vary depending on the type of aspiration, these values must be interpreted with caution. The primary indication for VFSS is for aspiration from swallowing dysfunction. The radionuclide salivagram has been shown to have a wide range of sensitivity, around 26–28% when compared to other diagnostic tests for aspiration, though again, there is no universal gold standard for detecting salivary aspiration [1, 3]. Gastroesophageal scintigraphy has been shown to have poor sensitivity compared to other measures of aspiration, with only 6% of patients with severe CP that have been shown to have high rates of aspiration with other tests [6]. The poor sensitivity of radionuclide salivagrams and gastroesophageal scintigraphy has limited the utility and clinical use of these studies, though they may be useful in select patients. Since chest radiograph and CT are not used specifically for diagnosis of chronic aspiration, their performance as a test for this is unknown, but studies have shown chest CT to be more sensitive in detecting diffuse changes from aspiration in children and adults. Knowledge of indications and key findings of imaging studies for diagnosis and management of aspiration is important in providing optimal patient care.

Conclusions

The imaging studies described above can all be useful in the diagnosis of aspiration from dysphagia in children. Imaging studies can be used specifically to establish a diagnosis of chronic aspiration, including VFSS, radionuclide salivagram, gastro-esophageal scintigraphy, and in specific cases barium esophagram. Other imaging studies, including chest radiograph and chest CT, are not typically used for diagnosis of chronic aspiration, but may show findings suggestive of aspiration, and can help determine the degree of lung injury from aspiration. Other modalities such as chest MR and lung ultrasound may have a role in evaluating aspiration in the future but currently have a minimal role in the diagnosis of aspiration. Further research is required to establish a gold standard in the diagnosis of aspiration, particularly in children.

References

1. Boesch RP, Daines C, Willging JP, Kaul A, Cohen AP, Wood RE, et al. Advances in the diagnosis and management of chronic pulmonary aspiration in children. Eur Respir J. 2006;28(4):847–61.
2. Marik PE. Aspiration pneumonitis and aspiration pneumonia. N Engl J Med. 2001; 344(9):665–71.
3. Tutor JD, Gosa MM. Dysphagia and aspiration in children. Pediatr Pulmonol. 2012; 47(4):321–37.
4. Colombo JL. Pulmonary aspiration. In: Hillman BC, editor. Pediatric respiratory disease: diagnosis and treatment. Philadelphia: WB Saunders; 1993. p. 429–36.
5. Hansell DM, Bankier AA, MacMahon H, McLoud TC, Müller NL, Remy J. Fleischner Society: glossary of terms for thoracic imaging. Radiology. 2008;246(3):697–722.
6. Rossi UG, Owens CM. The radiology of chronic lung disease in children. Arch Dis Child. 2005;90(6):601–7.
7. De Benedictis FM, Carnielli VP, de Benedictis D. Aspiration lung disease. Pediatr Clin N Am. 2009;56:173–90.
8. Baikie G, South MJ, Reddihough DS, Cook DJ, Cameron DJ, Olinsky A, et al. Agreement of aspiration tests using barium videofluoroscopy, salivagram, and milk scan in children with cerebral palsy. Dev Med Child Neurol. 2005;47(2):86–93.
9. Heyman S, Respondek M. Detection of pulmonary aspiration in children by radionuclide "salivagram". J Nucl Med. 1989;30(5):697–9.
10. Baez JC, Ciet P, Mulkern R, Seethamraju RT, Lee EY. Pediatric chest MR imaging: lung and airways. Magn Reson Imaging Clin N Am. 2015;23(2):337–49.
11. Supakul N, Karmazyn B. Ultrasound of the pediatric chest – the ins and outs. Semin Ultrasound CT MR. 2013;34(3):274–85.

Chapter 10
Oromotor Therapy

Tsu-Hsin Howe

Introduction

Feeding and swallowing disorders are common in infants and young children. Some reports claim that between 25% and 45% of typically developing children and up to 80% of children with developmental disorders demonstrate feeding and swallowing problems [2]. Within specific groups of patients, the prevalence of feeding and swallowing disorders is estimated at 20–45% of premature infants in the first 2 years of life [21, 42, 57, 59] and up to 70–80% in children with cerebral palsy [15].

Children can develop difficulties with feeding and swallowing as a result of a wide spectrum of medical conditions, congenital problems, developmental issues, or through a combination of any of these factors [28, 79]. Oral-motor problems are seen frequently in children with global neuromuscular impairments caused by cerebral palsy [1, 15], traumatic brain injury [66], prematurity, genetic conditions such as Down syndrome [46], craniofacial anomalies such as clefts in the lips and/or palate [76], craniofacial macrosomia, Pierre Robin sequence [65], and ankyloglossia [8] or in children with autistic spectrum disorders [58]. Children without neuromuscular impairments may also demonstrate oral-motor problems as a comorbidity of other medical conditions such as congenital cardiac diseases [22] or bronchopulmonary disorders/chronic lung diseases.

Depending on an infant or a young child's medical conditions and developmental status, he or she may demonstrate a unique constellation of oral-motor problems. For example, impaired oral sensorimotor function in children with cerebral palsy exhibits reduced lip closure, poor tongue function, tongue thrust, exaggerated bite reflex, tactile hypersensitivity, delayed swallow initiation, reduced pharyngeal motility, and drooling [3, 15]. On the other hand, problems with feeding and swallowing that occur as a result of cleft and craniofacial anomalies would manifest a

T.-H. Howe
Department of Occupational Therapy, New York University,
New York, NY, USA
e-mail: tsuhsin.howe@nyu.edu

© Springer International Publishing AG, part of Springer Nature 2018
J. Ongkasuwan, E. H. Chiou (eds.), *Pediatric Dysphagia*,
https://doi.org/10.1007/978-3-319-97025-7_10

different clinical picture [65]. Moreover, children with sensory-based feeding disorders, who experience oral aversion or food restriction, may demonstrate unique behavioral characteristics that require different treatment strategies [25].

Interventions for Oral-Motor and Sensory-Based Feeding Disorders

Because feeding and swallowing disorders are influenced by multiple factors, interventions for oral-motor and sensory-based feeding disorders are often conducted under a multifactorial framework. Oral-motor therapy is the most common therapeutic intervention for children with dysphagia. Oral-motor therapy can be used as a component of feeding therapy. It can be carried out alone or incorporated with other interventions such as positioning and swallow therapy. Clinicians use a variety of techniques to achieve a broad range of goals including increased oral awareness, improved separation and grading of oral-motor movements to enhance feeding skills, promotion of normal sensory oral experiences during mealtime, and improved oral-facial muscle tone to assist in oral structure stability [29, 74]. In order to create an oral-motor feeding plan individualized for the child, a comprehensive evaluation is warranted.

Oral-Motor Assessments

The oral-motor clinical assessment typically consists of a physical examination, oral structure, and oral-motor function examination. Many different clinical assessments are used to assess a child's feeding or swallowing function [45]. Assessments that consist of oral-motor components are discussed in this chapter.

Physical Examination

The purpose of physical examinations is to assess a child's general neuromotor control by analyzing elements of muscle tone, primitive reflex activity, and the development of antigravity postural control. Clinicians should always perform at least a brief assessment of the child's overall neuromotor control as problems in oral-motor control may be related to larger neuromotor control issues [90]. Clinicians should always keep in mind that resting postures or active movements may affect the status of muscle tone and primitive reflexes or vice versa. Providing proper support to facilitate adequate body alignment and optimal postural tone may be the first step before proceeding on to oral-motor therapy. Please refer to Chapter 11 for more details about positioning.

Oral Structure Assessment

Alteration of orofacial structures is common to some congenital syndromes and craniofacial anomalies. Knowledge of these syndromes and anomalies is foundational to consider any impact on swallowing and feeding for both short- and long-term prognoses. Clinicians should examine the oral cavity prior to any functional tests to evaluate each component of oral structure, including the lips, jaw, and tongue.

Lips

The lips should appear soft at rest. Clinicians should observe if an infant can seal around the artificial nipple or breast while sucking. When appropriate, clinicians should also observe if a child can use the upper lip to remove food from a spoon successfully or to keep lips closed while swallowing. Tight, retracted lips may be observed in children with abnormal muscle tone, such as those with cerebral palsy [90].

Jaw

At rest, clinicians should observe a neutral jaw position with loose upper and lower jaws. Common deviations of jaw position that might require intervention include a recessed jaw, in which the lower gum ridge is posterior to the upper gum ridge, or a depressed jaw, where the mouth is typically open. Asymmetries or lateral deviations of the jaw can also observed [90].

During sucking, normal jaw movement is smooth, in small and rhythmical excursion. When presenting food in a spoon or liquid in a cup to a child, he or she should open his or her mouth to receive the spoon or cup and close the jaw under the nipple, spoon, or cup to control the flow of the liquid or food into the mouth. Jaw movements during chewing should also be observed and assessed, taking into consideration a child's developmental stage, for appropriateness. The development of chewing occurs in three stages. Children start chewing with a munching, up-and-down movement of the jaw. They progress by adding lateral jaw motion to the vertical movements. Finally, they develop rotary motion [89]. Large or excessive excursion, which may cause the oral seal during sucking and eating to break, could indicate jaw instability. Lack of range of jaw movement, clenching, clonus, and tremors may also be observed in the jaw [90].

Tongue

Clinicians should examine the general appearance of the tongue and its resting position. A normally functioning tongue should appear soft, with a well-defined shape that is relatively thin and flat, and have a moderately rounded tip. There should be evidence of a slight central groove in the anterior-posterior direction. The tongue should lie in the bottom of the mouth between the lower gum ridges. It should not protrude over the lips and should not be seen when the mouth is closed [90]. Common deviations of the tongue include elevated tongue tip or humped, bunched, or retracted tongues. Lingual hypertonia in children with low muscle tone (e.g., children with Down syndrome) [61] or macroglossia (e.g., children with Beckwith-Wiedemann syndrome) can also be observed.

Clinicians should also assess tongue movements and mobility, including tongue lateralization, extension, cupping, and peristalsis. Tongue lateralization can be assessed by eliciting the transverse tongue reflex. To do so, clinicians may trace the lower gum ridge and brush the lateral edge of the tongue with a gloved finger. Extension of the tongue can be assessed by eliciting the tongue extrusion reflex. To do so, clinicians can either brush the lower lip downward toward the chin or push the tip of the tongue so the tongue will push out. Cupping assesses the degree to which the tongue hugs the finger while sucking. Peristalsis is the backward, wave-like motion of the tongue during sucking that should originate at the tip of the tongue and be felt with the back of the examiner's finger. Snapback is heard as a chucking sound when the tongue loses it grasp on the finger or nipple when an infant tries to generate negative pressure [8].

Oral-Motor Function Assessment

In addition to examining the components of oral structure individually, clinicians should also evaluate overall oral-motor control by conducting a functional exam to assess how these components work together to produce smooth and coordinated movements. Oral-motor skills are usually evaluated as part of feeding assessment to determine the child's ability to feed safely by mouth since they are a key aspect of this process. There are a wide range of approaches used in clinical practice to assess children's oral-motor skills. These range from the non-standardized general observation of children while feeding to the use of standardized assessments, which are in various stages of development and continue to be tested for psychometric soundness. Current assessment methods are predominantly subjective and are often not based on standardized assessment [78]. When possible, clinician should always incorporate standardized assessments alongside clinical observations of oral-motor skills in order to provide objective and measureable data.

Oral-Motor Assessment for Infants Less than 6 Months Old

Based on the reports that examine the psychometric properties of currently available oral-motor feeding assessments, the Neonatal Oral-Motor Assessment Scale (NOMAS) is the most widely tested for psychometric soundness in infants less than 6 months [16, 48].

The NOMAS [70] is designed to identify and quantify oral-motor patterns in neonates during non-nutritive and nutritive sucking. The NOMAS contains a 28-item checklist of tongue and jaw movement behaviors and categorizes them as of normal, disorganized, and dysfunctional [18]. The oral-motor components in the checklist include the rate, rhythmicity, and consistency of the degree of jaw excursion; the direction, range of motion, and timing of tongue movements; and tongue configuration.

Oral-Motor Assessments for Pediatric Populations

Barton and colleague identified eight assessments that are designed to assess oral-motor skills in the pediatric population [11]. The eight assessments are (1) the Ability for Basic Feeding and Swallowing Scale for Children (ABFS-C; [52]), (2) the Brief Assessment of Motor Function-Oral Motor Deglutition (BAMF-OMD; [85]), (3) the Behavioral Assessment Scale of Oral functions in Feeding (BASOFF; [69, 86]), (4) the Dysphagia Disorder Survey (DDS; [19, 81]), (5) the Functional Feeding Assessment Modified (FFAm; [40, 91]), (6) the Gisel Video Assessment (GVA; [39, 40]), (7) the Oral-Motor Assessment Scale (OMAS; [23]), and (8) the Schedule for Oral-Motor Assessment (SOMA; [83]). Among these assessments, three assessments (BAMF-OMD, GVA, and SOMA) are used to evaluate different textures, including liquid, puree, and chewable solids. Four assessments are designed for children with cerebral palsy (FFAm, GVA, OMAS, SOMA). Four are designed for children with developmental disabilities (ABFS-C, BAMF-OMD, BASOFF, DDS). Many reports analyze and discuss the pros and cons of these commonly used clinical assessments [11, 16, 45, 49]. Table 10.1 presents a summary of these eight assessments. Clinicians can refer to this information before choosing assessment(s) that best fit their desired clinical purposes.

Oral-Motor Intervention

Oral-motor intervention is an umbrella term. It comprises many different techniques and can be utilized in many different clinical manifestations and for varied purposes. Oral-motor strategies are used to increase functional strength and control of movement for feeding [14], to promote the onset of oral feeding, and to improve oral feeding performance [5]. They also can be used as a preventative measure, providing positive experiences that minimize the risk of oral aversion [25] and reduced oral hypersensitivity [43].

In the section that follows, the different areas in which clinicians might consider the use of oral-motor intervention will be discussed. Clinicians should understand the functional goals achievable through oral-motor intervention as well as the specific methods and techniques that may be used to achieve these goals. All of the

Table 10.1 Pediatric oral-motor assessments

Assessment	Purpose/description	Population/age range	Assessment type/items	Comments
Ability for Basic Feeding and Swallowing Scale for Children (ABFS-C)	Evaluation of children's feeding and swallowing ability	Developmental disabilities/2 months–14 years	Observational/five items (wakefulness, head control, hypersensitivity, oral-motor ability, saliva control)	
Brief Assessment of Motor Function-Oral Motor Deglutition (BAMF-OMD)	Evaluation of oral-motor deglutition	Developmental disabilities/6 months–18 years	Observational/11 items	
Behavioral Assessment Scale of Oral functions in Feeding (BASOFF)	Document strengths and weaknesses of oral function in relation to feeding difficulties	Developmental disabilities/10–38 months	Observational/14 items (jaw closure, lip closure over spoon and while swallowing, tongue control, chewing, sips liquid, etc.)	
Dysphagia Disorder Survey (DDS)	Screen the swallowing and feeding function for eating and drinking using three food types (solids that do and do not require chewing and liquid)	Intellectual and developmental disabilities/children and adults	Observational/15 items	
Functional Feeding Assessment Modified (FFAm)	Evaluation of oral-motor skills during feeding tasks	Cerebral palsy/pediatrics	Seven domains of ingestion, each domain contains 4–9 behaviors (spoon feeding, biting, chewing, cup drinking, straw drinking, swallowing, and clearing)	
Gisel Video Assessment (GVA)	Evaluation of ingestive skills	Cerebral palsy	Observational Four textures of food: hard solid-wheat biscuit, viscous-raisin, soft solid-processed cheese, and puree-applesauce offered and observed	

Oral-Motor Assessment Scale (OMAS)	Assesses oral-motor skills using functional tasks. To determine oral-motor impairment through feeding each texture (soft, solid, liquid)	Neurological damages/2–20 years	Observational/seven items (mouth closure, lip closure on utensil, lip closure during deglutition, control of the food during swallowing, mastication, straw suction, and control of liquid during deglutition)	The psychometric study reported that the OMAS is an accurate and reliable tool. It is sensitive to changes and useful for interventional studies [6]
Schedule for Oral-Motor Assessment (SOMA)	To record oral-motor skills and identify oral-motor dysfunction. It assesses children's oral-motor function in terms of discrete oral-motor movements including jaw, lip, and tongue control, across a range of food textures and fluids. The SOMA predominantly tests oral phase dysfunction; however, some items pertain to the pharyngeal phase	Cerebral palsy/8–24 months postnatal	Video recording of a structured feeding session. Seven different categories (liquid, puree, semisolid, sold, biscuits, dried fruit)	The psychometric properties of the SOMA including test-retest and interrater reliability, criterion, and predictive validity were reported to be excellent [53, 82]

intervention techniques should initially be delivered by qualified professionals with advanced training. Clinicians may consider teaching primary caregivers modified versions of oral-motor therapy to carry out at home with their children when appropriate. Safely delivering a home program is a great challenge for all professionals in the field. In addition, readers should be mindful that oral-motor therapy is often implemented alongside other approaches. A comprehensive perspective should always be adopted when managing children with dysphagia.

Facilitate Nutritive Sucking in Premature Infants

One of the major goals of implementing oral-motor therapy in premature infants is to facilitate nutritive sucking. Techniques used to facilitate feeding performance include oral stimulation, non-nutritive sucking, orocutaneous stimulations, and oral support. Oral stimulation strategies are used to promote the onset of oral feeding or to improve oral feeding performance for premature infants [26, 31, 32, 36, 62]. Oral stimulation is traditionally defined as stroking and/or pressure to the perioral and intraoral structures in a specific way. It can be delivered informally or following a protocol. For example, Fucile and her colleague described an oral stimulation program used for premature infants to enhance the oral feeding performance [31]. Their protocol uses a pre-feeding finger stimulation that includes 12 min of structured finger stroking on the cheeks, lips, gums, and tongue, followed by 3 min of pacifier sucking (i.e., 15 min once a day for one consecutive day, 1–30 min before a tube feeding).

Investigators reported a range of oral stimulation interventions that appear beneficial for preterm infants in terms of reducing the length of hospital stay and promoting earlier transitions to oral feeding, with reduced lengths of time on parenteral nutrition [43]. Greene, O'Donnell, and Walshe conducted a systematic review to determine the effectiveness of oral stimulations in attaining oral feeding in preterm infants born before 37 weeks postmenstrual age (PMA) [43]. Their results showed that in general, oral stimulation reduced the time it took to transition to oral feeding in comparison to standard care and another non-oral intervention [43].

The effectiveness of two oral-motor interventions for preterm infants [31, 60] was examined and shown to have positive outcomes [43]. The effectiveness of Gisel's pre-feeding oral stimulation protocol has been studied by many researchers as a primary oral stimulation intervention because of its clear description [4, 5, 32–34, 44, 62, 71, 77, 92]. Lessen [60] modified the Beckman Oral Motor Intervention (BOMI) program to a 5-min program for premature infants called Premature Infant Oral Motor Intervention (PIOMI). Strong evidence supports its effects on feeding progression and length of hospital stay [60, 67].

Non-nutritive sucking (NNS) refers to those sucking movements induced by a pacifier or a finger in the absence of fluids. It has been used regularly as a form of oral stimulation in oral-motor therapy. Moderate to strong evidence shows that NNS interventions demonstrate significant effects on the transition from gavage to full oral feeding, the transition from start of oral feeding to full oral feeding, weight gain

[4, 87], and the length of hospital stay for preterm infants [30, 72, 87]. The findings regarding the effects of NNS on other clinical variables such as feeding performance, intestinal transit time, and behavioral state during tube feedings and before, during, and after bottle feeding are inconclusive [47, 64]. None of the studies report negative outcomes. Studies also demonstrate that sensory-motor oral stimulation combined with either NNS or oral support can enhance the oral feeding performance of preterm newborns and lead to a decreased length of hospital stay [17, 77].

Other forms of oral-motor therapy including orocutaneous stimulation and oral support have been used to facilitate non-nutritive and nutritive sucking. Researchers demonstrated that frequency-modulated orocutaneous stimulation (e.g., NTrainer, pulsating pacifier) was effective in facilitating NNS in preterm infants with or without respiratory distress syndrome or chronic lung diseases [9, 10, 73]. Oral support, including that of the cheek and jaw, was reported as an effective technique in improving feeding performance in preterm infants [26, 50].

Facilitate Feeding Performance in Children with Cerebral Palsy

Sensorimotor approaches as a form of oral-motor therapy are conducted in children with cerebral palsy with the intent of increasing the efficiency of eating. Sensorimotor approaches are defined as any techniques used to facilitate lip closure, tongue lateralization, and rotary chewing, to inhibit tongue thrust, to decrease tactile hypersensitivity, and to encourage swallowing [37]. Detailed descriptions of these techniques can be found in research articles by Gisel [38] and Baghbadorani et al. [6].

One article provided evidence that a tactile stimulus to the posterior tongue and sequential tactile stimuli to varied locations on the lingual surface may induce independent swallowing in pediatric patients with lingual dysphagia [56]. Snider and colleagues [84] conducted a study examining the evidence pointing to the effectiveness of sensorimotor approaches as a part of feeding interventions in children with cerebral palsy. They concluded that there is conflicting evidence as to whether sensorimotor facilitation techniques are more effective than alternative treatments or no treatment in enhancing feeding safety and efficiency. However, readers should be reminded that oral sensorimotor approach is rarely implemented as a single model approach. Studies that evaluate the effectiveness of multimodal approaches including medical, oral-motor, behavioral, and environmental intervention and adaptations to improve feeding performance should be emphasized.

Preparation for Proper Muscle Tone

Oral-motor therapy can also be used to prepare proper muscle tone for feeding. Infants and toddlers with low muscle tone tend to have open mouth posture and subsequently have drooling problems, difficulty with jaw and lip closure, or difficulty forming a tight oral seal for sucking. They may also have difficulty with dynamic jaw and tongue stability, as well as graded jaw, lips, and tongue movements which may directly influence their ability to eat and drink [55]. Kumin and colleague presented a comprehensive home treatment protocol that includes oral massage, oral facilitation techniques, and non-speech oral exercises for addressing oral-motor issues in young children who exhibit low muscle tone as a result of Down syndrome [55]. Oral massages are used to increase sensory awareness and decrease hypersensitivity or tactile defensiveness. This sequence generally involves manual massage of the facial musculature and massaging inside the mouth with an implement such as a NUK oral massage brush or electric toothbrush. Oral exercises to improve graded movements of the jaw, lip, and tongue, including specific jaw exercises to improve jaw alignment, strength, and stability, are documented by many clinicians on the web [7, 12, 54].

Beckman Oral Motor Intervention (BOMI) [13] is one of the most commonly used oral-motor protocols in clinical settings. It can be used in conjunction with oral massage. Beckman developed this oral-motor program to provide assisted movement that activates muscle contractions and provides resistance training to build strength. The focus of these interventions is to increase functional responses to pressure and movement, range, strength, variety, and the control of lip, cheek, jaw, and tongue movement. The 15-min intervention consists of 25 manipulations of the oral and facial surface tissue and musculature. It is designed for term infants and children and adults with developmental delays that result in feeding difficulties [55, 60]. Even though it is a commonly used protocol, there is limited evidence supporting its effectiveness. Only one study reported positive outcome of using BOMI post-surgery in infants born with complex univentricle anatomy [20].

Another technique used to improve muscle tone is Castillo-Morales' therapy. The program combines manual stimulation with the facilitation of palatal plates [61, 63]. This approach has resulted in improved mimetic muscles, tongue retraction, and lip closure in children with Down syndrome [61, 63].

Improve Jaw Stability and Chewing

Since the early 1980s, many clinicians have proposed different strategies designed to improve jaw stability and chewing skills [68]. For example, Farber suggested the use of vibration over the temporalis, pterygoid, and masseter muscles combined with a quick stretch in the opposite direction of desired jaw movement to treat jaw instability [68]. However, the descriptions and research on interventions for jaw instability and chewing problems have been limited. No empirical studies reported the efficacy of these described techniques, and only a few structured approaches to teach children with feeding problems to chew have been documented in the literature. Eckman and colleague documented a structured intervention that combined oral-motor and behavioral components to teach chewing [24]. Positive outcomes were reported when implemented in two children with special needs. Arslan and colleagues [80] proposed a functional chewing training program for children with cerebral palsy. The protocol includes positioning the child and food, sensory stimulation, and chewing exercises. They placed a chewing tube in the child's molar area to facilitate chewing. In their initial report, the proposed chewing training was found to be effective in comparison to traditional oral-motor exercise. However, more evidence is needed to support their claims.

Decrease Drooling

Drooling is a problem in approximately 15–78% of children with cerebral palsy (CP) [1, 75]. Oral-motor therapy used to address drooling strives to improve oral-facial tone, increase oral-facial awareness, facilitate jaw and lip closure, and subsequently improve swallowing. A number of descriptive reports are available and outline various techniques to decrease drooling, which include the brushing, vibration, quick stretch, icing, and rubbing of the gums, the application of pressure to the oral-facial area for lip closure, and jaw support [51]. However, there is little published research that confirms any long-term effects on drooling control [27].

Decrease Tongue Thrusting and Tonic Bite Reflex

Abnormal oral reflexes, such as tongue thrusting and the tonic bite reflex, create feeding challenges for children with severe and profound disabilities [35]. Tongue thrusting is defined as a strong extension and protraction of the tongue before or during feeding. For children with neurological impairments, tongue thrusting may be observed as part of a generalized extensor pattern [37]. The tonic bite reflex is the tight closure of the jaw in response to an oral tactile stimulus placed in or around the mouth. An individual with a tonic bite reflex has trouble opening the mouth when the reflex has been elicited. Ganz [37] described an oral-motor intervention used to decrease tongue thrusting and the tonic bite reflex. Manual vibration and pressure techniques are used to decrease tongue thrusting. Manual vibration is applied around the mouth and to the area under the midline of the tongue on the either side of the frenulum to stimulate the tongue retrusion muscles. Pressure is applied to the anterior portion of the tongue and slowly moved posterior along the midline of the tongue. Both techniques were reported to decrease tongue thrusting for an 8-year-old girl with severe cerebral palsy [37]. Gum massage and pressure techniques are used to reduce the tonic bite reflex. The inner and outer gums are massaged from midline to the back of mouth and then back to midline while maintaining jaw control. Pressure is applied to the teeth using a tongue depressor wrapped in gauze and is designed to decrease a child's hypersensitivity and thereby decrease the tonic bite reflex. The techniques described in the article are commonly implemented by clinicians; however, little evidence can be found to support the effectiveness of these interventions.

Improve Oral Aversions

Some children with feeding problems have issues relating to accepting food and may be diagnosed with oral aversions [25, 41, 88]. The severity of oral aversions ranges from phases of pickiness to complete food refusal. Medical conditions such as gastroesophageal reflux or food allergy, mechanical/structural abnormalities including congenital anomalies (e.g., CHARGE or VATER syndrome), neurological impairments, and behavioral causes all can contribute to oral aversion. For children who show the signs and symptoms of oral aversion, oral-motor therapy may be used as preventative or preparatory technique to build oral sensory tolerance, as well as to provide positive oral experiences. Oral-motor therapy can also be used to treat oral-motor deficits as underlying reasons causing oral aversions. For example, children who have inadequate chewing skills may gag when attempting to swallow large chunks of food, and since gagging is a powerful aversive event, this may lead to further refusals of solid textured food. Teaching chewing skills in this incidence may result in the increased acceptance of food and decreased signs and symptoms of oral aversion. In summary, to achieve the best results when treating oral aversions, oral-motor therapy should combine behavioral modifications and medical interventions.

Conclusion

Children with feeding difficulties are a highly heterogeneous population with diverse etiologies and underlying strengths and weaknesses that promote or prevent skilled feeding [25]. There is strong to moderate evidence supporting the positive effects of oral-motor therapy on feeding performance in infants and young children with feeding problems [47]. However, most of the evidence gathered is from studies with a small sample size and limited intervention techniques. In addition, the interventions were often without sufficient descriptions. Further development of standard protocols and specific treatment regimens for target behaviors in different populations are warranted.

References

1. Aggarwal S, Chadha R, Pathak R. Feeding difficulties among children with cerebral palsy: a review. *Children*. 2015;1(7):9–12.
2. Arvedson JC. Assessment of pediatric dysphagia and feeding disorders: clinical and instrumental approaches. Dev Disabil Res Rev. 2008;14(2):118–27.
3. Arvedson JC. Feeding children with cerebral palsy and swallowing difficulties. Eur J Clin Nutr. 2013;67:S9–S12.
4. Asadollahpour F, Yadegari F, Soleimani F, Khalesi N. The effects of non-nutritive sucking and pre-feeding oral stimulation on time to achieve independent oral feeding for preterm infants. Iran J Pediatr. 2015;25(3):e809.

5. Bache M, Pizon E, Jacobs J, Vaillant M, Lecomte A. Effects of pre-feeding oral stimulation on oral feeding in preterm infants: a randomized clinical trial. Early Hum Dev. 2014;90(3):125–9.

6. Baghbadorani MK, Soleymani Z, Dadgar H, Salehi M. The effect of oral sensorimotor stimulations on feeding performance in children with spastic cerebral palsy. Acta Med Iran. 2014;52(12):899–904.

7. Bahr D. Ages and stages: resources for feeding, speech, and mouth function. 2017. Retrieved from http://www.agesandstages.net/courses.php

8. Ballard JL, Auer CE, Khoury JC. Ankyloglossia: assessment, incidence, and effect of frenuloplasty on the breastfeeding dyad. Pediatrics. 2002;110(5):e63.

9. Barlow SM, Lee J, Wang J, Oder A, Hall S, Knox K, et al. Frequency-modulated orocutaneous stimulation promotes non-nutritive suck development in preterm infants with respiratory distress syndrome or chronic lung disease. J Perinatol. 2014;34(2):136–42.

10. Barlow SM, Lee J, Wang J, Oder A, Oh H, Hall S, et al. Effects of oral stimulus frequency spectra on the development of non-nutritive suck in preterm infants with respiratory distress syndrome or chronic lung disease, and preterm infants of diabetic mothers. J Neonatal Nurs. 2014;20(4):178–88.

11. Barton C, Bickell M, Fucile S. Pediatric oral motor feeding assessments: a systematic review. *Phys Occup Ther Pediatr*. 2018;38(2):190–209.

12. Beckman D. Beckman oral motor. 2014. Retrieved from http://www.beckmanoralmotor.com/about.php

13. Beckman D. Oral motor intervention. 2017. Retrieved from http://www.beckmanoralmotor.com/about.php

14. Beckman D, Neal C, Phirsichbaum J, Stratton L, Taylor V, Ratusnik D. Range of movement and strength in oral motor therapy: a retrospective study. Fla J Commun Disord. 2004;21:7–14.

15. Benfer K, Weir K, Bell K, Ware R, Davies P, Boyd R. Oropharyngeal dysphagia in preschool children with cerebral palsy: oral phase impairments. Res Dev Disabil. 2014;35(12):3469–81.

16. Bickell M, Barton C, Dow K, Fucile S. A systematic review of clinical and psychometric properties of infant oral motor feeding assessments. Dev Neurorehabil. 2017:1–11. https://doi.org/10.1080/17518423.2017.1289272.

17. Boiron M, Da Nobrega L, Roux S, Henrot A, Saliba E. Effects of oral stimulation and oral support on non-nutritive sucking and feeding performance in preterm infants. Dev Med Child Neurol. 2007;49(6):439–44.

18. Braun MA, Palmer MM. A pilot study of oral-motor dysfunction in "at-risk" infants. Phys Occup Ther Pediatr. 1985;5(4):13–26.

19. Calis EA, Veugelers R, Sheppard JJ, Tibboel D, Evenhuis HM, Penning C. Dysphagia in children with severe generalized cerebral palsy and intellectual disability. Dev Med Child Neurol. 2008;50(8):625–30.

20. Coker-Bolt P, Jarrard C, Woodard F, Merrill P. The effects of oral motor stimulation on feeding behaviors of infants born with univentricle anatomy. J Pediatr Nurs. 2013;28(1):64–71.

21. Crapnell T, Rogers C, Neil J, Inder T, Woodward L, Pineda R. Factors associated with feeding difficulties in the very preterm infant. Acta Paediatr. 2013;102(12):e539–45.

22. da Rosa Pereira K, Firpo C, Gasparin M, Teixeira AR, Dornelles S, Bacaltchuk T, Levy DS. Evaluation of swallowing in infants with congenital heart defect. Int Arch Otorhinolaryngol. 2015;19(01):055–60.

23. De Oliveira Lira Ortega A, Ciamponi A, Mendes F, Santos M. Assessment scale of the oral motor performance of children and adolescents with neurological damages. J Oral Rehabil. 2009;36(9):653–9.

24. Eckman N, Williams KE, Riegel K, Paul C. Teaching chewing: a structured approach. Am J Occup Ther. 2008;62(5):514–21.

25. Edwards S, Davis AM, Ernst L, Sitzmann B, Bruce A, Keeler D, et al. Interdisciplinary strategies for treating oral aversions in children. J Parenter Enter Nutr. 2015;39(8):899–909.

26. Einarsson-Backes LM, Deitz J, Price R, Glass R, Hays R. The effect of oral support on sucking efficiency in preterm infants. Am J Occup Ther. 1994;48(6):490–8.

27. Fairhurst C, Cockerill H. Management of drooling in children. Arch Dis Child Educ Pract Ed. 2011;96(1):25–30.

28. Field D, Garland M, Williams K. Correlates of specific childhood feeding problems. J Paediatr Child Health. 2003;39(4):299–304.
29. Flanagan MA. Improving speech and eating skills in children with autism spectrum disorders: an oral-motor program for home and school. Shawnee Mission: AAPC Publishing; 2008.
30. Foster JP, Psaila K, Patterson T. Non-nutritive sucking for increasing physiologic stability and nutrition in preterm infants. Cochrane Database Syst Rev. 2017;(10):CD001071.
31. Fucile S, Gisel E, Lau C. Oral stimulation accelerates the transition from tube to oral feeding in preterm infants. J Pediatr. 2002;141(2):230–6.
32. Fucile S, Gisel E, Lau C. Effect of an oral stimulation program on sucking skill maturation of preterm infants. Dev Med Child Neurol. 2005;47(03):158–62.
33. Fucile S, Gisel E, McFarland DH, Lau C. Oral and non-oral sensorimotor interventions enhance oral feeding performance in preterm infants. Dev Med Child Neurol. 2011;53(9):829–35.
34. Fucile S, McFarland DH, Gisel EG, Lau C. Oral and nonoral sensorimotor interventions facilitate suck–swallow–respiration functions and their coordination in preterm infants. Early Hum Dev. 2012;88(6):345–50.
35. Fung EB, Samson-Fang L, Stallings VA, Conaway M, Liptak G, Henderson RC, et al. Feeding dysfunction is associated with poor growth and health status in children with cerebral palsy. J Am Diet Assoc. 2002;102(3):361–73.
36. Gaebler CP, Hanzlik JR. The effects of a prefeeding stimulation program on preterm infants. Am J Occup Ther. 1996;50(3):184–92.
37. Ganz SF. Decreasing tongue thrusting and tonic bite reflex through nueromotor and sensory facilitation techniques. Phys Occup Ther Pediatr. 1988;7(4):57–76.
38. Gisel EG. Oral-motor skills following sensorimotor intervention in the moderately eating-impaired child with cerebral palsy. Dysphagia. 1994;9(3):180–92.
39. Gisel EG, Patrick J. Identification of children with cerebral palsy unable to maintain a normal nutritional state. Lancet. 1988;331(8580):283–6.
40. Gisel EG, Alphonce E, Ramsay M. Assessment of ingestive and oral praxis skills: children with cerebral palsy vs. controls. Dysphagia. 2000;15(4):236–44.
41. González ML, Stern K. Co-occurring behavioral difficulties in children with severe feeding problems: a descriptive study. Res Dev Disabil. 2016;58:45–54.
42. Gouyon J-B, Iacobelli S, Ferdynus C, Bonsante F. Neonatal problems of late and moderate preterm infants. Semin Fetal Neonatal Med. 2012;17(3):146–52. https://doi.org/10.1016/j.siny.2012.01.015.
43. Greene Z, O'Donnell CP, Walshe M. Oral stimulation for promoting oral feeding in preterm infants. Cochrane Database Syst Rev. 2016;9:CD009720.
44. Harding C, Frank L, Van Someren V, Hilari K, Botting N. How does non-nutritive sucking support infant feeding? Infant Behav Dev. 2014;37(4):457–64.
45. Heckathorn D-E, Speyer R, Taylor J, Cordier R. Systematic review: non-instrumental swallowing and feeding assessments in pediatrics. Dysphagia. 2016;31(1):1–23.
46. Hennequin M, Faulks D, Veyrune JL, Bourdiol P. Significance of oral health in persons with down syndrome: a literature review. Dev Med Child Neurol. 1999;41(4):275–83.
47. Howe T-H, Wang T-N. Systematic review of interventions used in or relevant to occupational therapy for children with feeding difficulties ages birth–5 years. Am J Occup Ther. 2013;67(4):405–12.
48. Howe T-H, Sheu C-F, Hsieh Y-W, Hsieh C-L. Psychometric characteristics of the Neonatal Oral-Motor Assessment Scale in healthy preterm infants. Dev Med Child Neurol. 2007;49(12):915–9.
49. Howe T-H, Lin K-C, Fu C-P, Su C-T, Hsieh C-L. A review of psychometric properties of feeding assessment tools used in neonates. J Obstet Gynecol Neonatal Nurs. 2008;37(3):338–49.
50. Hwang Y-S, Lin C-H, Coster WJ, Bigsby R, Vergara E. Effectiveness of cheek and jaw support to improve feeding performance of preterm infants. Am J Occup Ther. 2010;64(6):886–94.
51. Iammatteo PA, Trombly C, Luecke L. The effect of mouth closure on drooling and speech. Am J Occup Ther. 1990;44(8):686–91.
52. Kamide A, Hashimoto K, Miyamura K, Honda M. Assessment of feeding and swallowing in children: validity and reliability of the Ability for Basic Feeding and Swallowing Scale for Children (ABFS-C). Brain Dev. 2015;37(5):508–14.

53. Ko MJ, Kang MJ, Ko KJ, Ki YO, Chang HJ, Kwon J-Y. Clinical usefulness of Schedule for Oral-Motor Assessment (SOMA) in children with dysphagia. Ann Rehabil Med. 2011;35(4):477–84.
54. Kumin L. Resource guide to oral motor skill difficulties in children with down syndrome. 2015.
55. Kumin L, Von Hagel KC, Bahr D. An effective oral motor intervention protocol for infants and toddlers with low muscle tone. Infant Toddler Intervention. 2001;11(3/4):181–200.
56. Lamm NC, De Felice A, Cargan A. Effect of tactile stimulation on lingual motor function in pediatric lingual dysphagia. Dysphagia. 2005;20(4):311–24. https://doi.org/10.1007/s00455-005-0060-7.
57. Laptook AR. Neurologic and metabolic issues in moderately preterm, late preterm, and early term infants. Clin Perinatol. 2013;40(4):723–38. https://doi.org/10.1016/j.clp.2013.07.005.
58. Laud R, Girolami P, Boscoe J, Gulotta C. Treatment outcomes for severe feeding problems in children with autism spectrum disorder. Behav Modif. 2009;33(5):520–36.
59. Leone A, Ersfeld P, Adams M, Meyer Schiffer P, Bucher HU, Arlettaz R. Neonatal morbidity in singleton late preterm infants compared with full-term infants. Acta Paediatr. 2012;101(1):e6–e10. https://doi.org/10.1111/j.1651-2227.2011.02459.x.
60. Lessen BS. Effect of the premature infant oral motor intervention on feeding progression and length of stay in preterm infants. Adv Neonatal Care. 2011;11(2):129–39.
61. Limbrock GJ, Fischer-Brandies H, Avalle C. Castillo-Morales' orofacial therapy: treatment of 67 children with down syndrome. Dev Med Child Neurol. 1991;33(4):296–303.
62. Lyu T-C, Zhang Y-X, Hu X-J, Cao Y, Ren P, Wang Y-J. The effect of an early oral stimulation program on oral feeding of preterm infants. Int J Nurs Sci. 2014;1(1):42–7.
63. Matthews-Brzozowska T, Cudziło D, Walasz J, Kawala B. Rehabilitation of the orofacial complex by means of a stimulating plate in children with down syndrome. Adv Clin Exp Med. 2015;24(2):301–5.
64. McCain GC. Promotion of preterm infant nipple feeding with nonnutritive sucking. J Pediatr Nurs. 1995;10(1):3–8.
65. Miller CK, Madhoun LL. Feeding and swallowing issues in infants with craniofacial anomalies. Perspect ASHA Spec Interest Groups. 2016;1(5):13–26.
66. Morgan A, Mei C, Anderson V, Waugh M-C, Cahill L, the TBI Guideline Expert Working Committee. Clinical practice guideline for the management of communication and swallowing disorders following paediatric traumatic brain injury. Melbourne: Murdoch Childrens Research Institute; 2017.
67. Osman A, Ahmed E, Mohamed H, Hassanein F, Brandon D. Oral motor intervention accelerates time to full oral feeding and discharge. Int J Adv Nurs Stud. 2016;5(2):228–33.
68. Ottenbacher K, Bundy A, Short MA. The development and treatment of oral-motor dysfunction: a review of clinical research. Phys Occup Ther Pediatr. 1983;3(2):1–13.
69. Ottenbacher K, Dauck BS, Gevelinger M, Grahn V, Hassett C. Reliability of the behavioral assessment scale of oral functions in feeding. Am J Occup Ther. 1985;39(7):436–40.
70. Palmer MM, Crawley K, Blanco IA. Neonatal Oral-Motor Assessment scale: a reliability study. J Perinatol. 1992;13(1):28–35.
71. Pimenta HP, Moreira ME, Rocha AD, Junior G, Clair S, Pinto LW, Lucena SL. Effects of non-nutritive sucking and oral stimulation on breastfeeding rates for preterm, low birth weight infants: a randomized clinical trial. J Pediatr. 2008;84(5):423–7.
72. Pinelli J, Symington A. Non-nutritive sucking for promoting physiologic stability and nutrition in preterm infants. *Evid Based Child Health*. 2011;6:1134–69. https://doi.org/10.1002/ebch.808.
73. Poore M, Zimmerman E, Barlow S, Wang J, Gu F. Patterned orocutaneous therapy improves sucking and oral feeding in preterm infants. Acta Paediatr. 2008;97(7):920–7.
74. Quitadamo P, Thapar N, Staiano A, Borrelli O. Gastrointestinal and nutritional problems in neurologically impaired children. Eur J Paediatr Neurol. 2016;20(6):810–5.
75. Reddihough D. Management of drooling in neurological disabilities: more evidence is needed. Dev Med Child Neurol. 2017;59:454–61.

76. Reid J. A review of feeding interventions for infants with cleft palate. Cleft Palate Craniofac J. 2004;41(3):268–78.
77. Rocha AD, Moreira MEL, Pimenta HP, Ramos JRM, Lucena SL. A randomized study of the efficacy of sensory-motor-oral stimulation and non-nutritive sucking in very low birthweight infant. Early Hum Dev. 2007;83(6):385–8.
78. Rogers B, Arvedson J. Assessment of infant oral sensorimotor and swallowing function. Dev Disabil Res Rev. 2005;11(1):74–82.
79. Rommel N, De Meyer A, Feenstra L, Veereman-Wauters G. The complexity of feeding problems in infants and young children presenting to a tertiary care institution. J Pediatr Gastroenterol Nutr. 2003;37:75–84.
80. Serel Arslan S, Demir N, Karaduman AA. Effect of a new treatment protocol called Functional Chewing Training on chewing function in children with cerebral palsy: a double-blind randomised controlled trial. J Oral Rehabil. 2017;44(1):43–50.
81. Sheppard JJ, Hochman R, Baer C. The dysphagia disorder survey: validation of an assessment for swallowing and feeding function in developmental disability. Res Dev Disabil. 2014;35(5):929–42.
82. Skuse D, Stevenson J, Reilly S, Mathisen B. Schedule for oral-motor assessment (SOMA): methods of validation. Dysphagia. 1995;10(3):192–202.
83. Skuse D, Wolke D, Reilly S. Schedule for oral motor assessment. London: Whurr; 2000.
84. Snider L, Majnemer A, Darsaklis V. Feeding interventions for children with cerebral palsy: a review of the evidence. Phys Occup Ther Pediatr. 2011;31(1):58–77.
85. Sonies BC, Cintas HL, Parks R, Miller J, Caggiano C, Gottshall SG, Gerber L. Brief assessment of motor function: content validity and reliability of the oral motor scales. Am J Phys Med Rehabil. 2009;88(6):464–72.
86. Stratton M. Behaviorial assessment scale of oral functions in feeding. Am J Occup Ther. 1981;35(11):719–21.
87. Tian X, Yi L-J, Zhang L, Zhou J-G, Ma L, Ou Y-X, et al. Oral motor intervention improved the oral feeding in preterm infants: evidence based on a meta-analysis with trial sequential analysis. Medicine. 2015;94(31):e1310. https://doi.org/10.1097/md.0000000000001310.
88. Williams KE, Seiverling L. Assessment and treatment of feeding problems among children with autism spectrum disorders. In: Patel VB, Preedy VR, Martin CR, editors. *Comprehensive guide to autism*. New York: Springer; 2014. p. 1973–93.
89. Wilson EM, Green JR. The development of jaw motion for mastication. Early Hum Dev. 2009;85:303–11.
90. Wolf LS, Glass RP. Feeding and swallowing disorders in infancy: assessment and management. Tucson: Therapy Skill Builders; 1992.
91. Yilmaz S, Basar P, Gisel EG. Assessment of feeding performance in patients with cerebral palsy. Int J Rehabil Res. 2004;27(4):325–9.
92. Younesian S, Yadegari F, Soleimani F. Impact of oral sensory motor stimulation on feeding performance, length of hospital stay, and weight gain of preterm infants in NICU. Iran Red Crescent Med J. 2015;17(7):e13515.

Chapter 11
Adaptive Feeding Techniques and Positioning: An Occupational Therapist's Perspective

Cheryl Mitchell and Stacey L. Paluszak

Introduction

Feeding is a highly complex and multifaceted activity with which many infants and children struggle [1, 2]. Oral-motor development can be affected by multiple factors including medical diagnoses, environment, developmental delay, food sensitivities, and negative oral experiences, to name a few. Infants and children who present with feeding difficulties can be referred to an occupational therapist (OT) or speech-language pathologist (SLP) who specializes in the evaluation and treatment of pediatric feeding disorders. Therapists will gather information using patient/family report and chart reviews to obtain pertinent information in the areas of medical, developmental, and feeding history. Along with clinical observation of feeding and developmental skills, these areas can give insight into the underlying medical, motor, sensory, and/or social causes for feeding difficulties [3]. Based on these findings, a treatment plan will be developed to address specific feeding skills. There are a variety of adaptive feeding techniques and positioning options that will be utilized during treatment sessions to address deficits and improve feeding success.

Although feeding and swallowing difficulties may arise any time along the feeding continuum, these difficulties often occur during the neonatal period when babies are just beginning to develop oral-motor and feeding skills. Initially, many infants are followed in the neonatal intensive care unit (NICU) or soon after discharge from the NICU. Preterm and medically complex infants often struggle with suck-swallow-breathe coordination leading to physiological instability during feeds and an increased risk for aspiration. The acquisition of skills required for successful feeding can be further impeded by medical comorbidities, hospital equipment, environment, poor postural alignment, and poor pulmonary functioning. Feeding issues

C. Mitchell (✉) · S. L. Paluszak
Physical Medicine and Rehabilitation, Texas Children's Hospital,
Houston, TX, USA
e-mail: crmitche@texaschildrens.org; slpalusz@texaschildrens.org

© Springer International Publishing AG, part of Springer Nature 2018
J. Ongkasuwan, E. H. Chiou (eds.), *Pediatric Dysphagia*,
https://doi.org/10.1007/978-3-319-97025-7_11

that go unaddressed may negatively impact the child's ability to transition to age-appropriate stages of feeding. Feeding specialists can provide guidance on managing feeding and swallowing difficulties in the hospital, home environment, or outpatient setting. There are a variety of treatment strategies to address feeding deficits including the use of therapeutic equipment, modified feeding utensils, and positioning techniques.

Adaptive Feeding Techniques

Prefeeding Skills and Taste Trials

Infants may not possess the skills needed to progress to bottle feeds due to neurodevelopmental immaturity, delayed oral-motor development, medical factors, poor state regulation, or poor physiologic stability [4]. Though the infant may not be safe to progress to oral feeding, it is important that they receive treatment to address deficit areas in oral-motor development. This treatment will assist with preparation for progression to oral feeds to reduce the impact on long-term health and nutrition. In these instances, prefeeding treatment options are available. Non-nutritive oral stimulation can be utilized to normalize responses to sensory input and to facilitate oral-motor coordination without the use of food for infants at risk for choking and aspiration. There are many commercially available tools for use in non-nutritive therapy. A feeding therapist can help guide patients and their families on appropriate selection and use of therapeutic oral-motor tools.

Once an infant demonstrates improved non-nutritive skills, but is not quite ready for advancement to a bottle, treatment can be progressed to include therapeutic taste trials. Although only offering minimal volumes, this may require the approval of a physician. Active sucking on a pacifier has been shown to improve feeding outcomes [5, 6]. Taste trials pair small, controlled tastes of expressed breast milk (EBM) or formula with active sucking on the pacifier. A binky trainer (Fig. 11.1) is one option for providing taste trials. It can be constructed by a therapist using a standard pacifier, a feeding tube, and a syringe, which are typically available in a hospital or clinic setting. An alternative to the binky trainer is the MediPop® (Fig. 11.2a and b), which is a pacifier molded to include a channel through which liquid can be directed. Both options allow the therapist to provide controlled tastes; however, there are aspects of each to consider. When deciding which tool to use, the therapist will consider availability of supplies, tolerance to the equipment, cost, and cleaning. The MediPop® is premade and shaped like a typical newborn pacifier, so no construction or modification by the therapist is required. Children with oral sensitivities sometimes have difficulty tolerating the binky trainer due to the feeding tube sticking out of the tip of the pacifier; however, the MediPop® is a single mold design with an internal channel which may be more easily tolerated. Whichever system is utilized, care should be taken to ensure the equipment is adequately cleaned between uses to prevent bacterial growth. If the patient is in the hospital

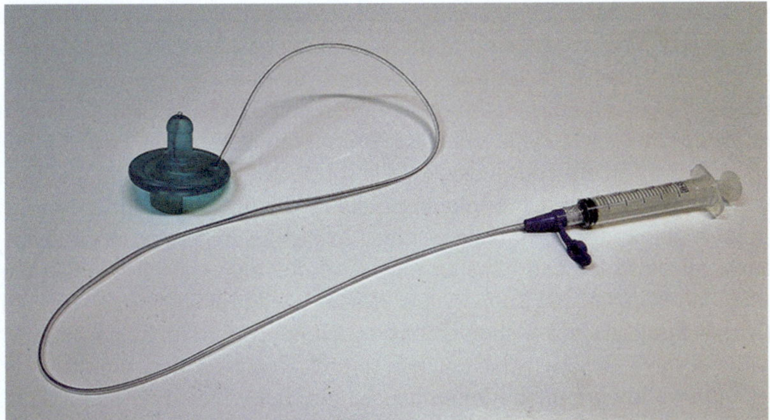

Fig. 11.1 A binky trainer constructed from a modified pacifier, small feeding tube, and syringe to provide small, controlled tastes

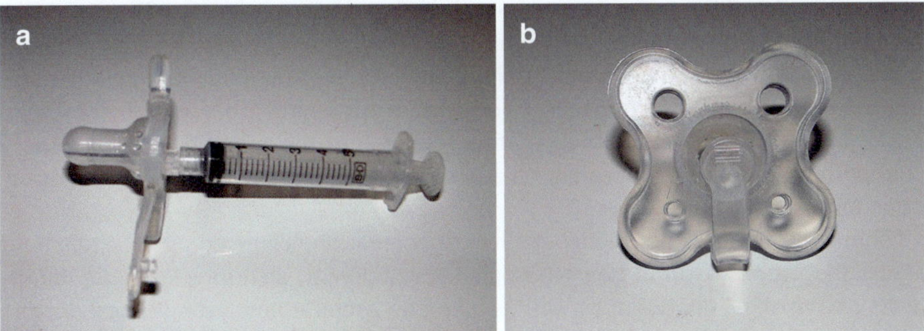

Fig. 11.2 (**a**) The valve on the MediPop® System can be opened, allowing a syringe to be attached for therapeutic tastes. (**b**) Once taste trials have been completed, the valve on the MediPop® can be closed. It can now be used as a pacifier without air intake

setting, the therapist will need to follow hospital guidelines for cleaning. Many hospitals require disposal of the feeding tube after each use, requiring a new tube every 24 h which can lead to increased costs. Both the binky trainer and the MediPop® can help facilitate control of bolus and coordination of swallow, thus improving feeding outcomes [7].

Bottle Feeding

Once the infant is demonstrating appropriate oral-motor control and managing an increase in bolus size, they can be progressed to bottle feeding. The length of time required to transition from taste trials to bottle feeding will vary depending upon the skills of the infant. Some infants may be able to transition quickly, within a session or two, while others may require multiple sessions before demonstrating readiness to advance. Once bottle feeding is introduced, there are several modifications or adaptive feeding techniques that may be implemented to address oral-motor limitations or incoordination. Nipple selection is a major consideration when addressing sucking and swallowing coordination. When selecting a nipple, the therapist will consider the attributes of the nipple, viscosity of the fluid, as well as the skills and coordination of the infant [8]. Nipples come in various materials, sizes, shapes, and flow rates, all of which can have an impact on feeding success. Due to the FDA recommendations from 2011 concerning risks related to thickening agents [9] (specifically that Simply Thick® should not be used in preterm infants or infants under 12 months of age), therapists have begun to look to slower flow nipples to address feeding and swallowing incoordination as an alternative to commercial thickeners. Several studies have looked at flow rates of both hospital-based and commercial nipples [10–12]. These studies suggest that there is a high level of variability between flow rates among disposable and commercial nipples. Variability between the same nipple type was also found which was thought to be due to the manufacturing process. In addition, commercial nipples advertised as "slow flow" have a large range of flow rates, from 5.6 to 46.3 mL/min. Although there were slightly different findings in flow rates, the results remain beneficial in guiding the therapist in making recommendations to transition the infant from hospital-based to home-based nipples. It is important to note that while selection of the appropriate bottle nipple is important, ultimately, coordination and safety will be closely monitored to determine tolerance to flow rate [13].

Nipple selection is not a one size fits all adaptation. The feeding specialist will assess the infant's overall neuromuscular development, anatomy, strength, endurance, and medical condition as well as take into account how each of these factors contribute to overall feeding expectations and needs. Considered together, these provide a baseline for determining proper nipple selection or need for use of a specialty bottle (Fig. 11.3). In the past, it was thought that fast flow was better as it helped to prevent feeding fatigue in preterm and medically complex patients. Now research has provided insight that faster flow rates can cause increased difficulty coordinating swallowing and breathing in infants who have baseline increased work of breathing or tachypnea, such as preterm infants or those with cardiac issues [14, 15]. In the end, it is the clinical presentation of the infant during both feeding assessment and treatment that will guide use of the appropriate equipment. This will enable the therapist to provide a safe and positive feeding experience that focuses on quality versus quantity of intake.

In addition to nipple selection, there are other adaptive feeding techniques to address decreased sucking and swallowing coordination. External pacing is a technique in which breaks are imposed after a certain number of sucks. This technique is utilized to address suck-swallow-breathe incoordination which may lead to apnea. Feeding induced apnea is more common in preterm infants; however, it can happen in term or older infants as well [16]. External pacing is achieved by lowering the

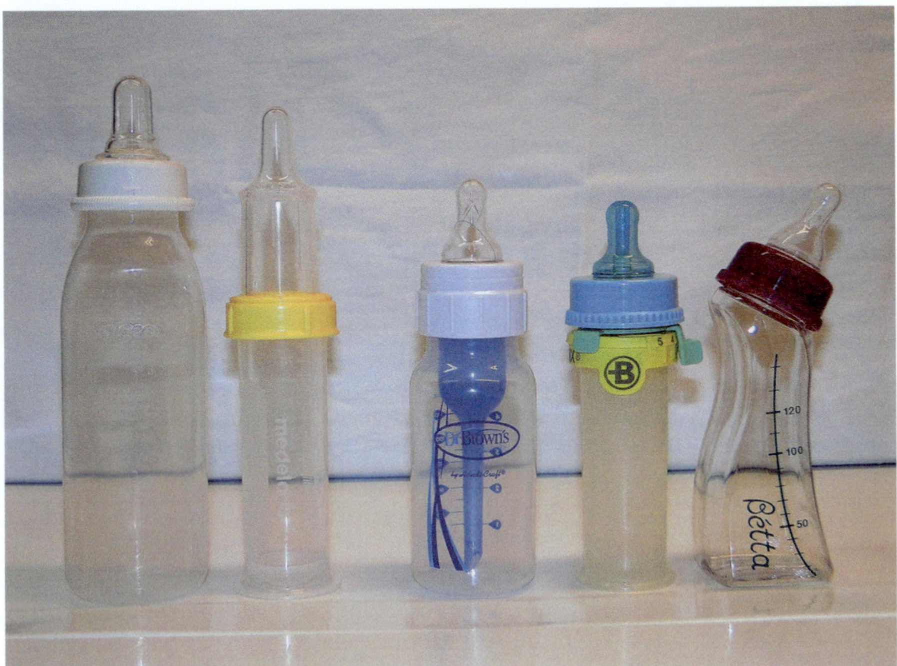

Fig. 11.3 Specialty bottles commonly used by therapists. From left to right: Pigeon bottle, Medela Special Needs Feeder (aka Haberman bottle), Dr. Brown's® Specialty Feeding System, Bionix Controlled Flow® Baby Feeder, and Betta Bottle

bottle to remove milk from the nipple or removing the nipple from the mouth entirely. The method, amount, and rate of pacing are varied depending upon the infant's tolerance and feeding cues. Over time, with maturity and practice, the infant should begin to self-pace independently, demonstrating improved suck-swallow-breathe coordination.

Thickening Feeds in Infancy

Altering the consistency of the liquid through thickening is another adaptive technique to consider when addressing infant dysphagia. Thickening should only be considered as a last resort after nipple flow rate, positioning, and pacing have been shown to be ineffective in preventing aspiration. It should only be utilized following instrumental evaluation of the swallow (VFSS or FES) per SLPs recommendations. For safest feeding practices, the consistency of the fluid as well as the choice of nipple to be used with the thickened liquid should be determined during the instrumental evaluation. No modifications in the nipple or consistency should be made without the guidance of a feeding specialist.

Cup Drinking

As the young infant progresses into late infancy, feeding therapists will assess readiness to transition from bottle feeds. When it is time to move from a bottle to a more mature drinking utensil, there are many commercially available cups that combine the therapeutic attributes with the convenient characteristics of the traditional sippy cups. When learning to drink from a cup, children often use neck extension to allow them to tip the cup to receive fluid. Cut-out cups, also known as nosey cups (Fig. 11.4), can be utilized to allow the child to maintain head and neck alignment from neutral to slightly flexed with cup drinking to improve the safety of the swallow. Nowadays, there are many sippy cup options that are available for purchase in stores which support maturation of oral-motor skills and allow a child to access the fluid with less assistance. There are also specialty cups which help to modify drinking requirements or allow the caregiver to assist more easily. Some cups are designed to assist with the flow of fluid in a more streamlined pattern toward midline which reduces the loss of fluid around the mouth. A squeeze bottle (Fig. 11.5) is a straw device that enables the caregiver to assist with priming the straw and modify for pressure changes required for straw drinking. It is very important to be under the care of a feeding specialist when children are using the squeeze bottle to ensure that families understand the risks associated with its use and are able to be educated in safe feeding techniques. A straw that only allows the fluid to travel in one direction would be beneficial to someone who had difficulty initiating and maintaining the intraoral pressure required for successful straw drinking. As with bottle feeding, the fluids offered with these cups can be modified by thickening the fluid to improve safety of swallow and allow improved bolus management.

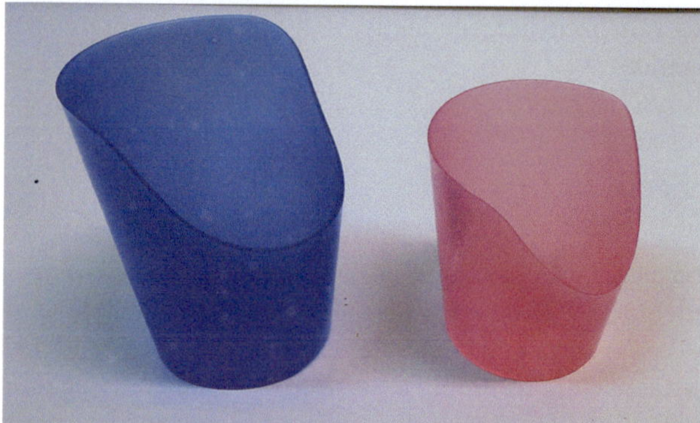

Fig. 11.4 Cut-out cups, also known as nosey cups, come in large and small sizes

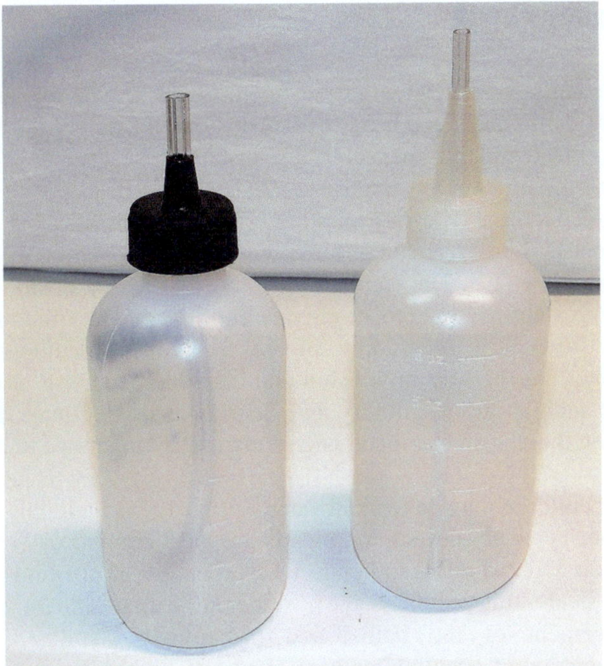

Fig. 11.5 Squeeze bottles adapted with tubing to address straw drinking

Use of Spoons

There is a wide assortment of spoons available to meet a variety of therapeutic needs and skill levels. When transitioning to purees, the choice of spoon can support the development of oral skills and feeding success. Spoons come in many sizes and shapes. It is important that the attributes of the spoon match with the skill level of a child. For example, for a child that has difficulty manipulating a bolus, a smaller-sized spoon will ensure a more manageable size bite with which to practice their skills. A feeding therapist may educate parents on specific spoon placement techniques to facilitate tongue and lip movements which would be achieved more easily with a smaller spoon. For children with decreased lip closure, a spoon with a shallower bowl would allow them to clear the bolus from the spoon more independently due to the decreased range of motion required to close their lips around the spoon. There are specialized spoons available as well. The Beckman E-Z spoon is a small flat spoon that can be used to easily place the bolus in the cheek. The maroon spoon is a specialty spoon that has a shallower bowl which will facilitate lip closure, address oral hypersensitivity, and decrease tongue thrust.

Positioning for Feeds

"A child's efficient use of the mouth for eating depends heavily on the steadiness or stability of the trunk, neck, and head" [17]. The effectiveness of the adaptive feeding techniques discussed thus far will be diminished in the absence of optimal positioning. Research supports the importance of a child's head position to improve swallowing and decrease risk for aspiration [18]. Proper positioning provides adequate alignment and postural support, allowing for improved coordination of the tongue, lips, and jaw [17]. The feeding therapist will provide positioning that provides symmetry, stability, and proper alignment of the pelvis, trunk, head, and jaw [19]. While positioning is important to support the skills of feeding, it is important to keep in mind that the way in which a child is positioned will also affect other body systems such as the respiratory and gastrointestinal systems. If positioning causes stress on these systems, it can negatively impact tolerance to and interest in feeding.

Infants and children may be fed in a variety of positions including upright, side-lying, or prone. Typically developing infants are most commonly bottle fed in the cradled position and can adapt to being fed in a variety of positions. However, in preterm or medically fragile infants, the position of the infant can impact respiratory effort, management of the bolus, and physiologic stability [20–22]. The semi-elevated sidelying position has been shown to be beneficial to address with oral-motor incoordination by allowing a slower feeding pace with improved bolus management for safe and effective swallowing, contributing to improved physiologic stability throughout the feed [23]. This study also found that infants were able to participate in feedings for longer periods in semi-elevated sidelying versus semi-elevated supine, suggesting that it is more supportive of the infant's motor and state development. Sidelying allows for decreased transit time by directing the fluid to the side of the mouth instead of directing it toward the airway, allowing increased time to manage the bolus. Prone positioning is another alternative and can assist with forward movement of the tongue and jaw in children with micrognathia, retracted tongue, oral hypertonicity, and certain craniofacial anomalies such as Pierre Robin. Gravity-assisted tongue protrusion and forward jaw excursion can ease bolus expression and management as well as clearing the airway for safe swallowing.

When working with a child, it is important to address positioning so that the child is able to attend to and learn from feeding-related tasks. If the child feels that he is adequately supported and not having to focus on balance and alignment, they are able to attend to stimulation and allow him to focus on the oral-motor skill being addressed.

The position of the infant or child greatly impacts proximal stability which is an important foundation for feeding. Positioning influences the effects of gravity on oral-motor movements as well as fluid flow rate. During a feeding evaluation, the therapist will assess overall alignment of the pelvis, trunk, neck, and head as well as positioning of upper and lower extremities to determine appropriate modifications to support proper alignment. The general position that is typically described for feeding a toddler or older child is in upright orientation with neutral alignment of the head and neck with slight neck flexion, along with hips, knees, and ankles each positioned at 90° of flexion with feet supported. However, positioning should be modified based on individual need. If postural control is compromised, equipment can be used to adjust alignment and provide stability which allows the child to focus his energy on oral-motor tasks. If the child feels that he is adequately supported and not having to focus on balance and alignment, he is able to attend to stimulation, and allow him to focus on the oral-motor skill being addressed.

A variety of seating devices can be utilized based upon the child's individual needs. A child who is more posturally challenged or who will have long-term positioning needs may benefit from specialty seating equipment which may include use of the child's custom wheelchair, a tumble form chair, or a Rifton Activity Chair. Some seating systems can be custom fit to provide varying degrees of support and will grow with the child. Commercially available high chairs and booster seats can also be used for support during feeding. These systems provide less postural support but can be modified with towel rolls or other external supports. Specialty seating is often ideal; however, this equipment can be very expensive and unobtainable for many families. There may also be a significant waiting period for custom equipment. In this instance, commercially available seating equipment may be more accessible.

Importance of Positioning the Neurologically Involved Patient

All children with feeding deficits will benefit from assessment of feeding posture. While a neurotypical child may be able to adapt to suboptimal positioning, this can compromise oral skills in the child with neurological impairments. "The normal child may readily compensate for misalignment during feeding. However, for the child with neurodisability any variation from the ideal head and trunk alignment may result in oral processing difficulties that will compromise eating and swallowing" [19]. This population typically requires custom equipment to address their positioning needs as appropriate alignment of the head, trunk, hips, and lower extremities is more challenging. Research has demonstrated that providing effective adaptive seating in this population, particularly custom-fit seating systems, promotes proper stabilization and improves functional feeding outcomes [24].

Positioning for Reflux

Children with gastroesophageal reflux (GER) may also benefit from specific positioning techniques as a non-pharmacological approach to reflux management. Infants and children with reflux often present clinically as disorganized feeders.

This presentation can be the result of the inability to engage in feeding due to discomfort caused by esophagitis. Studies have shown that reflux is frequently identified as the underlying medical condition in patients with feeding problems [25]. Over time, if left untreated, this may lead to further delays in oral-motor development due to feeding refusal and negative feeding experiences [26, 27]. Clinical signs and symptoms of reflux often present during feeds but can also present between feeds; therefore, it is important that positioning recommendations are followed throughout the day. Children with reflux often demonstrate decreased clinical signs and symptoms of reflux with use of upright positioning during and after feeds resulting in increased comfort level. Following feeds, this can be achieved by physically holding the patient upright or by using a positioning device which supports the child in an upright position, preferably with minimal hip flexion. Devices that position with increased hip flexion may increase abdominal pressure exacerbating reflux symptoms. There are also positioning devices, such as reflux wedges, that can be used for positioning patients on an incline following feeds and while sleeping to assist with reflux management.

Conclusion

When an infant or child is noted to have any concerns related to feeding development, it is very important that they are referred to a feeding specialist in a timely manner [28]. Delayed referral and initiation of therapy can negatively impact feeding development and outcomes. The efficiency of treatment will be diminished, and length of ongoing treatment will likely be extended. A feeding therapist can provide ongoing guidance regarding developmentally appropriate, individualized adaptive feeding techniques and positioning devices which, together with hands on therapy, can improve feeding outcomes.

References

1. Udall JN. Infant feeding: initiation, problems, approaches. Curr Probl Pediatr Adolesc Health Care. 2007;37(10):374–99.
2. Sullivan PB, Lambert B, Rose M, Ford-Adams M, Johnson A, Griffiths P. Prevalence and severity of feeding and nutritional problems in children with neurological impairment: Oxford Feeding Study. Dev Med Child Neurol. 2000;42(10):674–80.
3. Arvedson JC. Assessment of pediatric dysphagia and feeding disorders: clinical and instrumental approaches. Dev Disabil Res Rev. 2008;14:118–27.
4. Kish MZ. Oral feeding readiness in preterm infants: a concept analysis. Adv Neonatal Care [Internet]. 2013;13(4):230–7. Available from: http://www.ncbi.nlm.nih.gov/pubmed/23912014
5. Asadollahpour F, Yadegari F, Soleimani F, Khalesi N. The effects of non-nutritive sucking and pre-feeding oral stimulation on time to achieve independent oral feeding for preterm infants. Iran J Pediatr. 2015;25(3):e809.

 6. Rocha AD, Moreira MEL, Pimenta HP, Ramos JRM, Lucena SL. A randomized study of the efficacy of sensory-motor-oral stimulation and non-nutritive sucking in very low birthweight infant. Early Hum Dev. 2007;83(6):385.
 7. Bridwell M, Grimshaw J. The effects of a slow and controlled feeding protocol for the introduction of oral feeding for infants. Am J Occup Ther [Internet]. 2015 Jul 1 [cited 2017 Jul 31];69(Suppl. 1):6911515162p1. Available from: http://ajot.aota.org/article.aspx?doi=10.5014/ajot.2015.69S1-PO4094
 8. Ross E, Fuhrman L. Supporting oral feeding skills through bottle selection. Perspect Swallowing Swallowing Disord. 2015;24(April):50–7.
 9. Office of the Commissioner. Consumer updates – FDA expands caution about SimplyThick. [cited 2017 Aug 1]. Available from: https://www.fda.gov/ForConsumers/ConsumerUpdates/ucm256250.htm
10. Pados BF, Park J, Thoyre SM, Estrem H, Nix WB. Milk flow rates from bottle nipples used for feeding infants who are hospitalized. Am J Speech Lang Pathol. 2015;24(4):671–9.
11. Jackman KT. Go with the flow: choosing a feeding system for infants in the neonatal intensive care unit and beyond based on flow performance. Newborn Infant Nurs Rev. 2013;13(1):31–4.
12. Damian LA, Johnson K. Dr. Brown's Medical » Nipple flow rates: what are they really and how does this affect our clinical practice? [Internet]. [cited 2017 Jul 30]. Available from: https://www.drbrownsbaby.com/medical/clinical-evidence/nipple-flow-rates-what-are-they-really-and-how-does-this-affect-our-clinical-practice/
13. Scheel CE, Schanler RJ, Lau C. Does the choice of bottle nipple affect the oral feeding performance of very-low-birthweight (VLBW) infants? Acta Paediatr [Internet]. 2005;94(9):1266–72. Available from: http://www.ncbi.nlm.nih.gov/pubmed/16203676; http://www.pubmedcentral.nih.gov/articlerender.fcgi?artid=PMC2386985
14. Shaker C. Problem-solving cardiac babies: slow flow vs standard nipple? – Shaker 4 Swallowing and Feeding [Internet]. [cited 2017 Jul 30]. Available from: https://shaker4swallowingandfeeding.com/2016/09/02/problem-solving-cardiac-babies-slow-flow-vs-standard-nipple/
15. Chang Y-J, Lin C-P, Lin Y-J, Lin C-H. Effects of single-hole and cross-cut nipple units on feeding efficiency and physiological parameters in premature infants. J Nurs Res. 2007;15(3):215–23.
16. Wolf LS, Glass RP. Feeding and swallowing disorders in infancy. San Antonio: Therapy Skill Builders; 1992.
17. Morris SE, Klein MD. Pre-feeding skills. 2nd ed. Austin: pro-ed; 2000. 297 p
18. Larnert G, Ekberg O. Positioning improves the oral and pharyngeal swallowing function in children with cerebral palsy. Acta Paediatr. 1995;84(6):689–92.
19. Redstone F, West JF. The importance of postural control for feeding. Pediatr Nurs [Internet]. 2004;30(2):97–100. Available from: http://www.ncbi.nlm.nih.gov/pubmed/15185730
20. Clark L, Kennedy G, Pring T. Improving bottle feeding in preterm infants: investigating the elevated side-lying position. Infant [Internet]. 2007;3(4):154–8. Available from: http://www.infantgrapevine.co.uk/pdf/inf_016_ife.pdf
21. McFarland DH, Lund JP, Gagner M. Effects of posture on the coordination of respiration and swallowing. J Neurophysiol. 1994;72(5):2431–7.
22. Mizuno K, Inoue M, Takeuchi T. The effects of body positioning on sucking behaviour in sick neonates. Eur J Pediatr [Internet]. 2000;159(11):827–31. Available from: http://www.ncbi.nlm.nih.gov/pubmed/11079195
23. Park J, Thoyre S, Knafl GJ, Hodges EA, Nix WB. Efficacy of semielevated side-lying positioning during bottle-feeding of very preterm infants: a pilot study. J Perinat Neonatal Nurs. 2014;28(1):69–79.
24. Hulme JB, Shaver J, Acher S, Mullette L, Eggert C. Effects of adaptive seating devices on the eating and drinking of children with multiple handicaps. Am J Occup Ther. 1987;41(2):81–9.
25. Rommel N, De Meyer A-M, Feenstra L, Veereman-Wauters G. The complexity of feeding problems in 700 infants and young children presenting to a tertiary care institution. J Pediatr Gastroenterol Nutr. 2003;37(1):75–84.

                                                    C. Mitchell and S. L. Paluszak

26. Hyman PE. Gastroesophageal reflux: one reason why baby won't eat. J Pediatr. 1994;125(6 Part 2):S103.
27. Field D, Garland M, Williams K. Correlates of specific childhood feeding problems. J Paediatr Child Health. 2003;39(4):299–304.
28. Manno C, Fox C, Eicher P, Kerwin M. Early oral-motor interventions for pediatric feeding problems: what, when and how. J Early Intensive Behav Interv [Internet]. 2005;2(3):45–159. Available from: http://psycnet.apa.org/journals/eib/2/3/145/

Chapter 12
Treatment for Dysphagia: A Speech Language Pathologist's Perspective

Laura Brooks

Management of pediatric dysphagia is extremely complex and often requires a multidisciplinary approach. Children with dysphagia are at increased risk for developing respiratory compromise, failure to thrive, feeding refusal, and stressful interactions with their caregivers [1]. Etiologies of dysphagia may evolve from five broad diagnostic categories:

Neurologic (i.e., prematurity, central nervous system conditions)
Respiratory and other conditions impacting suck-swallow-breathe coordination (i.e., respiratory syncytial virus, bronchopulmonary dysplasia, cardiac disease)
Gastrointestinal (i.e., reflux)
Anatomic abnormalities of the aerodigestive tract (i.e., craniofacial abnormalities, vocal fold hypomobility, laryngeal cleft)
Other or unknown [1–4]

When planning treatment for an individual with dysphagia, it is critical to understand the medical history as it impacts feeding. The treatment strategies must target the etiology of the impairment as well as the symptoms that are associated with the dysphagia diagnosis/etiology. The therapist must ask: Why do these impairments exist? What is my rationale for therapy? What impact does the underlying disease have? What is developmentally appropriate for this child?

The primary goals of feeding and swallowing intervention for children are:

- Treat the impairment or cause of aspiration or laryngeal penetration.
- Minimize the risk of pulmonary complications.
- Prevent future feeding issues by maximizing positive experiences.
- Help promote the safest and least restrictive diet with adequate nutrition and hydration.
- Empower caregivers to carryover strategies.

L. Brooks
Department of Rehabilitation, Children's Healthcare of Atlanta, Atlanta, GA, USA

© Springer International Publishing AG, part of Springer Nature 2018
J. Ongkasuwan, E. H. Chiou (eds.), *Pediatric Dysphagia*,
https://doi.org/10.1007/978-3-319-97025-7_12

- Attain age-appropriate eating skills in the most normal or functional manner possible.
- Maximize quality of life [1, 5, 6].

In medicine, a physician prescribes medication to *reduce* adverse events, as the risk can rarely, if ever, be eliminated. Similarly, for patients with dysphagia, the clinician implements evidence-based strategies to *reduce* the risk of complications from dysphagia, preserve pulmonary integrity, and identify the method of intervention which is least likely to cause an adverse event (i.e., aspiration or pneumonia) [7]. Although the impact of recurrent aspiration on the developing airways is not clear, it is believed that some adult lung diseases originate from childhood lung disorders such as pneumonia [8–12]. Therefore it is critical that we intervene to reduce potential complications.

The following sections will first review common treatment questions/controversies specific to three different age groups and then address other issues applicable to all ages.

Treatment Strategies for Infants

Cue-Based Feeding Versus Volume-Driven Feeding

Oral feeding is considered the most complex sensorimotor task the infant performs [13]. Clinicians and caregivers may experience pressure from physicians to reach a target volume in order to maintain oral feeds, which at times can compromise the quality of the feed. Volume is an important goal and measure of feeding ability, and volume goals are often necessary for the infant to discharge from a hospital without an enteral feeding tube. However volume is a by-product of a "quality feeding" where there is physiologic stability, good state regulation, and endurance. Facilitating cue-based feeding during which the infant guides the caregiver helps establish ongoing communication as the infant's feeding needs change [14, 15]. Long-term feeding problems can be a consequence of neonatal conditions, with over 50% of parents reporting feeding difficulties 6 months after NICU discharge and almost half at 12 months [16]. These numbers emphasize the need to support parent-infant communication from the start.

Suck/swallow/breathe sequence is the ideal rhythm for bottle feeding [17]. In addition to premature infants, infants with CLD, cardiac anomalies, injury to the CNS, and some healthy term infants can have delays in this maturation process [10, 18]. Pacing is an intervention that can be implemented by the clinician if the infant demonstrates three to five sucks without taking a breath. The goal of pacing is to *prevent* a stressful situation (as opposed to responding after the fact), as lack of breathing while feeding, or apneic swallows, can lower blood oxygen concentration and cause hypoxia [14, 19]. Pacing has been shown to decrease bradycardic episodes, shorten NICU length of stay, improve sucking efficiency, promote more mature feeding behaviors, and thus prepare the family for success at discharge [20]. Similar to pacing is a co-regulated, dynamic approach where the infant guides the caregiver as to the timing, frequency, and length of the pause rather than the caregiver offering a break every set number of swallows [15, 19].

How Does the Clinician Know if an Infant Is Ready to Feed?

Taking a moment to monitor the infant prior to a feed can give valuable information about the readiness for oral intake. The clinician can make adjustments to help the baby become more engaged and supported such as reducing distractions, adjusting lighting, and swaddling. It is important to look at the following parameters before the feeding and note if any changes occur during or after a feed:

- Color
- State (alert, drowsy)
- Respiratory rate counted over 60 s
- Vocal quality (weak cry, stridor)
- Oxygen requirements
- Tolerance of tube feeding
- Secretion management
- Work of breathing
- Heart rate
- Oxygen saturation

What Position Is Best for Feeding?

Many studies have supported elevated sidelying as a position for feeding, as it promotes improved oxygen saturations, decreased heart rate and respiratory rate changes, briefer apneic events, and reduced work of breathing [21, 22]. In addition, the oral transit time of milk from the oral cavity, through the pharynx, to the esophagus is influenced by gravity, and the sidelying position may allow for more time to manage the flow more efficiently, possibly allowing infants with higher respiratory rates more opportunity for breaths [19]. If the infant extracts too much milk from the nipple, they can spill the milk anteriorly in the sidelying position more easily than if positioned upright or cradled.

In contrast, other studies reported minimal differences between sidelying and cradle position in terms of maintaining physiologic stability and reaching full oral feeds [23, 24]. The feeder should be cautious when feeding the infant in cradle position as apnea and bradycardia can occur in premature infants when positioned with the neck in flexed position, i.e., chin tuck position [25]. Babies with nasal regurgitation may benefit from positioning near upright to reduce material entering the nasopharynx [26].

Modifying the infant's position is an effective strategy to achieve immediate improvement in an infant's feeding ability. Clinically, adjusting an infant from cradle to elevated sidelying seems to have the greatest impact, and the safety of this position can be confirmed in an instrumental swallow study.

Which Position Is Best After the Feeding? Is Upright All Wrong?

Studies have shown that most acid reflux events occur in the supine position [27]. "Right sidelying" has been suggested to facilitate gastric emptying and "left sidelying" or "prone" reduces reflux [27, 28]. One study suggested the right sidelying position for the first hour after feeds with a position change to the left thereafter to promote gastric emptying and reduce reflux [29]. Prone position is considered a good option for infants with reflux or digestive problems [27, 28]. However the American Academy of Pediatrics (AAP) recommends that infants sleep exclusively on their back for the first 6–12 months of life [30] so the family may be receiving contradictory recommendations from their providers. It has also been reported that 30° incline did not influence reflux events [27] although this continues to be used as a strategy to reduce reflux events. Some believe that positioning upright allows gravity to assist in reducing reflux events; however, this position could actually increase intra-abdominal pressure and reflux [27].

Given these findings in the setting of the conflicting AAP recommendations, the caregiver should discuss the options with the infant's medical team to determine the safest position for his/her baby.

Bottles/Nipples: Is There Such a Thing as a "Right" One for Each Baby?

Given the variety of nipple sizes, shapes, and flow rates, parents try to search for the "best" bottle for their baby. This effort can be futile and expensive. One of the most important parameter to consider is flow rate.

Does a Baby Have to Work Harder to Get the Milk Out of a Slow-Flow Nipple?

A caregiver might offer a faster-flow nipple to "help" the infant finish the bottle, but this larger bolus delivery could result in misdirection of the milk into the airway and/or physiologic instability [15]. Infants fed with a slower-flow nipple have been shown to consume larger volumes, demonstrate shorter feeding times, and demonstrate better sucking efficiency [31]. Interestingly, Chang's study found that infants fed with a crosscut nipple (fast flow) had significantly higher respiratory rates *with higher* SpO_2 (oxygen saturations) during the feeding than infants fed with a slower-flow nipple, although SpO_2 was still within a safe range, >94% [31].

It is also important to note that there is often no consistency across brands as to "slow flow," "medium flow," and "fast flow"; additionally there may be inconsistencies within a single brand.

Chin/Cheek Support: Is It Really Supportive?

Chin and cheek support may be used with caution for the appropriate infant. For inefficient feeders, one study showed that application of oral support (chin or cheek) decreased leakage and increased rate of intake without increasing additional physiological distress [32]. But before implementing this support, the feeder should compare the baby's pacifier suck to the bottle suck. A baby with strong suction on the pacifier and weak suction with the bottle may be self-limiting, which is an appropriate response to inappropriate demands (i.e., too much flow). In such case, increasing the flow is counterproductive.

Eliciting a Nutritive Suck Versus Over-prodding

There are gentle stimulation techniques to promote initiation of a nutritive suck for the patient who is awake and alert but not orienting to the nipple, such as triggering a rooting reflex, tilting the bottle down so the nipple touches the palate, or gently twisting the bottle. The feeder should be mindful of the difference between gentle re-engagement versus prodding when a baby is communicating that he/she is not ready to feed. If milk flow is introduced passively, it can lead to adverse reactions like choking and/or physiologic instability [15].

Oral Stimulation, Non-nutritive Suck (NNS), and Oromotor Exercises for Infants: Which Intervention Is Actually Beneficial?

NNS intervention (pacifier dry or dipped in milk) is generally considered a positive pre-feeding intervention, with some studies showing a decrease in hospitalization length of stay, quicker transition from tube to bottle feeds, and better bottle feeding performance [33]. However, there is less consensus on the benefits of oral exercises and stimulation techniques in infants such as strength building and stroking. One study did find that the combination of NNS (pacifier) + OS (stroking the cheeks, lips, gums, and tongue) intervention reduced the transition time from introduction to independent oral feeding and enhanced the milk transfer rate [34]. However, another study showed that 9 out of 16 infants experienced instability including "mild apnea/bradycardia episodes" during oral motor intervention which included techniques such as stroking [35]. Although the infants "self-corrected" after pausing the intervention, the feeder needs to be thoughtful about whether a task should be performed which results in any instability.

Should an Infant with Baseline Tachypnea Still Feed Orally?

Some babies with certain medical diagnoses such as cardiac anomalies have baseline tachypnea, which is the infant's "norm." Others may have transient tachypnea post intubation as the child weans from oxygen support. Given the close temporal relation between the respiratory cycle and swallow apnea during oral feeding, successful coordination can be difficult for some infants [36]. Infants commonly swallow as often as 60 times a minute during feeding, and suck-swallow-breathe coordination is the ideal pattern. Thus, if an infant needs to breathe much more than 60 times a minute, feeding may result in misdirection of milk flow [37]. Therefore, infants with tachypnea associated with cardiac anomalies or upper respiratory infections can have difficulty with oral feeds. Therefore parameters can be placed on feeding recommendations such as "only feed if respiratory rate is less than 70."

One solution may be to offer only small therapeutic trials which can give the patient some pleasure and exposure while supporting the priority need which is to maintain respiratory stability and successfully wean from supplemental oxygen. Caregivers may be tempted to increase oxygen for a feed; however oxygen is a drug [38] and the goal should be weaning from oxygen rather than increasing it for difficult tasks.

Treatment Strategies for the Toddler and Younger Child

Presentations of feeding/swallowing disorders are variable for toddlers, such as a new-onset dysphagia as a result of an acute medical diagnosis, change in status of underlying medical condition, or unresolved dysphagia from infancy.

One of the challenges with this age group is that some children may require behaviorally based interventions to treat feeding refusal secondary to learned aversions, even after the underlying conditions have been corrected [1]. Even more challenging can be the population of children with limited food repertoire or presence of dysphagia with aspiration without a known medical etiology despite thorough workup (i.e., MRI, microlaryngoscopy with bronchoscopy) [39].

Swallowing therapy for children can involve alteration of temperature, bolus size, consistency, and feeding equipment [5, 40] as these changes can impact swallowing physiology [6, 41].

Basic treatment principles of sensorimotor therapy:

1. Therapeutic strategies should be selected to address the specific neuromuscular impairments clinically judged to be interfering with function.
2. Optimum postural alignment and postural control are essential (i.e., upright 90° hip, knee, and ankle flexion, head in neutral position, or chin tuck).
3. Therapy strategies should be applied just prior to or during the performance of a target task, i.e., "specificity of training."
4. Train according to the developmental skill sequence in which they are typically acquired.
5. As the patient advances, task demands should be increased and facilitation strategies reduced [42, 43].

Intensive Feeding Programs Versus Forced Feeding?

Forced feeding seldom leads to feeding success. Complications are more apt to follow (e.g., food refusal, failure to thrive, and/or other more maladaptive behavior) [5]. However, there are sensory-behavioral feeding programs, which target improved oral intake by gradually working with the child's acceptance and empowering them to allow or reject progression of food offerings. Positive reinforcement and escape extinction are two commonly used interventions to treat behavioral-based feeding problems, although escape extinction has been criticized for possible undesirable side effects, including initial increases in problem behavior, aggression, and emotional responses [44]. Shaping, modeling, and prompting are also strategies that may improve oral intake [5].

How Can the Clinician Wean Toddlers Off Thickened Liquids on Which They Were Placed as an Infant?

Clinicians should strive to recommend the least thickened liquids required for safe swallowing and actively work toward return to unthickened liquids [45]. For the toddler on a prolonged thickened liquid diet, common sense suggests that a gradual approach to weaning is best rather than jumping from honey-thick to nectar-thick liquids to allow for training pharyngeal and laryngeal neuromusculature coordination. Signs and symptoms of aspiration are the best predictors of success, and the medical team must closely monitor coughing, congestion, and worsening respiratory status [39].

Are Oromotor Exercises Helpful?

Choosing evidence-based oral motor techniques to improve swallowing activity can be difficult for clinicians given the challenges in understanding how neuromuscular dysfunctions affect movement and how motor-based treatments influence underlying impairments [42]. For example, Clark 2003 found that slow stretching, tapping (for hypertonicity), and vibration are not likely to benefit the lips and tongue but could potentially benefit jaw closing muscles. Massage was noted to have potential for relaxation of oral musculature. However, others suggest that tapping, vibration, and/ or stroking improve function for children with a variety of oromotor deficits such as limited upper lip movement, lingual retraction, and limited lingual movement [46].

One study implemented a variety of oromotor exercises and found that oral motor treatment consisting of oral massage, Beckman facilitation techniques, therapeutic feeding techniques, jaw/bubbles/horn/straw exercises improved eating and drinking skills for children with low muscle tone [47].

Treatment Strategies for the Older Child

Compensatory swallowing maneuvers, changes in posture, and exercises which are used with adults may be appropriate for the older child, such as the supraglottic swallow or chin-down position [41]. However, because the child's neurological system is developing, further research is needed to determine the propriety of treating pediatric patients with techniques that have been validated in adults [1].

Can the 3 oz Swallow Screening Be Used with Children?

The 3 oz swallow screening initially was studied with adults but now has been tested for children ages 2–18 with results revealing that its sensitivity for predicting aspiration status during FEES was 100%. There was a high false-positive rate of 48.4% [48]. This screening can be highly useful for the clinician conducting a bedside assessment and/or treatment sessions as it can help determine candidacy for and/or timing of an instrumental swallow study.

Can the Free Water Protocol Be Adapted to the Older Pediatric Population?

The free water protocol established for adult patients has obvious benefits, and adaptations have been applied to pediatrics. The protocol suggests that with good oral hygiene, aspiration of water poses little risk to the patient, and aspirated water will be reabsorbed into the bloodstream. This may be an appealing option for patients with dysphagia who refuse thickened liquids [49].

Special Populations/Consideration/Controversies that Can Be Applied to All Ages

Thickening: Is It Really a "Last Resort?"

Thin liquids may be difficult to swallow safely due to impaired timing and coordination. In an effort to preserve pulmonary integrity, thickened liquids (if proven to be swallowed safely) may be recommended. Thickening liquids slows oropharyngeal transit time while creating a more cohesive bolus, which makes the liquid easier to control and minimizes the risk of aspiration before the swallow. In addition, thickening can increase timing/duration of UES opening and amount of hyolaryngeal movement [50]. One study showed that infants with silent aspiration who were placed on thickened liquids demonstrated a decrease in subsequent acute respiratory illnesses [51].

However, the products that are offered to thicken formula and expressed breast milk can have a negative impact on the child's immature digestive tract. Some of the gum-based thickeners (xanthan gum, carob bean, cellulose) have been linked with NEC in infants, and the FDA has recommended some thickeners not to be introduced to babies under 12 months of age. The increased risk may be associated with the product itself or bacterial contamination in the production line [52]. Rice or oat cereals can be used for thickening formula but are not effective in thickening breast milk as the enzymes in expressed breast milk break down the cereal. It is important, however, to consider the high degree of variability when using thickening as a strategy based on a modified barium swallow study. In addition to cereals lacking consistency across brands and types (rice, oatmeal), cornstarch and gum-based thickeners have been shown to be highly variable depending on the brand of thickener, time allowed to thicken, and the composition of the base liquid to which the thickener is added [53]. The clinician who is recommending thickened liquids for a patient based on a modified barium swallow study needs to have an understanding of the various viscosity measurements for each liquid and thickener combination. For example, some commercial thickeners added to orange juice and apple juice become thicker than those added to water and milk. Conversely, certain thickeners added to milk are twice as thick as those added to water, apple juice, and orange juice [53]. Additionally, "honey-thick Varibar" tested in fluoroscopy is at least 2× thicker than many of the "honey-thick" marketed commercial thickeners and is actually considered "spoon thick."

The child's gastrointestinal status must be considered before recommending thickening liquids for infants and children [54]. Young children who aspirate thin liquids may have difficulty maintaining adequate hydration with thickened liquids due to the changes in texture and taste, providing a dilemma for both families and health professionals [55]. Foods such as applesauce for water or juice and yogurt for milk have been suggested to improve acceptance. Adults placed on thickened liquids may perceive their drinks to be more filling and may consume less than those on thin liquids – this could be the case for infants and children [56].

Given these valid concerns on both sides of the argument, a clinician can be left feeling stuck between two undesirable outcomes when considering the pulmonary damage that can come from the recurrent aspiration that results from dysphagia versus the need for extreme caution when prescribing thickened fluids [52].

High-Flow Nasal Cannula (HFNC) and Nasal Continuous Positive Airway Pressure (NCPAP): To Feed or Not to Feed

A competent coordination of breathing and swallowing is critical as these functions share the pharynx as a common pathway [10]. Patients who are on HFNC or NCPAP need this increased level of respiratory support in order to maintain adequate respiration, so the priority of feeding needs to be questioned as it can place the patient at risk for aspiration or penetration [57]. Additionally there is the possibility that increased pressure or flow could make it difficult to close the airway adequately during a swallow and/or misdirect part of the bolus into the airway. However, one study showed that "developmentally and medically appropriate neonates" who were on lower levels of O_2 between 2 and 3 L via NC were able to tolerate introduction of oral feeding with physiologic stability, although supplemental feeds were still required [58].

Should the Patient Ever Be Placed on "Strict NPO" (Nil Per Os, Nothing by Mouth)?

In situations where it is deemed unsafe to allow the child to continue an oral diet and an enteral feeding tube is placed, it is generally recommended that the patient practice *some* oral feeding in order to maintain oromotor skills and interest in oral feeding. The volume and consistencies recommended by the clinician will be based on the patient's overall respiratory health, clinical or instrumental swallow assessment results, and current medical status.

Since swallowing is the best exercise for swallowing, small PO trials will address the pharyngeal phase of swallow [59] rather than focusing on techniques that target the oral phase only. If there are unique instances where the physician feels that the medical condition is too grave for any PO such as severe pulmonary hypertension in a child with a cardiac anomaly, it is important that at least the oral skills are maintained.

It has been suggested that there is a critical period during late gestation and early postnatal life where treatment of respiratory distress syndrome may significantly alter the structure and function of the developing brain and possibly negatively impact the transition to oral feeds [36].

There seems to be a critical and sensitive period for development of normal feeding behaviors, particularly for introduction of solid foods. The longer the delay in the introduction of solids, the more difficult it can be for children to enjoy exploring a variety of food tastes and textures [5, 60].

When swallowing dysfunction is present, it may interrupt normal development at critical or sensitive times, possibly interfering with development of feeding/swallowing skills, and eventually lead to feeding aversions [1]. Therefore, providing at least some amount of exposure and practice can help avoid these future challenges.

Is Anything "Safe" to Aspirate?

Repeated episodes of aspiration can contribute to a variety of lung disorders such as pneumonia [61]. It is critical that a child's lungs are protected from aspiration. In infants, smaller and more compliant airways have a higher likelihood of being obstructed by a small amount of aspirated material, in turn making it more difficult for the infant to clear material from the lungs [62]. There are no simple or well-defined answers to the questions: "How much aspiration is too much? How will aspiration affect long term respiratory health"? [10] "Is there anything safe to aspirate?"

One study has associated milk aspiration with wheezing in young children and found it to be a potential risk factor for asthma [61]. Studies have looked into the impact of formula, breast milk, water, secretions, and saline on the lungs. Milk in considered to be toxic to the lower airway and is associated with chemical pneumonitis. Aspiration of oropharyngeal secretions can also cause lower airways infections. More inert fluids, such as saline and water, are considered not inherently toxic to the lungs but can cause laryngeal chemoreflex (LCR) response [63]. This is a response to material entering the airway such as apnea, laryngeal constriction, hypertension, and bradycardia [64].

In animal studies, water, cow's milk, and glucose induced apnea when applied to the laryngeal entrance, whereas normal saline did not [65].

There is conflicting evidence regarding the impact of thin versus thicker liquids/purees on the lungs when aspirated. One study showed that aspiration of thin liquids (compared to thickened liquids and purees) was the only consistency associated with an increased risk of pneumonia [66]. In contrast, another study reported that the risk of developing pneumonia was significantly greater when thickened liquids and purees were aspirated as opposed to thin liquids [67]. A more recent study on rabbits tested the impact of water, cornstarch (CS)-thickened water, and xanthan gum (XG)-thickened water on the lungs. Only 12.5% of rabbits whose lungs were instilled with CS-thickened water survived the 4-day study. All animals instilled with water and XG-thickened water survived, but the animals given XG-thickened water did present with greater pulmonary inflammation, pulmonary interstitial congestion, and alveolar edema than animals instilled with water. The authors concluded that aspiration of CS-based thickener can be fatal, and aspiration of XG-thickened water causes greater lung injury than aspiration of water alone [68].

Advancing the Child to an Oral Diet

For the clinician trying to advance the infant's oral intake, the transition needs to be made in a controlled manner. Management decisions for children with dysphagia with or without respiratory compromise may be based on each child's presumed ability to tolerate aspiration and the sequelae associated with the swallowing dysfunction, which can be subjective [10].

Additionally, the decision to advance a child's diet may address the goals of one specialty while counteracting those of another, which is why a team approach is critical. Close monitoring of signs and symptoms of aspiration is recommended. However, the high frequency of silent aspiration in children, reportedly >90%, can compromise the ability to detect aspiration [69]. Thus, clinicians often look at other signs, such as new-onset chest congestion, wet/gurgly vocal quality, subtle stress signs, or refusal, as possible signs of dysphagia. Worsening asthma, increased use of respiratory medications, new-onset pneumonia, or respiratory infections can be a sign of unsuccessful weaning from enteral feeding [39].

Endotracheal Intubation and Considerations

Significant concerns surround the risk of swallowing dysfunction post intubation including damage to the larynx or trachea [7] and/or palate remodeling leading to velopharyngeal incompetence [54, 70]. Several factors to be considered when treating a patient post intubation:

1. Was the intubation emergent or was it planned for surgery? Patients who were emergently intubated have a higher risk of trauma to larynx or trachea [7].
2. How long was the patient intubated? Duration of ventilation and continuous positive airway pressure are associated with delayed attainment of full enteral or oral feeding for infants [71, 72].
3. How large was the endotracheal tube and were there multiple attempts to establish an airway?
4. Did the patient self-extubate?

References

1. Lefton-Greif MA. Pediatric dysphagia. Phys Med Rehabil Clin N Am. 2008;19(4):837–51.
2. Gewolb IH, Vice FL. Abnormalities in the coordination of respiration and swallow in preterm infants with bronchopulmonary dysplasia. Dev Med Child Neurol. 2006;48(07):595–9.
3. Khoshoo V, Edell D. Previously healthy infants may have increased risk of aspiration during respiratory syncytial viral bronchiolitis. Pediatrics. 1999;104(6):1389–90.
4. Sheikh S, Allen E, Shell R, Hruschak J, Iram D, Castile R, McCoy K. Chronic aspiration without gastroesophageal reflux as a cause of chronic respiratory symptoms in neurologically normal infants. Chest J. 2001;120(4):1190–5.
5. Arvedson JC. Swallowing and feeding in infants and young children. GI Motil. 2006; https://doi.org/10.1038/gimo17.
6. Martin-Harris B, Brodsky MB, Michel Y, Castell DO, Schleicher M, Sandidge J, Maxwell R, Blair J. MBS measurement tool for swallow impairment—MBSImp: establishing a standard. Dysphagia. 2008;23(4):392–405.
7. Coyle JL. Dysphagia following prolonged endotracheal intubation: is there a rule of thumb? Dysphagia. 2014;23(2):80–6.
8. Eber E, Zach MS. Long term sequelae of bronchopulmonary dysplasia (chronic lung disease of infancy). Thorax. 2001;56(4):317–23.
9. Johnston ID, Strachan DP, Anderson HR. Effect of pneumonia and whooping cough in childhood on adult lung function. N Engl J Med. 1998;338(9):581–7.
10. Lefton-Greif MA, McGrath-Morrow SA. Deglutition and respiration: development, coordination, and practical implications. InSemin Speech Lang. 2007;28(03):166–79.
11. Shaheen SO, Barker DJ, Shiell AW, Crocker FJ, Wield GA, Holgate ST. The relationship between pneumonia in early childhood and impaired lung function in late adult life. Am J Respir Crit Care Med. 1994;149(3):616–9.
12. Von Mutius E. Paediatric origins of adult lung disease. Thorax. 2001;56(2):153–7.
13. Rogers B, Arvedson J. Assessment of infant oral sensorimotor and swallowing function. Dev Disabil Res Rev. 2005;11(1):74–82.
14. Ross ES, Philbin MK. Soffi: an evidence-based method for quality bottle-feedings of preterm, ill, and fragile infants. J Perinat Neonatal Nurs. 2011;25(4):349–59.
15. Shaker C. Cue-based feeding in the NICU: using the infant's communication as a guide. Neonatal Netw. 2013;32(6):404–8.
16. Hawdon JM, Beauregard N, Slattery J, Kennedy G. Identification of neonates at risk of developing feeding problems in infancy. Dev Med Child Neurol. 2000;42(4):235–9.
17. Van der Meer A, Holden G, Van der Weel R. Coordination of sucking, swallowing, and breathing in healthy newborns. J Pediatr Neonatol. 2005;1(2):69–72.
18. Bamford O, Taciak V, Gewolb IH. The relationship between rhythmic swallowing and breathing during suckle feeding in term neonates. Pediatr Res. 1992;31(6):619–24.
19. Thoyre SM, Holditch-Davis D, Schwartz TA, Roman CR, Nix W. Coregulated approach to feeding preterm infants with lung disease: effects during feeding. Nurs Res. 2012;61(4):242–51; Thurlbeck WM. Postnatal human lung growth. Thorax. 1982;37(8):564–71
20. Law-Morstatt L, Judd DM, Snyder P, Baier RJ, Dhanireddy R. Pacing as a treatment technique for transitional sucking patterns. J Perinatol. 2003;23(6):483–8.
21. Clark L, Kennedy G, Pring T, Hird M. Improving bottle feeding in preterm infants: investigating the elevated side-lying position. Infant. 2007;3(4):154–8.
22. Park J, Thoyre S, Knafl GJ, Hodges EA, Nix WB. Efficacy of semielevated side-lying positioning during bottle-feeding of very preterm infants: a pilot study. J Perinat Neonatal Nurs. 2014;28(1):69–79.
23. Dawson JA, Myers LR, Moorhead A, Jacobs SE, Ong K, Salo F, Murray S, Donath S, Davis PG. A randomised trial of two techniques for bottle feeding preterm infants. J Paediatr Child Health. 2013;49(6):462–6.

24. Lau C. Is there an advantage for preterm infants to feed orally in an upright or sidelying position? J Neonatal Nurs. 2013;19(1):28–32.
25. Thach BT, Stark AR. Spontaneous neck flexion and airway obstruction during apneic spells in preterm infants. J Pediatr. 1979;94(2):275–81.
26. Kummer A. Cleft palate & craniofacial anomalies: effects on speech and resonance. Nelson Educ. 2013:149.
27. Tobin JM, McCloud P, Cameron DJ. Posture and gastro-oesophageal reflux: a case for left lateral positioning. Arch Dis Child. 1997;76(3):254–8.
28. Elser HE. Positioning after feedings: what is the evidence to reduce feeding intolerances? Adv Neonatal Care. 2012;12(3):172–5.
29. van Wijk MP, Benninga MA, Dent J, Lontis R, Goodchild L, McCall LM, Haslam R, Davidson GP, Omari T. Effect of body position changes on postprandial gastroesophageal reflux and gastric emptying in the healthy premature neonate. J Pediatr. 2007;151(6):585–90.
30. Task Force on Sudden Infant Death Syndrome. SIDS and other sleep-related infant deaths: updated 2016 recommendations for a safe infant sleeping environment. Pediatrics. 2016;138:e20162938.
31. Chang YJ, Lin CP, Lin YJ, Lin CH. Effects of single-hole and cross-cut nipple units on feeding efficiency and physiological parameters in premature infants. J Nurs Res. 2007;15(3):215–23.
32. Hwang YS, Lin CH, Coster WJ, Bigsby R, Vergara E. Effectiveness of cheek and jaw support to improve feeding performance of preterm infants. Am J Occup Ther. 2010;64(6):886–94.
33. Foster JP, Psaila K, Patterson T. Non-nutritive sucking for increasing physiologic stability and nutrition in preterm infants. Cochrane Database Syst Rev. 2016;10:CD001071.
34. Zhang Y, Lyu T, Hu X, Shi P, Cao Y, Latour JM. Effect of nonnutritive sucking and oral stimulation on feeding performance in preterm infants: a randomized controlled trial. Pediatr Crit Care Med. 2014;15(7):608–14.
35. Lessen BS. Effect of the premature infant oral motor intervention on feeding progression and length of stay in preterm infants. Adv Neonatal Care. 2011;11(2):129–39.
36. Barlow SM. Oral and respiratory control for preterm feeding. Curr Opin Otolaryngol Head Neck Surg. 2009;17(3):179.
37. Da Costa SP, van Den Engel-Hoek L, Bos AF. Sucking and swallowing in infants and diagnostic tools. J Perinatol. 2008;28(4):247–57.
38. Omer IM, Ibrahim NG, Nasr AM. Oxygen therapy in neonatal intensive care units in Khartoum State. Sudan J Paediatr. 2015;15(2):49–51.
39. Richter GT. Management of oropharyngeal dysphagia in the neurologically intact and developmentally normal child. Curr Opin Otolaryngol Head Neck Surg. 2010;18(6):554–63.
40. Prasse JE, Kikano GE. An overview of pediatric dysphagia. Clin Pediatr. 2009;48(3):247–51.
41. Logemann JA. Behavioral management for oropharyngeal dysphagia. Folia Phoniatr Logop. 1999;51(4–5):199–212.
42. Clark HM. Neuromuscular treatments for speech and swallowing: a tutorial. Am J Speech Lang Pathol. 2003;12(4):400–15.
43. Sheppard JJ. The role of oral sensorimotor therapy in the treatment of pediatric dysphagia. Dysphagia. 2005;14(2):6–10.
44. Bachmeyer MH. Treatment of selective and inadequate food intake in children: a review and practical guide. Behav Anal Pract. 2009;2(1):43.
45. Cichero JA. Thickening agents used for dysphagia management: effect on bioavailability of water, medication and feelings of satiety. Nutr J. 2013;12(1):54.
46. Arvedson JC. Management of pediatric dysphagia. Otolaryngol Clin N Am. 1998;31(3):453–76.
47. Kumin L, Von Hagel KC, Bahr DC. An effective oral motor intervention protocol for infants and toddlers with low muscle tone. Infant Toddler Intervention. 2001;11(3/4):181–200.
48. Suiter DM, Leder SB, Karas DE. The 3-ounce (90-cc) water swallow challenge: a screening test for children with suspected oropharyngeal dysphagia. Otolaryngol Head Neck Surg. 2009;140(2):187–90.
49. Bronson-Lowe C, Leising K, Bronson-Lowe D, Lanham S, Hayes S, Ronquillo A, Blake P. Effects of a free water protocol for patients with dysphagia. Dysphagia. 2008;23(4):430.

50. Dantas RO, Kern MK, Massey BT, Dodds WJ, Kahrilas PJ, Brasseur JG, Cook IJ, Lang IM. Effect of swallowed bolus variables on oral and pharyngeal phases of swallowing. Am J Physiol. 1990;258(5):G675–81.
51. Coon ER, Srivastava R, Stoddard GJ, Reilly S, Maloney CG, Bratton SL. Infant videofluoroscopic swallow study testing, swallowing interventions, and future acute respiratory illness. Hosp Pediatr. 2016;6(12):707–13.
52. Gosa MM, Corkins MR. Necrotizing enterocolitis and the use of thickened liquids for infants with dysphagia. Dysphagia. 2015;24(2):44–9.
53. Garcia JM, Chambers E, Matta Z, Clark M. Viscosity measurements of nectar-and honey-thick liquids: product, liquid, and time comparisons. Dysphagia. 2005;20(4):325–35.
54. Tutor JD, Gosa MM. Dysphagia and aspiration in children. Pediatr Pulmonol. 2012;47(4):321–37.
55. Weir K, McMahon S, Chang AB. Restriction of oral intake of water for aspiration lung disease in children. Cochrane Database Syst Rev. 2005;(4):CD005303.
56. Cichero JA, Nicholson TM, September C. Thickened milk for the management of feeding and swallowing issues in infants: a call for interdisciplinary professional guidelines. J Hum Lact. 2013;29(2):132–5.
57. Ferrara L, Bidiwala A, Sher I, Pirzada M, Barlev D, Islam S, Rosenfeld W, Crowley CC, Hanna N. Effect of nasal continuous positive airway pressure on the pharyngeal swallow in neonates. J Perinatol. 2017;37:398–403.
58. Leder SB, Siner JM, Bizzarro MJ, McGinley BM, Lefton-Greif MA. Oral alimentation in neonatal and adult populations requiring high-flow oxygen via nasal cannula. Dysphagia. 2016;31(2):154–9.
59. Perlman AL, Luschei ES, Du Mond CE. Electrical activity from the superior pharyngeal constrictor during reflexive and nonreflexive tasks. J Speech Lang Hear Res. 1989;32(4):749–54.
60. Illingworth RS, Lister J. The critical or sensitive period, with special reference to certain feeding problems in infants and children. J Pediatr. 1964;65(6):839–48.
61. Janahi IA, Elidemir O, Shardonofsky FR, Abu-Hassan MN, Fan LL, Larsen GL, Blackburn MR, Colasurdo GN. Recurrent milk aspiration produces changes in airway mechanics, lung eosinophilia, and goblet cell hyperplasia in a murine model. Pediatr Res. 2000;48(6):776–81.
62. Simon M, Collins MS. The pediatric lung and aspiration. Dysphagia. 2013;22(4):142–54.
63. Karim RM, Momin IA, Lalani II, Merchant SS, Sewani AA, Hassan BS, Mahmood N. Aspiration pneumonia in pediatric age group: etiology, predisposing factors and clinical outcome. JPMA. 1999;49(4):105–8.
64. Thach BT. Maturation and transformation of reflexes that protect the laryngeal airway from liquid aspiration from fetal to adult life. Am J Med. 2001;111(8):69–77.
65. Mizuno K, Ueda A, Takeuchi T. Effects of different fluids on the relationship between swallowing and breathing during nutritive sucking in neonates. Neonatology. 2002;81(1):45–50.
66. Weir K, McMahon S, Barry L, Ware R, Masters IB, Chang AB. Oropharyngeal aspiration and pneumonia in children. Pediatr Pulmonol. 2007;42(11):1024–31.
67. Taniguchi MH, Moyer RS. Assessment of risk factors for pneumonia in dysphagic children: significance of videofluoroscopic swallowing evaluation. Dev Med Child Neurol. 1994;36(6):495–502.
68. Nativ-Zeltzer N, Kuhn MA, Imai DM, Traslavina RP, Domer AS, Litts JK, Adams B, Belafsky PC. The effects of aspirated thickened water on survival and pulmonary injury in a rabbit model. Laryngoscope. 2018;128(2):327–31.
69. Arvedson J, Rogers B, Buck G, Smart P, Msall M. Silent aspiration prominent in children with dysphagia. Int J Pediatr Otorhinolaryngol. 1994;28(2–3):173–81.
70. Tutor JD. Dysphagia and aspiration in the pediatric patient. Dysphagia. 2001;10(2):6–9.
71. Jadcherla SR, Wang M, Vijayapal AS, Leuthner SR. Impact of prematurity and co-morbidities on feeding milestones in neonates: a retrospective study. J Perinatol. 2010;30(3):201–8.
72. Park J, Knafl G, Thoyre S, Brandon D. Factors associated with feeding progression in extremely preterm infants. Nurs Res. 2015;64(3):159–67.

Part II
Special Topics and Controversies in Pediatric Dysphagia

Chapter 13
Ankyloglossia and Dysphagia

Jeffrey Cheng and Eileen Raynor

Anatomy

Congenital ankyloglossia or tongue-tie refers to an anomaly of the lingual frenulum, which may result in decreased oral tongue mobility affecting latching for breast-feeding, feeding, and speech. There have been notable public health campaigns promoting the health, social, and economic benefits of breastfeeding, perhaps raising awareness of congenital tongue-ties [1]. The membrane or tissue that makes up the lingual frenulum lies on the ventral surface of the tongue and connects it to the floor of the mouth. This may range in its clinical characteristics from thin and membranous to a thick and diffuse band of tissue (Fig. 13.1). This can affect a newborn's ability to breastfeed or a child's ability to spoon-feed as well as impact speech articulation.

The tongue-tie entity most commonly encountered and referred to is an anterior attachment. This is often easily identified and well recognized by the general public and healthcare providers. Most of the clinical investigations evaluating frenotomy as an intervention for breastfeeding difficulty are targeted at this type of tongue-tie. Frenotomy can be performed in a number of ways, including with cold steel or laser division, and primarily refers to simply dividing the lingual frenulum. More complex lingual frenulum issues may be addressed by frenuloplasty, which involves

J. Cheng (✉)
Pediatric Otolaryngology, Division of Head and Neck Surgery and Communication Sciences,
Duke University Medical Center, Durham, NC, USA
e-mail: jeffrey.cheng@duke.edu

E. Raynor
Pediatric Otolaryngology, Division of Head and Neck Surgery and Communication Sciences,
Duke University Medical Center, Durham, NC, USA

Duke University Medical Center, Durham, NC, USA
e-mail: Eileen.raynor@duke.edu

© Springer International Publishing AG, part of Springer Nature 2018
J. Ongkasuwan, E. H. Chiou (eds.), *Pediatric Dysphagia*,
https://doi.org/10.1007/978-3-319-97025-7_13

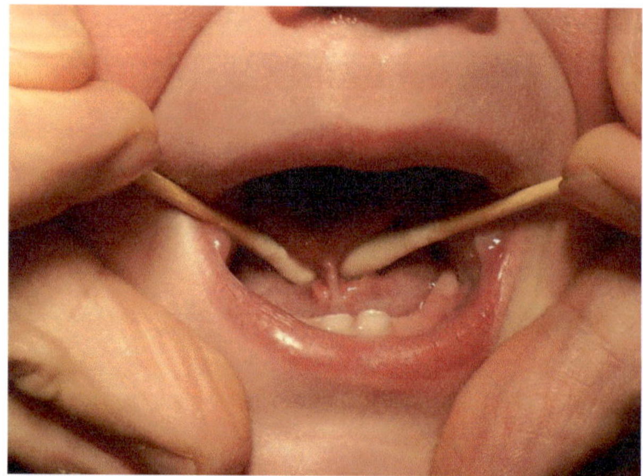

Fig. 13.1 Anteriorly attached thick frenulum (type II); note heart-shaped deformity of the tongue above the cotton applicators. (Reprinted from O'Callahan et al. [2], Copyright 2013, with permission from Elsevier)

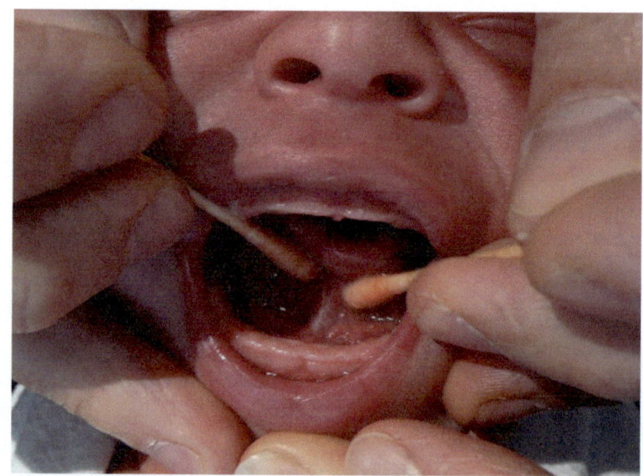

Fig. 13.2 Posteriorly attached frenulum (type III); note thickened fibrous-type band under the tongue (Reprinted from O'Callahan et al. [2], Copyright 2013, with permission from Elsevier)

rearrangement of the local tissue and closure with sutures. Risks include minor bleeding, and in rare cases, cautery may be necessary to achieve hemostasis. Other less frequent risks are potential injury to the submandibular ducts, scarring which can lead to retethering of the tongue. Additionally, with the use of a laser, there is a risk of untintentional burn to surrounding tissues.

There is limited information and less recognition regarding posterior ankyloglossia. It does not have the usual appearance of anterior ankyloglossia and is a relatively newly recognized clinical entity. Anterior ankyloglossia can be generally categorized as type I or type II. Type I has an insertion point extending up to the anterior tip of the oral tongue, and type II attaches slightly posterior to the anterior tip at the anterior third of the oral tongue. Posterior ankyloglossia has been categorized into types III and IV. Type III has been described as a thickened lingual frenulum (Fig. 13.2), and type IV is a submucosal frenulum, which appears as a broad and flat area of mucosal tissue that is void of any typical frenular tissue and results in restricted mobility of the tongue especially with tongue elevation [2].

Most commonly, posterior ankyloglossia is identified by lactation consultants and is not as well recognized or known by most healthcare providers [3]. Posterior ankyloglossia is generally thicker and attached further back from the tongue tip. Addressing this problem is gaining in popularity and has been demonstrated to be effectively managed in the office setting with frenotomy similar to anterior ankyloglossia [2].

Controversy

Ankyloglossia has been implicated in a variety of newborn and infant feeding problems, mostly commonly with difficulty with latching or staying attached to the nipple for breastfeeding. Issues may include problems affecting both the mother and the baby. The family may report maternal and newborn/infant concerns including but not limited to nipple pain and discomfort, development of plugs and mastitis, difficulty with latching, maintaining hold of the nipple, and poor effectiveness of extracting breast milk.

Goals of frenotomy in newborns are primarily twofold: first is the improvement in comfort and effectiveness of breastfeeding, and second is avoidance of the potential for development of speech impairment and/or dysphagia arising from poor tongue mobility. Consultation is often sought during the newborn period for both of these issues. Frenotomy can be performed safely and effectively without the need for local or general anesthesia in the newborn and early infant time period. Most studies recommend in-office frenotomy up to about age 3 months. This is true for posterior tongue-tie as well. Delay in seeking evaluation and management for frenotomy later in infancy or as a toddler may cause the family to miss this time window and technically may not be advisable to perform in an office or non-operative room setting due to risk of bleeding or injury to surrounding structures while trying to restrain an active baby. Frenotomy has been demonstrated to be a very well-tolerated and safe procedure [4].

Breastfeeding

With regard to the first objective of improvement in the breastfeeding experience for the dyad of the newborn and breastfeeding mother, there has been conflicting evidence in the literature regarding the effectiveness of frenotomy in the newborn period. It may difficult to ascertain if there is a direct causal relationship between performing frenotomy and improvement in breastfeeding symptoms. Breastfeeding is a complex and multifactorial activity. Improvement post-frenotomy may simply be related to the natural clinical history of breastfeeding with improvement over time as observed with expectant management. In cases of thin anteriorly attached frenulae, some babies can stretch their frenulum over time, thereby resolving early breastfeeding problems. Latch scores, however, have been demonstrated to be lower in tongue-tied newborns than in normal controls [5]. Latch scores are a breastfeeding assessment tool: L is for how the baby latches onto the breast, A is for audible swallowing, T is for nipple type,

C is for mother's comfort, and H is for how much head support is needed to hold the infant to the breast. This is rated on a 0–2 scale, and higher is more favorable. A few studies eliminated the "C" and only looked at the four other factors [6]. A randomized control trial with a sham procedure control group performed by Buryk et al. demonstrated that there were immediate improvements in breastfeeding and decreases in nipple pain in the frenotomy group. The authors advocated that their results provide relatively convincing evidence that mothers with breastfeeding issues and newborns with congenital ankyloglossia should seek consultation for frenotomy [7]. However, a systematic review performed several years later by Francis et al. found that only a small body of evidence supported frenotomy for mother-based improvements in breastfeeding but that the strength of evidence was low to insufficient [8]. Others have also commented on the conflicting evidence supporting improvement in latching and breastfeeding after frenotomy, as up to half of all breastfeeding babies with ankyloglossia will not encounter any problems [9, 10]. Recently, a prospective cohort study was performed by Ghaheri et al., and the authors demonstrated that there was a significant improvement in breastfeeding outcomes from surgical release of a tongue-tie. In 78% of their cohort, an isolated posterior tongue-tie was identified. Benefits have been noted to be immediate and within the first week after surgical division and continue to persist for months [11]. Benoiton et al. also reported similar findings regarding posterior tongue-tie release and continued improvements at 2 weeks of follow-up [12].

Objective clinical predictors have not yet been identified to help guide patient selection for those newborns who would most benefit and improve chances of success for sustained breastfeeding [13]. Drawing conclusions from prior reports is challenging, as there are few reported clinical predictors to help in decision-making and may often include newborns who underwent thickened, tethered upper labial/maxillary frenum as well, and there are likely multifactorial contributors to breastfeeding challenges in difficulties for dyads of breastfeeding mothers and newborns. Albeit, it appears that in general, most authors conclude that early identification and tongue-tie release within the first few weeks of life improve the breastfeeding experience and prevent poor breastfeeding outcomes [14–16]. In conclusion, it does appear that current clinical evidence supports the use of frenotomy in newborns to improve maternal nipple pain and breastfeeding problems. It may also be beneficial to raise awareness and identification of the less clinically obvious posterior tongue-tie. In addition, there is little, if any, evidence currently regarding the effects of ankyloglossia on swallowing function beyond breastfeeding. Decreased tongue mobility may contribute to ineffective and inefficient movement and transfer of the food bolus from the oral phase of mastication to the initial oropharyngeal phase of swallowing. Further investigation in this area may be warranted.

Speech Outcomes

Speech articulation in infants and toddlers is a complex orchestra and requires coordination of oral, oropharyngeal, nasal, nasopharyngeal, and laryngeal musculature and structures. One of the components that has been implicated as impairing developmentally appropriate acquisition of speech articulation comes from potential limitations in tongue mobility due to a restrictive lingual frenulum. With regard to the speech outcomes and tongue mobility, there appears to be a long-term benefit to early frenotomy during the newborn period. This is supported by Walls et al., who evaluated articulation in children at 3 years of age with a history of congenital ankyloglossia. They compared those who underwent frenotomy and those who did not and found that those who underwent frenotomy had better intelligibility scores [17]. However, these results differ than the conclusions drawn from a systematic review by Webb et al.; their findings suggested that there is no significant data to support a link between congenital ankyloglossia and speech articulation problems [4].

Conclusion

To date, there is still controversy within the literature regarding the role of early frenotomy on later speech and articulation outcomes. There is evidence, however, to support frenotomy to improve breastfeeding for the dyad of newborn babies and their mothers. Informed and shared medical decision-making between the clinical care provider and the mother and family should be undertaken; the available evidence presented should be considered, along with the family's perspective and values, when deciding whether or not to proceed with frenotomy in the newborn for congenital ankyloglossia. Unfortunately, there are currently no reliable clinical predictors of success for newborn frenotomy to help guide patient selection; therefore, each case must be evaluated on an individual basis. In addition, there is considerable variation in the surgical technique and procedure; thus, it is difficult to make definitive conclusions at this time about the optimal technical approach.

References

1. Joseph KS, Kinniburgh B, Metcalfe A, Razaz N, Sabr Y, Lisonkova S. Temporal trends in ankyloglossia and frenotomy in British Columbia, Canada, 2004-2013: a population-based study. CMAJ Open. 2016;4:E33–40.
2. O'Callahan C, Macary S, Clemente S. The effects of office-based frenotomy for anterior and posterior ankyloglossia on breastfeeding. Int J Pediatr Otorhinolaryngol. 2013;77: 827–32.
3. Pransky SM, Lago D, Hong P. Breastfeeding difficulties and oral cavity anomalies: the influence of posterior ankyloglossia and upper-lip ties. Int J Pediatr Otorhinolaryngol. 2015;79: 1714–7.
4. Webb AN, Hao W, Hong P. The effect of tongue-tie division on breastfeeding and speech articulation: a systematic review. Int J Pediatr Otorhinolaryngol. 2013;77:635–46.
5. Puapornpong P, Raungrongmorakot K, Mahasitthiwat V, Ketsuwan S. Comparisons of the latching on between newborns with tongue-tie and normal newborns. J Med Assoc Thail. 2014;97:255–9.
6. Lau Y, Htun TP, Lim PI, Ho-Lim S, Klainin-Yobas P. Psychometric evaluation of 5- and 4-item versions of the LATCH breastfeeding assessment tool during the initial postpartum period among a multiethnic population. PLoS One. 2016;11(5):e0154331.

 7. Buryk M, Bloom D, Shope T. Efficacy of neonatal release of ankyloglossia: a randomized trial. Pediatrics. 2011;128:280–8.
 8. Francis DO, Krishnaswami S, McPheeters M. Treatment of ankyloglossia and breastfeeding outcomes: a systematic review. Pediatrics. 2015;135:e1458–66.
 9. Cawse-Lucas J, Waterman S, St Anna L. Clinical inquiry: does frenotomy help infants with tongue-tie overcome breastfeeding difficulties? J Fam Pract. 2015;64:126–7.
10. Power RF, Murphy JF. Tongue-tie and frenotomy in infants with breastfeeding difficulties: achieving a balance. Arch Dis Child. 2015;100:489–94.
11. Ghaheri BA, Cole M, Fausel SC, Chuop M, Mace JC. Breastfeeding improvement following tongue-tie and lip-tie release: a prospective cohort study. Laryngoscope. 2017;127:1217–23.
12. Benoiton L, Morgan M, Baguley K. Management of posterior ankyloglossia and upper lip ties in a tertiary otolaryngology outpatient clinic. Int J Pediatr Otorhinolaryngol. 2016;88:13–6.
13. Dollberg S, Marom R, Botzer E. Lingual frenotomy for breastfeeding difficulties: a prospective follow-up study. Breastfeed Med. 2014;9:286–9.
14. Riskin A, Mansovsky M, Coler-Botzer T, et al. Tongue-tie and breastfeeding in newborns-mothers' perspective. Breastfeed Med. 2014;9:430–7.
15. Todd DA, Hogan MJ. Tongue-tie in the newborn: early diagnosis and division prevents poor breastfeeding outcomes. Breastfeed Rev. 2015;23:11–6.
16. Toner D, Giordano T, Handler SD. Office frenotomy for neonates: resolving dysphagia, parental satisfaction and cost-effectiveness. ORL Head Neck Nurs. 2014;32:6–7.
17. Walls A, Pierce M, Wang H, Steehler A, Steehler M, Harley EH Jr. Parental perception of speech and tongue mobility in three-year olds after neonatal frenotomy. Int J Pediatr Otorhinolaryngol. 2014;78:128–31.

Chapter 14
Type 1 Laryngeal Clefts

Prasad John Thottam and Deepak K. Mehta

Introduction

As healthcare provider and parental awareness of swallowing dysfunction has increased over the past several years, the identification of laryngeal cleft (LC) anomalies has also increased. Previously, the incidence of laryngeal cleft was estimated to be 1:10,000–1:20,000 patients, but it is now estimated that laryngeal clefts are present in 5–7.6% of patients with chronic aspiration/penetration with swallowing [1, 2]. With this new mindfulness, treatment options have increased to benefit patients with these anomalies.

Benjamin and Inglis first proposed the classification of laryngeal clefts most frequently utilized in current medical literature in 1989. Type 1 clefts are the most common form of LC. They are described as a notch limited to the interarytenoid region and extend no further than to the level of the true vocal folds. They do not extend into the cricoid cartilage and are thought to be a result of dysfunctional interarytenoid muscular development or lack of normal arytenoid cartilage formation. Type 2 clefts extend into the upper portion of the cricoid cartilage, type 3 clefts extend through the entire cricoid cartilage, and type 4 clefts extend into the trachea to the thoracic inlet [3]. Patients with type 3 and 4 clefts often present at birth or early in life with significant respiratory events and/or aspiration. Type 3 and 4 LC are rare, often life-threatening, and repaired soon after birth. Some disorders associated with LCs are Opitz syndrome, Pallister-Hall syndrome, CHARGE syndrome, and VACTERL association.

P. J. Thottam (✉)
Pediatric Otolaryngology, Beaumont Children's Hospital, Royal Oak, MI, USA
e-mail: prasad.thottam@beaumont.org

D. K. Mehta
Department of Otolaryngology, Texas Children's Hospital, Houston, TX, USA
e-mail: dkmehta@texaschildrens.org

© Springer International Publishing AG, part of Springer Nature 2018
J. Ongkasuwan, E. H. Chiou (eds.), *Pediatric Dysphagia*,
https://doi.org/10.1007/978-3-319-97025-7_14

Type 1 and 2 laryngeal clefts often identified after more common causes have been ruled out or when they are identified as a co-contributor. Oropharyngeal swallowing disorders are most commonly identified as neurological in nature, but as multifactorial causes have become more easily identified, LCs are increasing in recognition and treatment [4].

Evaluation and Diagnosis

True type 1 and 2 laryngeal clefts are diagnosed intraoperatively during direct laryngoscopy and bronchoscopy (DLB) through palpation and visualization, but there are signs and tests that can be conducted in an outpatient setting that can assist in diagnosis. It is theorized that the majority of patients with type 1 LC are asymptomatic but that they can be encountered in as high as 7.6% of children with ongoing respiratory symptoms [1, 5, 6]. The most common presenting complaint is choking and coughing which is exacerbated with drinking [7]. These patients in particular struggle with thinner liquids and will often present from their primary care physician on a thickened diet. Children may also present with chronic wet cough, stridor, recurrent croup, or difficulty with weight gain secondary to food aversion.

The ideal evaluation tool of children with feeding symptomatology is fiberoptic endoscopic evaluation of swallowing (FEES). This test allows anatomic examination of larynx and supraglottic structures while providing dynamic information on a patient's swallow. Through this examination the interarytenoid pattern of aspiration and/or penetration of different consistencies can assist the physician in their diagnosis of a potential LC (Fig. 14.1). If FEES is not tolerated or an option, then modified barium swallow (MBS) studies are utilized. MBS studies are excellent to confirm aspiration but do expose the patient to radiation and offer limited anatomical information.

In order to confirm suspicion of a LC, a DLB is required. During this procedure the supraglottic, glottis, subglottic, trachea, and bronchi are evaluated and directly visualized. This allows the surgeon to directly palpate and examine the extent of the laryngeal cleft (aiding in proper classification) as well as examine for coexisting airway lesions that could also be contributing to the patient's symptoms. Laryngomalacia has been reported to be present in up to 35% of patients with type 1 LC [7].

Treatment

The management and treatment of a LC can range from diet modification to open surgical repair depending on the patient, comorbidities, and type of LC. Type 1 and 2 LCs are often managed endoscopically with injection or suture, while types 3 and 4 are traditionally performed open. Recently repair of type 3 and 4 LCs has been described through both endoscopic and robotic approaches, but at the current time, this is still considered experimental [8–10].

Fig. 14.1 Interarytenoid penetration/aspiration of thin liquids through laryngeal cleft

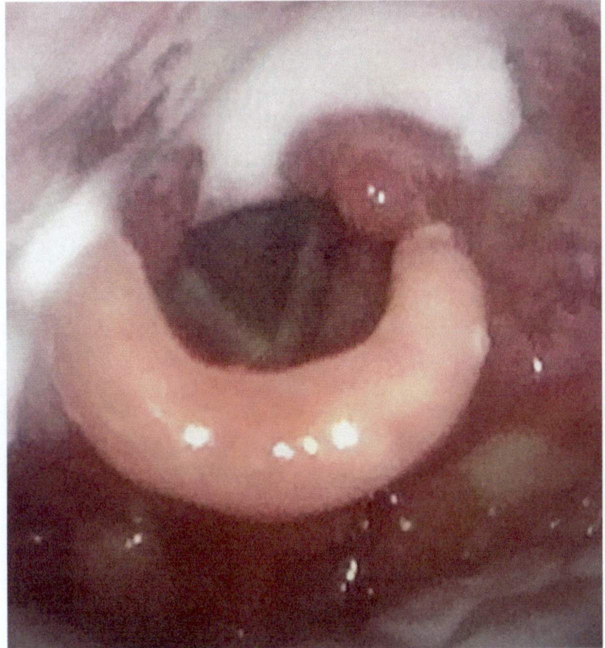

Laryngeal Cleft Injection

Injection laryngoplasty of the interarytenoid region for type 1 laryngeal cleft associated swallowing dysfunction is currently the mainstay surgical treatment. In a recent study, 75% of patients with swallowing dysfunction and type 1 laryngeal cleft demonstrated improved swallowing after injection laryngoplasty [7], while another study demonstrated improved swallowing in 50% of patients with normal anatomy and chronic post-interarytenoid injection [2].

The injection laryngoplasty of the interarytenoid region is performed utilizing the standard suspension microlaryngeal positioning with the patient supine and spontaneous ventilation. A microscope or zero-degree endoscope can be used for visualization. Once the patient is suspended, the interarytenoid region is palpated and isolated (vocal fold spreaders can be utilized if needed), and the endoscopic needle is then primed with aqueous/glycerin/carboxymethyl cellulose gel (Prolaryn gel). The needle is then placed into the interarytenoid space until the cricoid is felt. Then the 0.2–0.4 cc is injected into the interarytenoid space as the needle is slowly withdrawn. A submucosal elevation of this region should be observed if this is performed properly. Care is taken to not inject into the subglottis or cricopharyngeal region (Fig. 14.2).

Once this is completed, the patient is admitted overnight and observed. It is our practice to maintain the patient on their current diet until they are evaluated and cleared by speech and language for an advancement of their diet.

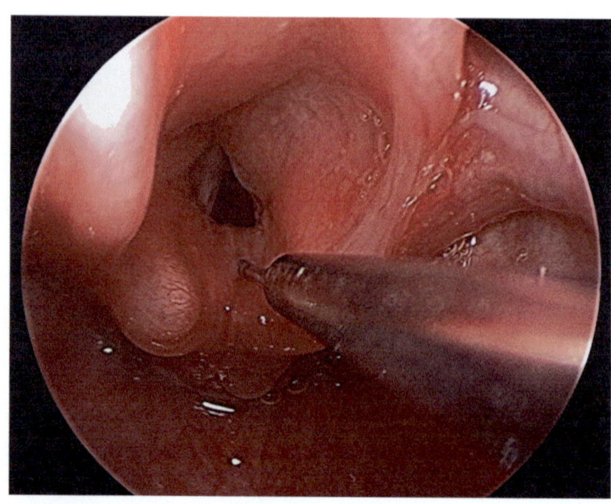

Fig. 14.2 Injection of interarytenoid region using laryngeal needle

Endoscopic Surgical Repair

Endoscopic surgical repair of type 1 LC is predominately reserved after injection laryngoplasty failure or return of symptoms after injection. It is also routinely performed for type 2 LC and, more recently, for types 3 and 4. Success rate for endoscopic formal repair of type 1 LC has been reported to be as high as 90% [7].

The injection laryngoplasty of the interarytenoid region is performed utilizing the standard suspension microlaryngeal positioning with the patient supine and spontaneous ventilation. A microscope or zero-degree endoscope can be used for visualization. The patient is suspended, and the interarytenoid region is isolated (vocal fold spreaders can be utilized if needed). Using laser or sickle knife, the interarytenoid region is incised from the apex to the corniculate cartilage (Fig. 14.3). Then using microlaryngeal instrumentation, submucosal flaps are elevated on both the esophageal and laryngeal side of the interarytenoid region. Once this is completed, the esophageal portion is re-approximated using 4-0 PDS suture on a P2 needle with the knot facing the esophageal inlet (Fig. 14.4). Then using the same suture, this technique is carried out in the same fashion on the laryngeal side, but care is taken to bury the knot in the mucosa to avoid irritation. Though some surgeons advocate keeping the patient intubated overnight, the authors do not routinely do this.

The patient is admitted and observed overnight. It is our practice to maintain the patient on their current diet until they are evaluated and cleared by speech and language for an advancement of their diet.

Challenges and Controversies

As diagnosis and treatment of pediatric swallowing disorders has increased, so has the attention to laryngeal clefts and the interarytenoid region in general. More recently, pattern of aspiration and repeat penetration through the interarytenoid region has

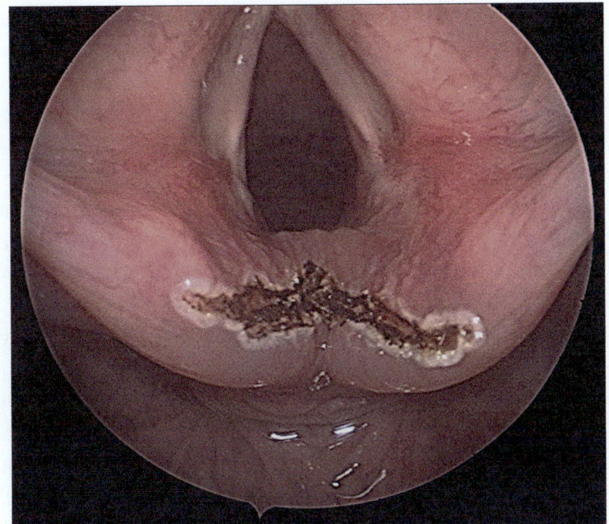

Fig. 14.3 Incised interarytenoid region with CO_2 laser

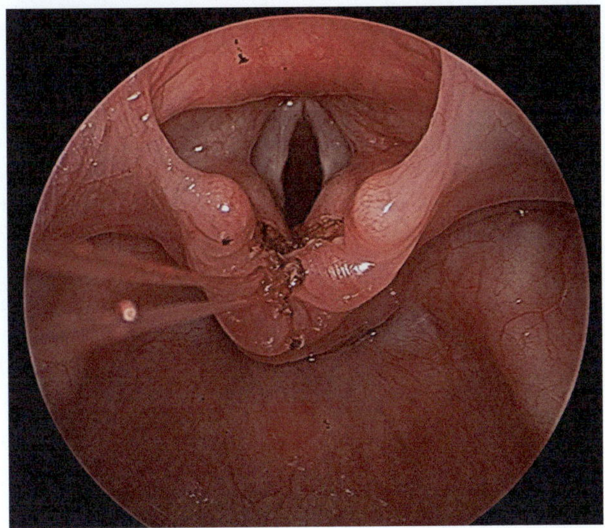

Fig. 14.4 Sutures closure of esophageal facing portion of interarytenoid defect

become a guide for possible augmentation even in normal anatomy, as opposed to the traditional definition and physical findings of a true laryngeal cleft [2]. Some otolaryngologists have added the subclassification of "low interarytenoid height" to their investigation when examining those patients that have this pattern of aspiration but don't fully fit the classification of a type 1 laryngeal cleft [11].

Recent data and research examining laryngeal cleft and interarytenoid augmentation for patients with swallowing disorders related to this region have been favorable regardless the presence of a true cleft or not [2, 11]. In one study, a significant portion of patients with normal anatomy but chronic aspiration benefitted from injection of augmentin to the interarytenoid region [2]. Also, when compared to those with LC-1, patients with normal anatomy had longer-lasting and better results after augmentation [2]. These findings, though more recent and still being examined, have many examining laryngeal clefts now as functional and/or anatomical as opposed to traditional anatomical classification. Consequently, pediatric otolaryngologists are beginning to treat the pattern of swallowing disorder over the anatomical findings alone. It is the authors' practice to follow this algorithm of treatment and let the pattern of the swallowing disorder determine our management.

Laryngeal clefts are more frequently seen in patients with Opitz G/BBB syndrome, Pallister-Hall syndrome, VACTERL/VATER association, and CHARGE syndrome. These children often have underlying neurological conditions, which along with the laryngeal cleft, can lead to complex dysphagia. When treating patients with neurological conditions and laryngeal clefts, FEES becomes an even more important tool in management. It is the authors' practice to evaluate all of these children with both FEES and MBS to get a complete assessment of swallowing. If interarytenoid patterns of aspiration/ penetration are seen as well as diffuse translaryngeal aspiration/penetration and/or other motor related dysphagia, the option of laryngeal repair is given. Educating the caregivers on expectations is key with these patients as in our experience, the success rate is lower and repair of the interarytenoid region may only be partially effective. We often combine this with intense occupational and speech therapy.

Conclusion

With the increase of multidisciplinary clinics and informed parents and physicians, the incidence of type 1 laryngeal cleft has increased considerably [7, 11, 12]. As awareness of pediatric swallowing disorders has became more prevalent, the diagnosis and treatment of LCs have also increased. With this, new research into interarytenoid augmentation for functional patterns of swallowing disorders over just anatomical has gained interest. Research on the success of both injection laryngoplasty and endoscopic surgical repair has demonstrated promising results [2, 7, 11, 12].

References

1. Parsons DS, Stivers FE, Giovanetto DR, Phillips SE. Type I posterior laryngeal clefts. Laryngoscope. 1998;108:403–10.
2. Horn DL, DeMarre K, Parikh SR. Interarytenoid sodium carboxymethylcellulose gel injection for management of pediatric aspiration. Ann Otol Rhinol Laryngol. 2014;123:852–8.
3. Benjamin B, Inglis A. Minor congenital laryngeal clefts: diagnosis and classification. Ann Otol Rhinol Laryngol. 1989;98:417–20.
4. Beer S, Hartlieb T, Muller A, Granel M, Staudt M. Aspiration in children and adolescents with neurogenic dysphagia: comparison of clinical judgment and fiberoptic endoscopic evaluation of swallowing. Neuropediatrics. 2014;45:402–5.
5. Moungthong G, Holinger LD. Laryngotracheoesophageal clefts. Ann Otol Rhinol Laryngol. 1997;106:1002–11.

6. Eriksen C, Zwillenberg D, Robinson N. Diagnosis and management of cleft larynx. Literature review and case report. Ann Otol Rhinol Laryngol. 1990;99:703–8.
7. Thottam PJ, Georg M, Chi D, Mehta DK. Outcomes and predictors of surgical management in type 1 laryngeal cleft swallowing dysfunction. Laryngoscope. 2016;126:2838–43.
8. Leishman C, Monnier P, Jaquet Y. Endoscopic repair of laryngotracheoesophageal clefts: experience in 17 cases. Int J Pediatr Otorhinolaryngol. 2014;78:227–31.
9. Adil E, Al Shemari H, Rahbar R. Endoscopic surgical repair of type 3 laryngeal clefts. JAMA Otolaryngol Head Neck Surg. 2014;140:1051–5.
10. Leonardis RL, Duvvuri U, Mehta D. Transoral robotic-assisted laryngeal cleft repair in the pediatric patient. Laryngoscope. 2014;124:2167–9.
11. Jefferson ND, Carmel E, Cheng AT. Low inter-arytenoid height: a subclassification of type 1 laryngeal cleft diagnosis and management. Int J Pediatr Otorhinolaryngol. 2015;79:31–5.
12. Johnston DR, Watters K, Ferrari LR, Rahbar R. Laryngeal cleft: evaluation and management. Int J Pediatr Otorhinolaryngol. 2014;78:905–11.

Chapter 15
Laryngomalacia, Supraglottoplasty, and Feeding and Swallowing Disorders: Is There An Association?

Hamdy El-Hakim, Andre Isaac, and Wendy Johannsen

Introduction

Laryngomalacia (LM) is a commonly encountered entity in infants and children with stridor and other upper aerodigestive symptoms [1]. Although the presentation and functional deficits encompass stridor, cyanotic spells, failure to thrive, and feeding and swallowing disorders (FSD), traditionally, the main focus had been on the respiratory impairment. The earlier and majority of the literature has been concerned mainly with the most severe cases whose life or thriving was at risk and the assessment of surgical success to relieve them [2]. Later research examined the association of LM with sleep-disordered breathing (SDB) [3], and only relatively recently has interest been directed toward the impact of FSD.

This may have been in part due to the increase in active collaboration of pediatric otolaryngologists with the speech and language pathologists in the management of FSD. The innovation of fiberoptic endoscopic evaluation of swallowing (FEES) in the 1990s most certainly defined further the role of the laryngologist in that process [4]. However since research in pediatric FSD as a whole has been lagging behind [5], progress on that front has been relatively slow.

For the purpose of this review, we shall attempt to explore the information pertinent to the association between LM and its surgical treatment on one hand and FSD.

H. El-Hakim (✉)
Department of Surgery, Stollery Children's Hospital, Edmonton, AB, Canada
e-mail: Hamdy.elhakim@ahs.ca

A. Isaac
Otolaryngology-Head and Neck Surgery, Stollery Children's Hospital, Edmonton, AB, Canada
e-mail: aisaac@ualberta.ca

W. Johannsen
Speech and Audiology, Stollery Children's Hospital, Edmonton, AB, Canada
e-mail: wendy.johannsen@ahs.ca

© Springer International Publishing AG, part of Springer Nature 2018
J. Ongkasuwan, E. H. Chiou (eds.), *Pediatric Dysphagia*,
https://doi.org/10.1007/978-3-319-97025-7_15

Legitimate questions include:

- Is there a relation between LM and FSD? Is the relation etiological, consequential, or simply overlap of prevalence? Is the relationship discernible from the confounding comorbidities that may affect feeding and swallowing?
- Is there a relationship between supraglottoplasty and FSD? Does the former effectively treat the latter as part of managing LM? Can surgery cause new-onset FSD? Are there differences between techniques of surgery?

Laryngomalacia and Feeding and Swallowing Disorders

There are several mechanisms that may furnish a basis for a relation between LM and FSD. These are, namely, epidemiological variables, potential pathophysiological mechanisms, and etiologic factors and associations. We shall discuss these individually and also probe whether the literature provides some proof for an existing association.

Epidemiologic Characteristics

With the provision that LM is a distinct structural entity and FSD is a symptom complex, the epidemiology of both is poorly documented [2, 6]. However, there is good ground indicating that both are commonly encountered in the general population, which gives credence to the possibility of coexistence by mere chance in a substantial number of patients. For instance, in a large cohort study (*n* of 128) at our center, we identified that LM was the commonest structural airway diagnosis (26%) among non-neurologically impaired children presenting with FSD [7].

Despite the significant academic output on the surgical treatment of LM, there have been a much smaller number of large cross-sectional or longitudinal cohort studies describing its epidemiological features [2]. A systematic review in 2016 performed by Isaac et al. came to the conclusion that the common belief in spontaneous resolution of LM and its symptoms actually rested on very weak evidence [2]. We shall next comment on the documentation of symptoms of FSD in cohort studies of LM.

Using an updated search of the literature used for the referenced review, we examined the documentation of FSD among infants in children with LM in cohort studies. In a large cohort study, Thompson in 2007 reported that among 223 infants with congenital LM 71.5% presented with feeding difficulties, but the author did not specify a particular protocol for assessment of the patients nor indicated the type of feeding difficulty [8]. In 2012, Wright and Goudy reported a significantly smaller number of patients with feeding difficulties at baseline (16 patients only), in a 115 strong patient study (again with no mention of methods of assessment) [9]. There are, however, two studies that executed a more systematic evaluation of FSD among LM patients. The first is by Cooper et al. who found that through a combination of clinical assessment ($n = 56$) and VFSS ($n = 32$), they elicited abnormalities in 60 (68%) out of 88 patients, approaching the prevalence figure of Thompson [10]. They specified that 21 patients aspirated, and 8 had demonstrated penetration. The second study is probably the only one that sets its primary objective to investigate FSD in patients with LM. Simons et al. reported that symptoms of FSD were documented in nearly half of their cohort (163/324) [11]. Swallowing was assessed clinically in 53, VFSS in 72, and FEES in 130 patients. Interestingly, they claimed that at least one abnormal swallowing assessment was present in 97/120 (80.8%) patients who were symptomatic and in 43/65 (66.2%) patients who actually were not. Overall, 140/185 had at least one abnormal evaluation, thereby approaching the figure reported by Cooper et al. despite admitting they did not evaluate all the cohort nor in a homogenous fashion.

Etiology, Pathogenesis, and Associations

It is quite plausible that some relation or association exists between LM and FSD since both encompass some alteration of suck, swallow, and breath pattern in infants as indeed would any compromise in the large airways (e.g., subglottic stenosis, tracheomalacia, or bronchomalacia). This would be in line with the anatomical theory attempting to explain LM, which then would imply there is a correlation between the severities of both conditions. Thompson demonstrated that patients with moderate and severe LM choked and coughed while eating in 100% and 89%, respectively, whereas those with the mild condition did so in 55.1% only [8]. She also documented, separately, that feeding difficulties occurred in the moderate and severe disease in 93.7% and 91.7%, respectively, as opposed to 39.7% in the mild form. This observation was not replicated by Simons et al., and perhaps the explanation rests with the different definitions of FSD and the methods used to detect them in both papers [11]. In effect at this point in time, there is no proven or reproducible relation between the severity or magnitude of LM and FSD.

But since the etiology and comorbid factors associated with LM remain highly controversial and topical, the relation may have an alternative basis. Gastroesophageal reflux disease (GERD) has been proposed as a cause for dysphagia or FSD, although emerging evidence casts doubt about that in children and actually points that eosinophilic esophagitis (which is not uncommonly confused with GERD) is a more likely culprit. GERD still enjoys a significant interest in LM research. The specific relations studied were, namely, the prevalence of GERD among LM patients, its contribution as a cofactor in the severity of LM symptoms, the improvement imparted by anti-reflux therapy on these symptoms, and the etiological relation between the two conditions. Fortunately, the literature was systematically assessed in 2012 [12]. Overall the meta-analysis documented a prevalence of 59% in LM patients from 25 studies (*n* of 1295 patients). Out of these studies, four documented the prevalence of GERD in patients with other airway diagnoses, which turned out not to be different from that with LM. Upon stratifying the data by severity of LM, GERD was found to be more prevalent in the severe form (OR 9.86, *P* < 0.0001) compared to the mild one. The remaining evidence was inconclusive for the benefit of anti-reflux treatment, and there was no basis for an etiological relationship. This meta-analysis acknowledged the significant heterogeneity between the studies, low quality due to methodological flaws, and variable definition of GERD diagnosis. These studies also included children with multiple comorbidities. Thus, the role of the associated GERD with LM on FSD is hard to establish.

The etiological theory, which rests on some sound scientific basis, is based on altered sensorimotor integrative function. In her Triological thesis, Thompson studied systematically a large cohort of patients (*n* of 223), both retro- and prospectively, and after testing 134 children, she found that the laryngeal adductor reflex was impaired in proportion to the severity of LM and to the presence of comorbidity (specifically the presence of GERD) [8]. The impairment also improved commensurate with resolution of symptoms, whether spontaneously or after treatment. Ulualp et al. tested the laryngopharyngeal sensory threshold of 40 children and reviewed the data retrospectively [13]. The group came to the conclusion that abnormal swallowing parameters were more common among children and infants with abnormal laryngeal adductor reflex and that most children with swallowing abnormalities had an abnormal reflex. In adults, the threshold of the laryngeal adductor reflex has been claimed to correlate with the presence of dysphagia and GERD, although the agreement between sensory testing and that of objective swallowing assessment is not straightforward [14, 15]. Work on pediatric patients is very scarce in this area, but the principle that the test may be a surrogate for swallowing impairment is an attractive and scientifically attractive idea [16].

Most of the aforementioned sources from the literature reported on cohorts with a significant proportion of patients with comorbid factors that may affect FSD such as GERD, prematurity at birth, hypotonia, neurologic conditions, syndromes, and cardiac disease. As such one cannot imagine that these variables are not confounding the relationship between FSD and LM.

Currently there are no formal guidelines for assessing children with LM. However a group of experts (International Pediatric ORL Group – IPOG) recently advocated feeding and swallow assessment in children who manifest with cough, choking, regurgitation, feeding difficulties, or present with poor weight gain and/or failure to thrive [17]. The group also recommended evaluating children with evidence of aspiration or those who harbor a neurologic disease that may affect swallowing. They specifically supported undertaking a multidisciplinary process including a speech and language pathologist and a dietitian and considering instrumental assessment using VFSS and/or FEES. Lastly the recommendations also included considering acid suppression where penetration and/or aspiration was documented using objective measures.

Conclusion

The evidence points to a significant prevalence exceeding half of any consecutive cohort of patients with LM, regardless of the associated comorbid variables. This behooves us to at least screen regularly for FSD in this group of patients. Moreover, this problem can significantly affect the parents emotionally, as demonstrated in a quality of life study on LM patients [18]. Since most aspirating infants and children do so silently [7, 19, 20], we feel that the argument for resorting only to clinical assessment is a weak one and recourse to FEES or VFSS should be considered especially in this high-risk group. With respect to research into the topic, although it is feasible to stratify any given sizable cohort according to comorbid diagnoses that may affect feeding and swallowing, the single diagnosis that will prove difficult will be GERD given the prevalence and the fickle nature of proving the diagnosis beyond the shadow of doubt. But with this in mind, efforts should continue to clarify the pathogenesis of FSD associated with LM.

Supraglottoplasty and FSD

Supraglottoplasty (SGP), the endoscopic reference standard procedure for treating significant LM, has been widely claimed a consistently successful procedure [21]. Whereas its objectives have recently included correction of SDB [22], its original targets were the awake respiratory symptoms, cyanotic spells, and feeding difficulties. At this point in time, we have more literature on the surgery than the condition itself as previously alluded to.

Etiology/Mechanism

The relation between SGP and FSD could be *causative*, *coincidental*, or *a permutation* of both. Since the surgery interferes with supraglottic structures (aryepiglottic folds, supra-arytenoid tissue, glosso-epiglottic fold, and epiglottis or a permutation of the three) [23], it may affect even temporarily the sensory innervation from both the superior laryngeal and the recurrent laryngeal nerves, thereby interrupting the laryngeal adductor reflex [24]. According to individual preference, the surgeon may choose from a myriad of instruments (variety of lasers to cold steel and powered tools), and each will have a specific impact on the tissues which could affect the healing process in different ways. That may also predispose to supraglottic stenosis, which would compromise further the airway and negatively affect feeding and swallowing. The latter complication has been scarcely reported in the SGP literature and apparently may occur in 3.7% of cases [21], but even still without active search and proof of absence, it might be a variable to contend with. The coincidental relation is simply that the patient would harbor an unrelated etiology for the FSD (through an underlying comorbidity like neurological condition, esophagitis, etc.). This situation will only be ruled out if both the causative comorbidity and the status of feeding and swallowing are known and documented *before* the surgery is performed, and supraglottic stenosis is excluded postoperatively. In an effort to cater for comorbidities, Preciado and Zalzal undertook a systematic review (single search engine) to estimate surgical failure [21]. On the risk of aspiration postoperatively, the relative risk ratio for significant aspiration was 4.3 (95% CI 1.25–15.06), based on pooling data from three studies. The authors declared transparently that the literature used was heterogeneous in regard to the definition of failure, stratification of results by comorbidity, severity of LM, and instrument and techniques used and that the level of evidence generally was fairly low (level IV). We would add that there was no mention of the effect of concomitant secondary airway lesions nor other treatment of FSD that the systematic review objectives and inclusion criteria were actually less than well defined and that performing it on a single search engine limits its comprehensiveness.

There are no particular evidence-based guidelines for an evaluation process of feeding and swallowing for infants and children with LM before SGP. The IPOG recommendations indicate that candidates will, by proxy, require some form of assessment [17]; however postoperatively the paper did not push for a routine inquiry or tests for evaluating these problems. This likely reflects the current practice, as several large series of SGP did not specify pre- and/or postoperative prevalence of FSD nor the type of the problem, let alone the methods of assessment. It is not surprising then to notice that the baseline prevalence figures of FSD varied from 6% to 58%, reflecting heterogeneous, inconsistent processes [25–28], whereas Erickson et al., upon applying a fixed screening process to 90 patients, reported that 73 patients were symptomatic [29]. In that study, 67 were clinically assessed by SLP, and 30 had VFSS (30 had aspiration and 2 had penetration). These authors did not report objective postoperative data, unfortunately committing the same pervasive problem of retrospective studies.

However, there are several articles that set their objective to report on FSD after SGP. Two studies set out to confirm the effect of prematurity at birth on postoperative FSD. The first is by De Moreno and Matt who studied retrospectively 2360 patient charts, among whom 337 were premature, and stratified them by severity according to gestational age [30]. The authors excluded the patients who had evidence of aspiration before the operation but without specifying the method of assessment. Seventy-five patients aspirated postoperatively, 20 of whom were premature at birth and 55 were not. This left the prevalence rate at 5.9% for all the prematurely born, 2.7% for the term born, and 8.5% for the severely premature. The paper left some room for doubt as there was neither documentation nor calculations for any comorbid factors, and the authors never specified any protocols or basis for assessment and labeling the aspiration. Durvasula et al. tackled the same issue again in the same year [31]. The group compared the outcome after SGP of 40 prematurely born patients with 136 born at term. Their baseline dysphagia rates were 72% and 58.8%, respectively (statistically not significant), based on a definition that includes choking or cough during feeds, requirement for thickening oral liquids, penetration, or aspiration on VFSS. Postoperatively preterm patients were at 32.5% dysphagia rate as opposed to 6.6% (statistically significant) for the term born. The authors excluded all patients with other comorbid factors such as syndromes, neurological or cardiac conditions, and commendably documented the prevalence of other secondary airway lesions, which were more prevalent in the preterm group. Accordingly, although limited, the literature points that premature birth will predispose to residual FSD after SGP. Neither study suggested a new onset FSD.

The following analysis will concentrate on papers that addressed the issue of FSD following SGP be it residual or new onset. Schroeder et al. aimed at assessing postoperative aspiration and its risk factors after carbon dioxide laser techniques in 52 infants and children treated over 6 years [32]. They found that whereas 43 out of 52 did not have signs of aspiration before surgery, 37% aspirated postoperatively (out of these were 28% of the 43 who never had preoperative documentation of aspiration) and observed that the majority of those who aspirated preoperatively persistently did so postoperatively. All children were assessed before the operation *clinically* by SLP, and accordingly VFSS was recommended (only nine were performed). The newly diagnosed patients were treated (oral thickening or alternate route of feeding) for varying periods of time (up to 18 months). Synchronous secondary airway lesions were encountered in 58% of cases, and 14% were neurologically impaired. GERD was suspected in 79%. The authors noted that the swallowing status preoperatively was the main determinant for postoperative swallowing function. This assertion may not be fully vindicated owing to the sample size and the absence of preoperative testing on all the patients and multivariable analysis. But given the conditions of the practice, the message was actually an important call on the specialty to be alert to a significant clinical problem which may not only fail to resolve by the operation but also arise because of it. The question relating to whether the new onset FSD was related to the technique of the procedure also was raised. Subsequently, the same group published a retrospective review comparing cold steel and carbon dioxide laser [33]. They reported that new onset aspiration occurred in 3 out of 13 in the cold steel group versus 9 out of 16 in the laser group. The study however was underpowered to confirm the conclusion that the technique does not affect that outcome.

Following that, researchers from Cincinnati Children's Hospital reported on 50 of their patients who had undergone SGP over a period of 5 years [34]. The unique aspect of this work is the availability of pre- and postoperative objective swallowing assessment (FEES) which sets it aside from most other papers. Having demonstrated improvements in penetration (81.8%) and aspirations (86.1%) and the absence of new onset aspiration, the authors concluded that cold steel SGP is highly successful in achieving improvements in swallowing parameters and is safe to undertake with a minimal risk of postoperative aspiration. They also demonstrated a statistically significant improvement of the thresholds of the adductor reflex response. The caveat resides in two points. The first is the absence of data on the points in time of the pre- and postoperative testing and the concomitant medical treatment for GERD. This leaves some doubt on the true effective line of treatment, possibility of spontaneous resolution, and missing a new onset problem with swallowing that may have resolved before some of the FEES were done. One point worth noting is that despite the authors dividing their cohort by severity of LM using Thomson's description in 2007, they stated that the commonest reason for their intervention was swallowing and feeding problems.

Another series was published afterward (2011) from the United States on 75 infants who had undergone SGP over a 4-year period, examining the change in status of feeding and swallowing (specifically, nutritional intake and SLP reports to look for qualifications of feeding difficulties) [35]. In the abstract, the investigators' assertion was that 46 out of 48 patients had either an improvement or no deterioration of their oral intake status, with only two experiencing a transient deterioration which recovered within 2 months using conservative measures. In a subgroup of 27 infants who harbored other medical comorbidities (hydrocephalus, seizures, micrognathia, and others), 22% required other interventions as oral thickened feeds or alternate route of feeding. The subjection of the infants to objective assessment of swallowing (here specified as VFSS) was at the discretion of the surgeon and only if available and not overridden by urgency to control the airway distress. Unfortunately the results section did not include any details on the results of the VFSS.

Finally Chun and colleagues reported on 24 patients whom they qualified as normally developing infants and children without evidence of preoperative swallowing problems [36]. This group used two techniques, cold steel and carbon dioxide laser, according to the preference of the surgeon. Seventeen had clinical assessment for swallowing after surgery due to clinical concerns, and six exhibited clinical signs of swallowing dysfunction, ultimately three of which had undergone VFSS confirming aspiration. As stated by the authors, no children had undergone VFSS before surgery, and there was no comment on a screening process. The paper then asserts that the affected patients regained normal swallowing using a combination of conservative measures by the fourth week postoperatively.

Conclusion

SGP is usually performed on patients with significant LM. Given how prevalent FSD is among LM patients, we can deduce that these groups will harbor a higher risk. The literature implies that comorbid conditions like prematurity at birth, certain neurological diagnoses (not always specified), cardiac problems, and chromosomal abnormalities will be at a higher disadvantage preoperatively and might not be as hopeful for a resolution after surgery as their healthier counterparts. Otherwise healthy LM patients should be offered the possibility of improvement of the symptoms of feeding and swallowing difficulties, with the caveat that other variables may be at play and that those that are undergoing the surgery for breathing problems and sleep-disordered breathing may be at risk of acquiring some new difficulty after surgery albeit transiently. We cannot clearly decide at this point in time that certain techniques (steps or instruments) of SGP are riskier than others with respect to that or that certain steps of the surgery pose more likelihood of that development. With the ever-increasing indications for surgery, discussing FSD should be standard of practice.

Relevant Feeding and Swallowing Disorder Specifics

Earlier studies on LM and SGP grouped FSD under one topic: feeding difficulties. Later work used the term "dysphagia" more often. The parameters set to assess pre- and postoperatively are getting more specific, which is a healthy sign. Generally speaking, the terms feeding and swallowing are often used interchangeably; however, they can be more accurately separated into distinct issues where an infant or child can have one in the absence of the other. Upon quoting and analyzing the literature in this chapter, we have been careful to directly use the terms used in the individual papers. It is possible to see how difficult to compare or pool data concerning this subject.

Feeding disorders are defined as "problems in a broad range of eating activities that may or may not be accompanied by a difficulty with swallowing food or liquid." Swallowing disorders and dysphagia are synonymous terms. Dysphagia can occur in one or more phases of swallowing (oral, pharyngeal, and esophageal). Any disruption to any phase in swallowing can result in compromised airway protection [37].

The signs and symptoms of feeding and swallowing difficulties vary across developmental stages [38]. A feeding problem can exist without a swallowing problem, and sometimes a swallowing problem may be prevented if the feeding problem is addressed. For instance, an incorrect nipple shape and flow rate can cause a feeding problem, which can lead to a swallowing problem. An infant who is drinking from a nipple with a fast flow rate may have spillage from the lips, coughing, and increased work of breathing during feeding. Changing the nipple to a slower flow rate may eliminate the spillage from the lips. The infant would also be able to better coordinate his suck/swallow/breathe pattern resulting in less coughing. Feeding problems across ages can be characterized by lack of developmentally appropriate self-feeding skills, lengthy meal times, suboptimal weight gain and growth, selective eating, a restricted food repertoire, oral aversion, or food/liquid refusal. A learned aversion to eating due to an anatomical or functional disorder that may have made feeding difficult or uncomfortable may continue to persist even after the underlying problem is resolved. As such the community of pediatric otolaryngology should be more specific about the use of terms and methods of investigation in the future.

References

1. Holinger PH, Brown WT. Congenital webs, cysts, laryngoceles and other anomalies of the larynx. Ann Otol Rhinol Laryngol. 1967;76(4):744–52. https://doi.org/10.1177/000348946707600402.
2. Isaac A, Zhang H, Soon SR, Campbell S, El-Hakim H. A systematic review of the evidence on spontaneous resolution of laryngomalacia and its symptoms. Int J Pediatr Otorhinolaryngol. 2016;83:78–83. https://doi.org/10.1016/j.ijporl.2016.01.028.
3. Thevasagayam M, Rodger K, Cave D, Witmans M, El-Hakim H. Prevalence of laryngomalacia in children presenting with sleep-disordered breathing. Laryngoscope. 2010;120(8):1662–6. https://doi.org/10.1002/lary.21025.

4. Hartnick CJ, Miller C, Hartley BEJ, Willging JP. Pediatric fiberoptic endoscopic evaluation of swallowing. Ann Otol Rhinol Laryngol. 2000;109(11):996–9. https://doi.org/10.1177/000348940010901102.

5. Plowman EK, Mehdizadeh O, Leder SB, Martino R, Belafsky PC. A bibliometric review of published abstracts presented at the Dysphagia Research Society: 2001-2011. Dysphagia. 2013;28(2):123–30. https://doi.org/10.1007/s00455-012-9420-2.

6. Bhattacharyya N. The prevalence of pediatric voice and swallowing problems in the United States. Laryngoscope. 2015;125(3):746–50. https://doi.org/10.1002/lary.24931.

7. Svystun O, Johannsen W, Persad R, Turner JM, Majaesic C, El-Hakim H. Dysphagia in healthy children: characteristics and management of a consecutive cohort at a tertiary centre. Int J Pediatr Otorhinolaryngol. 2017;99:54–9. https://doi.org/10.1016/j.ijporl.2017.05.024.

8. Thompson DM. Abnormal sensorimotor integrative function of the larynx in congenital laryngomalacia: a new theory of etiology. Laryngoscope. 2007;117:1–33. https://doi.org/10.1097/MLG.0b013e31804a5750.

9. Wright CT, Goudy SL. Congenital laryngomalacia: symptom duration and need for surgical intervention. Ann Otol Rhinol Laryngol. 2012;121:57–60. https://doi.org/10.1016/j.otohns.2009.06.308.

10. Cooper T, Benoit M, Erickson B, El-Hakim H. Primary presentations of laryngomalacia. JAMA Otolaryngol Head Neck Surg. 2014;140:521–6. https://doi.org/10.1001/jamaoto.2014.626.

11. Simons JP, Greenberg LL, Mehta DK, Fabio A, Maguire RC, Mandell DL. Laryngomalacia and swallowing function in children. Laryngoscope. 2015;126:478–84. https://doi.org/10.1002/lary.25440.

12. Hartl TT, Chadha NK. A systematic review of laryngomalacia and acid reflux. Otolaryngol Head Neck Surg. 2012;147:619–26. https://doi.org/10.1177/0194599812452833.

13. Ulualp S, Brown A, Sanghavi R, Rivera-Sanchez Y. Assessment of laryngopharyngeal sensation in children with dysphagia. Laryngoscope. 2013;123(9):2291–5. https://doi.org/10.1002/lary.24024.

14. Aviv JE, Spitzer J, Cohen M, Ma G, Belafsky PC, Close LG. Laryngeal adductor reflex and pharyngeal squeeze as predictors of laryngeal penetration and aspiration. Laryngoscope. 2002;112(2):338–41. https://doi.org/10.1097/00005537-200202000-00025.

15. Phua SY, McGarvey LPA, Ngu MC, Ing AJ. Patients with gastro-oesophageal reflux disease and cough have impaired laryngopharyngeal mechanosensitivity. Thorax. 2005;60(6):488–91. https://doi.org/10.1136/thx.2004.033894.

16. Tabaee A, Johnson PE, Gartner CJ, Kalwerisky K, Desloge RB, Stewart MG. Patient-controlled comparison of flexible endoscopic evaluation of swallowing with sensory testing (FEESST) and videofluoroscopy. Laryngoscope. 2006;116(5):821–5. https://doi.org/10.1097/01.mlg.0000214670.40604.45.

17. Carter J, Rahbar R, Brigger M, et al. International Pediatric ORL Group (IPOG) laryngomalacia consensus recommendations. Int J Pediatr Otorhinolaryngol. 2016;86:256–61. https://doi.org/10.1016/j.ijporl.2016.04.007.

18. Thottam PJ, Simons JP, Choi S, Maguire R, Mehta DK. Clinical relevance of quality of life in laryngomalacia. Laryngoscope. 2016;126(5):1232–5. https://doi.org/10.1002/lary.25491.

19. Lefton-Greif MA, Carroll JL, Loughlin GM. Long-term follow-up of oropharyngeal dysphagia in children without apparent risk factors. Pediatr Pulmonol. 2006;41(11):1040–8. https://doi.org/10.1002/ppul.20488.

20. Sheikh S, Allen E, Shell R, et al. Chronic aspiration without gastroesophageal reflux as a cause of chronic respiratory symptoms in neurologically normal infants. Chest. 2001;120(4):1190–5. https://doi.org/10.1378/chest.120.4.1190.

21. Preciado D, Zalzal G. A systematic review of supraglottoplasty outcomes. Arch Otolaryngol Head Neck Surg. 2012;138(8):718–21. https://doi.org/10.1001/archoto.2012.1251.

22. White DR. Is supraglottoplasty underutilized? Laryngoscope. 2012;122(Suppl 4(S4)):S91–2. https://doi.org/10.1002/lary.23810.

23. Zalzal GH, Collins WO. Microdebrider-assisted supraglottoplasty. Int J Pediatr Otorhinolaryngol. 2005;69(3):305–9. https://doi.org/10.1016/j.ijporl.2004.10.009.
24. Olthoff A, Schiel R, Kruse E. The supraglottic nerve supply: an anatomic study with clinical implications. Laryngoscope. 2007;117(11):1930–3. https://doi.org/10.1097/MLG.0b013e318123f2e7.
25. Douglas CM, Shafi A, Higgins G, et al. Risk factors for failure of supraglottoplasty. Int J Pediatr Otorhinolaryngol. 2014;78(9):1485–8. https://doi.org/10.1016/j.ijporl.2014.06.014.
26. Toynton SC, Saunders MW, Bailey CM. Aryepiglottoplasty for laryngomalacia: 100 consecutive cases. J Laryngol Otol. 2001;115(1):35–8. https://doi.org/10.1258/0022215011906966.
27. Reddy DK, Matt BH. Unilateral vs. bilateral supraglottoplasty for severe laryngomalacia in children. Arch Otolaryngol Head Neck Surg. 2001;127(6):694–9. https://doi.org/10.1097/00132586-200204000-00032.
28. Whymark AD, Clement WA, Kubba H, Geddes NK. Laser epiglottopexy for laryngomalacia: 10 years' experience in the west of Scotland. Arch Otolaryngol Head Neck Surg. 2006;132(9):978–82. https://doi.org/10.1001/archotol.132.9.978.
29. Erickson B, Cooper T, El-Hakim H. Factors associated with the morphological type of laryngomalacia and prognostic value for surgical outcomes. JAMA Otolaryngol Head Neck Surg. 2014;140(10):927–33. https://doi.org/10.1001/jamaoto.2014.1843.
30. De Moreno LCA, Matt BH. The effects of prematurity on incidence of aspiration following supraglottoplasty for laryngomalacia. Laryngoscope. 2014;124(3):777–80. https://doi.org/10.1002/lary.21855.
31. Durvasula VSPB, Lawson BR, Bower CM, Richter GT. Supraglottoplasty in premature infants with laryngomalacia: does gestation age at birth influence outcomes? Otolaryngol Head Neck Surg. 2014;150(2):292–9. https://doi.org/10.1177/0194599813514370.
32. Schroeder JW, Thakkar KH, Poznanovic SA, Holinger LD. Aspiration following CO_2 laser-assisted supraglottoplasty. Int J Pediatr Otorhinolaryngol. 2008;72(7):985–90. https://doi.org/10.1016/j.ijporl.2008.03.007.
33. Rastatter JC, Schroeder JW, Hoff SR, Holinger LD. Aspiration before and after supraglottoplasty regardless of technique. Int J Otolaryngol. 2010;2010:912814. https://doi.org/10.1155/2010/912814.
34. Richter GT, Wootten CT, Rutter MJ, Thompson DM. Impact of supraglottoplasty on aspiration in severe laryngomalacia. Ann Otol Rhinol Laryngol. 2009;118(4):259–66. https://doi.org/10.1177/000348940911800404.
35. Eustaquio M, Lee EN, Digoy GP. Feeding outcomes in infants after supraglottoplasty. Dysphagia. 2012;27(3):442. https://doi.org/10.1007/s00455-012-9400-6.
36. Chun RH, Wittkopf M, Sulman C, Arvedson J. Transient swallowing dysfunction in typically developing children following supraglottoplasty for laryngomalacia. Int J Pediatr Otorhinolaryngol. 2014;78(11):1883–5. https://doi.org/10.1016/j.ijporl.2014.08.017.
37. American Speech-Language-Hearing Association. Feeding and swallowing disorders (dysphagia) in children. 2017. http://www.asha.org/public/speech/swallowing/Feeding-and-Swallowing-Disorders-in-Children/. Accessed 4 Aug 2017.
38. Arvedson JC. Assessment of pediatric dysphagia and feeding disorders: clinical and instrumental approaches. Dev Disabil Res Rev. 2008;14(2):118–27. https://doi.org/10.1002/ddrr.17.

Chapter 16
Vocal Fold Paralysis and Dysphagia: Challenges and Controversies

Ryan Belcher and Nikhila Raol

Introduction

The term vocal fold paralysis (VFP) has a spectrum of entities within literature that describe vocal fold motion impairment, including vocal fold immobility, adductor or abductor paralysis, and vocal fold paresis [1]. VFP is known to be a major cause of voice impairment, dysphagia, and respiratory problems. The degree by which these are manifested often depends on whether the patient has unilateral VFP or bilateral VFP, as well as etiology of the VFP, patient age, and other patient characteristics. While the majority of pediatric studies that have focused on the management of VFP have emphasized respiratory and voice outcomes, dysphagia and impaired swallowing function are important consequences of VFP. It is likely that the prevalence numbers for pediatric dysphagia are not accurately represented in the literature and that only a small fraction of the affected children receive services for their swallowing difficulties [2]. This chapter looks to describe the relationship between VFP and dysphagia in the pediatric patient, focusing specifically on the challenges the otolaryngologist faces in the workup and management of this entity.

R. Belcher (✉)
Otolaryngology-Head and Neck Surgery, Vanderbilt University School of Medicine, Children's Hospital at Vanderbilt, Nashville, TN, USA
e-mail: ryan.belcher@vumc.org

N. Raol
Otolaryngology-Head and Neck Surgery, Emory University School of Medicine, Children's Healthcare of Atlanta, Atlanta, GA, USA
e-mail: npraol@emory.edu

© Springer International Publishing AG, part of Springer Nature 2018
J. Ongkasuwan, E. H. Chiou (eds.), *Pediatric Dysphagia*,
https://doi.org/10.1007/978-3-319-97025-7_16

Epidemiology

It has been estimated that VFP, both unilateral and bilateral, represents roughly 10% of all congenital laryngeal lesions [3]. Both sexes are equally affected, and these children generally present before 2 years of age. Bilateral VFP has been reported to encompass between 30% and 62% of the VFP cases, [4] although the incidence of unilateral VFP is also increased at pediatric centers with pediatric cardiothoracic surgery. VFP is behind only laryngomalacia as the most common cause of neonatal stridor [5, 6]. With improved technology and advances in practice over the years, VFP is being diagnosed more accurately and frequently. Bilateral VFP patients most commonly present with dyspnea and stridor, and the airway becomes the primary focus of the management of these patients, though they may also have impairments of swallow function and voice. Unilateral VFP children are more likely to present with voice and swallowing problems than dyspnea, but both of these patient groups have additional morbidity due to their aspiration and dysphagia risk, with loss of airway protective mechanisms, including decreased laryngopharyngeal sensation and impaired glottal closure [7].

More than 500,000 children in the United States are diagnosed with dysphagia each year, although this is likely an underestimation of the true burden as parent reporting may not always be accurate, and it has been shown less than 25% of parents seek medical help for this issues [2]. The downstream effects of dysphagia with or without VFP can be significant including the need for gastrostomy tube in some patients. It has been shown the need for gastrostomy tube placement in patients with VFP ranges from 15% to 63% [8–11]. While gastrostomy tubes carry their own risk to the patients, they are also burdensome to the caregivers, as they have been shown to have a much lower quality of life and increased rates of depression [12]. This again highlights one of the many challenges otolaryngologists face when managing pediatric patients with VFP.

Presentation and Workup

Identifying the underlying etiology of VFP is essential and can often dictate the management of the patient. Although children and adults have some overlapping etiologies of VFP, including trauma, neoplasms, or neurologic causes, their frequencies and rates of incidence vary significantly. Previous studies have shown idiopathic causes [13] and iatrogenic trauma from cardiothoracic surgery as two of the most common etiologies of VFP in the pediatric population [11, 14]. The large majority of etiologies for VFP are encompassed by two broad categories: congenital and acquired. Table 16.1 summarizes the etiologies of VFP. The discussion and nuances of each etiology are beyond the scope of this chapter, but specific etiologies will be discussed in further detail later in the chapter in regard to their impact on the management.

Table 16.1 Etiologies of vocal fold paralysis in pediatric population

(I) Acquired
(A) Trauma
(a) Birth injury (e.g., forceps delivery)
(b) Iatrogenic via surgical correction of cardiovascular or esophageal abnormality
(c) Intubation related
(d) Vagal nerve stimulator
(e) Foreign body ingestion
(f) Thyroid surgery
(B) Infections
(a) Guillain-Barré syndrome
(b) Diphtheria
(c) Rabies
(d) Tetanus
(e) Syphilis
(f) Tuberculosis
(g) Botulism
(h) Pertussis encephalitis
(i) Polyneuritis
(j) Polioencephalitis
(C) Neurotoxicity
(a) Vincristine
(II) Inherited
(A) Genetic
(a) Isolated mutation
(b) Autosomal dominant
(c) Autosomal recessive
(d) X-linked
(B) Associated neurologic disease
(a) Charcot-Marie-Tooth disease
(III) Congenital
(A) Peripheral nervous system
(a) Congenital myasthenia gravis
(b) Skull base platybasia
(B) Central nervous system
(a) Meningocele
(b) Meningomyelocele
(c) Arnold-Chiari malformation
(d) Hydrocephalus
(e) Encephalocele
(f) Cerebral agenesis
(g) Nucleus ambiguous dysgenesis

(continued)

Table 16.1 (continued)

(C) Cardiovascular anomalies
(a) Patent ductus arteriosus
(b) Transposition of the great vessels
(c) Vascular ring
(d) Tetralogy of Fallot
(e) Dilated aorta
(f) Double aortic arch
(g) Interventricular septal defect
(D) Associated with other congenital anomalies
(a) Cricopharyngeal stenosis
(b) Esophageal cyst, duplication, atresia
(c) Bronchogenic cyst

Presentation

The signs and symptoms of unilateral or bilateral VFP in a pediatric patient are variable, given the range of effects of an abnormally functioning larynx. Due to their broad presentation of symptoms, the correct diagnosis of VFP is often not made for weeks or months, with symptoms attributed to other respiratory disorders including recurrent croup or asthma [15]. Symptoms of unilateral or bilateral VFP in children include stridor, dysphagia, aspiration, dysphonia, respiratory distress, apnea, ineffective cough, abnormal cry, among others [5, 6, 11]. There are notable differences in presentation between bilateral and unilateral VFP. In bilateral VFP the child's voice or cry is often near normal because his/her vocal folds are typically in a paramedian position. Respiratory symptoms are often much more severe in bilateral VFP cases, including persistent stridor, dyspnea, apneas, or cyanosis [16]. In contrast, unilateral VFP cases are more likely to present with dysphonia, including abnormal cry, breathiness of the voice, or decreased ability to project [16].

Dysphagia is prevalent in both populations of VFP with presenting symptoms including aspiration pneumonia, choking or coughing with feeds, or tachypnea with feeds. The index of suspicion should be high, and threshold for intervention should be low in these children, as a study of children with unilateral VFP suggests that even when aspiration is not seen on modified barium swallow (MBS), children with VFP are still at risk for aspiration pneumonia [14]. There have not been any studies to date that have investigated the discrete differences in dysphagia, aspiration rates, or components of the swallowing mechanisms between unilateral or bilateral VFP.

Workup

Given the wide variety of symptoms with which a child with VFP can present, a thorough history and physical are of utmost importance. During the evaluation of the child, it is important to note presence and degree of stridor, any abnormalities in their cry or voice, respiratory issues including retractions or tachypnea, and any feeding difficulties. Elicited history should including previous surgeries, particularly cardiac, neck, posterior fossa, or pulmonary surgeries. Other information that should be garnered includes the presence of neurologic disorders, congenital heart disease, congenital anomalies, and, although rare, any history of familial VFP [17].

In cases in which the etiology of the VFP is unclear or unknown, the focus should be on the anatomy of the child, including the brainstem, mediastinum, and vagus nerve (including the recurrent laryngeal nerves) [18]. Dedicated imaging should be performed for these structures, specifically computerized tomography (CT), which is preferred for the neck and chest. Magnetic resonance imaging (MRI) is preferred for the skull base, brain, and brainstem, as it can detect anatomical abnormalities of the brainstem, such as Arnold-Chiari malformation.

The otolaryngologist has a variety of tools at his/her disposal with which to evaluate the larynx and to identify and document VFP, including flexible laryngoscopy, rigid stroboscopy, direct laryngoscopy under general anesthesia, ultrasound, and pulmonary function tests [19–21]. The ideal examination is performed, while the patient is awake to fully assess vocal fold mobility, and flexible laryngoscopy has become the standard procedure for assessment (Fig. 16.1). Despite the advances in technology, evaluation of an infant or small child's larynx may be challenging due to edema, frequent laryngeal movement due to rapid respirations, copious secretions, or concomitant laryngomalacia. Therefore, the addition of the ability to record the examination with playback features that can slow down the video makes flexible laryngoscopy that much more valuable [19].

Laryngeal ultrasound to assess VFP has shown promise in its utility, particularly in low-resource settings where flexible laryngoscopy may not be available. A study comparing diagnosis of VFP with laryngeal ultrasound to direct laryngoscopy with

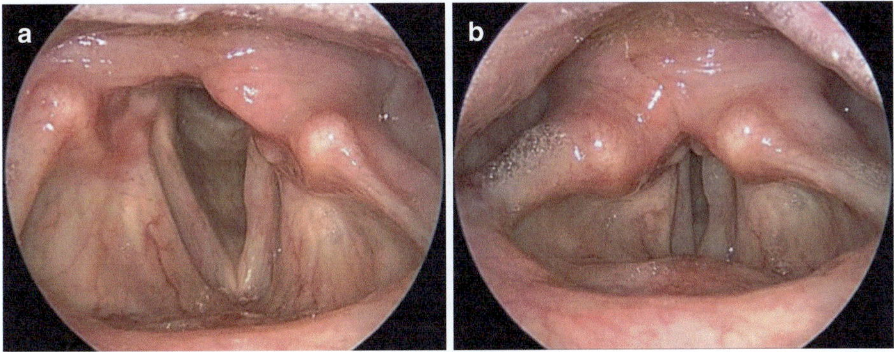

Fig. 16.1 Vocal fold paralysis as seen on flexible fiberoptic nasolaryngoscopy. (**a**) Left vocal fold paralysis results in a shortened and flaccid vocal fold, as compared to the right side during abduction. (**b**) Incomplete glottal closure is seen with adduction, as the left vocal fold remains in the paramedian position. This allows for a gap, resulting in dysphagia and potential aspiration with various consistencies of food/liquid

anesthesia found a concordance rate of 88.2% for unilateral VFP and 82.1% for bilateral VFP [21]. Transcutaneous laryngeal ultrasound can also be used in addition to or in lieu of flexible laryngoscopy to screen for VFP in challenging cases, thus avoiding the hemodynamic changes that may occur in children who do not tolerate flexible laryngoscopy well, as well as potentially avoiding the need for direct laryngoscopy with anesthesia [22]. The relative ease of operating an ultrasound machine and of learning the necessary technique to diagnose VFP makes the ultrasound an attractive option. The laryngeal anatomy of children makes them more ideal candidates for evaluation of VFP with laryngeal ultrasound compared to adults, given their lack of calcification of thyroid cartilage and shorter distance of ultrasound probe to the posterior larynx [22, 23]. Further studies are warranted to confirm its utility.

In certain instances, direct laryngoscopy and bronchoscopy under anesthesia are warranted to fully evaluate a child's larynx and confirm the diagnosis of VFP after noninvasive workup has been completed. Obtaining the appropriate anesthetic plane to evaluate vocal fold motion and the entire airway is of utmost importance with this procedure, so the assistance of a well-trained pediatric anesthesiologist is a necessity. Evaluation in the operating room is also recommended if other airway pathology is suspected, cases involving endolaryngeal trauma or endotracheal intubation, or bilateral VFP. If endolaryngeal trauma or endotracheal intubation is the suspected etiology of VFP, evaluation for cricoarytenoid fixation and posterior glottal stenosis is critical. Operative examination also provides the otolaryngologist with the ability to evaluate the larynx in children with concomitant feeding difficulties. Palpation for a laryngeal cleft, evaluation for tracheoesophageal fistula, or other laryngeal abnormalities is recommended. Assessment of the airway with direct laryngoscopy and bronchoscopy is also indicated in instances where children with suspected VFP cannot be examined at bedside or in the clinic with flexible laryngoscopy due to intolerance of exam, which may be behavioral or physiologic in nature.

Pediatric VFP patients will often have feeding difficulties at the time of diagnosis. While the airway should be the key focus on initial evaluation, dysphagia adds further morbidity to these patients, and swallowing function studies should be considered as an important and crucial component in the evaluation. Both a modified barium swallow (MBS) test and functional endoscopic evaluation of swallow (FEES) are commonly used studies to evaluate swallowing. An MBS can be helpful in characterizing dysphagia, as it can confirm the presence of aspiration, as well as help identify strategies to manage and prevent aspiration (Fig. 16.2). The information gained from an MBS can help determine the need for altering the rate of feeding and texture of feeds to improve the dysphagia or avoid aspiration and its associated complications [14]. Associated mediastinal anomalies, including vascular rings, can also be identified with an MBS. A FEES using the flexible laryngoscope is another option for evaluating swallowing in pediatric patients. Compared to an MBS, a FEES is able to examine swallowing function with multiple food/liquid consistencies, evaluate laryngeal sensation, and has no exposure to radiation. While it cannot distinguish penetration from aspiration due to a white out of

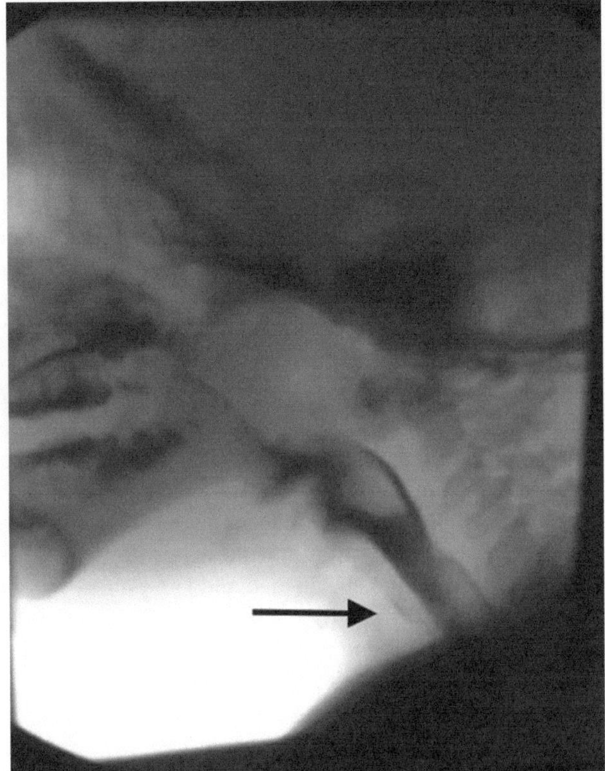

Fig. 16.2 Modified barium swallow demonstrating aspiration into the airway, as noted by the arrow. This can indicate incomplete glottal closure, as can be seen with unilateral vocal fold paralysis

the screen during swallowing, it can give more information regarding the path taken by the food/liquid, thereby giving more detail regarding the etiology of aspiration.

Another confirmatory test for unilateral or bilateral VFP that has been used more frequently in recent years is laryngeal electromyography (EMG). It is especially useful prior to performing a more permanent procedure such as laryngeal reinnervation or thyroplasty, although it does not seem to have much utility in predicting return of function in congenital VFP [24, 25]. In adults, this procedure is often performed in the awake setting, while in children, it typically requires a general anesthetic and is carried out at the time of endoscopy.

Management

Decisions for management strategies are multifactorial in children with VFP. Each case is unique, including their etiology, severity of symptoms, comorbidities, and whether there is unilateral or bilateral involvement. Obtaining and maintaining a safe and stable airway is universally agreed upon as top priority in these patients, especially if they present in respiratory distress. Other goals in management to be considered include the preservation and possible improvement of speech or voice and improving swallowing function. The management strategy for bilateral vs. unilateral VFP can also differ drastically.

The etiology of the VFP plays a large role in deciding how to manage the patient and especially on timing of interventions. Should the child have a progressive neuromuscular disease process, the spontaneous recovery from paralysis is much less likely than a child that has spontaneous idiopathic unilateral VFP. Children who present with bilateral VFP should be evaluated for a meningomyelocele or Arnold-Chiari malformation before decision is made whether or not to proceed with invasive procedures such as tracheostomy. In these cases, ventriculoperitoneal shunt or posterior fossa decompression procedure should be considered first in order to decrease morbidity and prevent complications [18, 26–28]. Some advocate for securing and supporting the airway for at least 4 weeks prior to tracheostomy, in order to give VFP patients who have a good chance of recovery of vocal fold movement adequate time for recovery prior to moving forward with tracheostomy [18].

There is no established timeframe for laryngeal procedures after diagnosis of VFP, particularly in children with an airway that is stabilized. Decision-making takes into account the child's age and symptoms, as well as the desires and wishes of the parents and the surgeon's experience level and skill [19]. Deciding on the correct time to intervene is also complicated by the fact that recovery of unilateral or bilateral VFP varies within the literature from 16% to 64%, with time to recovery varying from 6 weeks to 11 years [5, 11, 13, 27–30]. The etiology of the VFP also affects the recovery rate, as iatrogenic VFP from cardiothoracic surgery recovers at a rate much lower than idiopathic or congenital VFP [11]. It should be noted while vocal fold movement may recover, it is possible that the child's phonation, respiratory status, or swallowing function may not return to baseline. Laryngeal synkinesis, partial reinnervation, cross-innervation, compensatory mechanisms, or other patient factors may be responsible.

Another important aspect to consider is the urgency with which the procedure is needed based on symptoms. The Food and Drug Administration (FDA) has issued warnings on a number of anesthetic agents for pediatric patients. The associated neurodevelopmental risks have been found to be greater in children less than 3 years of age. Since thickened liquids, nasogastric feeds, and other feeding options can be used to temporize patients until they are at a safer age for intervention under general anesthesia, some have recommended waiting until the child is 3 years of age prior to proceeding with elective surgery [31].

In children who do not spontaneously recover either unilateral or bilateral vocal fold movement, their swallowing function can recover at rates that surpass return of their vocal fold movement [7, 11, 32]. However, children with developmental delay or central neurologic etiology of VFP do not show the same capacity to recover their swallowing function as those children without delay [7, 33]. Patients with multiple deficits in the swallowing mechanisms may have insurmountable obstacles to overcome to safely feed by mouth, regardless of vocal fold motion status [7].

Bilateral Vocal Fold Paralysis

Children with bilateral VFP present more often in respiratory distress than do children with unilateral VFP. The main challenge with these patients is the decision regarding tracheostomy placement. While tracheostomy was previously a common intervention for bilateral VFP, in as many as 67% of cases [28, 34, 35], more recent studies have demonstrated a decrease in the rate of tracheostomy in these patients, to as low as 33% [27, 29, 30, 36]. This is thought to be due to improved neonatal care, the use of positive pressure oxygenation via nasal cannula, and improvement in management and treatment of cardiovascular disorders, among other factors. One of the challenges when deciding whether or not tracheostomy is needed in these patients is deciding how long to wait following diagnosis of vocal fold motion impairment. While the measures described above buy more time prior to having to perform a tracheostomy, there is no consensus on how much time an otolaryngologist should wait prior to placing tracheostomy vs. observation and waiting for recovery. This is in part due to the lack of good evidence in literature and the retrospective nature of most of the case series.

While the decision on the correct time to intervene and place a tracheostomy on a child with bilateral VFP is difficult to determine, it is to be noted that the tracheostomy is a potentially reversible procedure that can allow time for spontaneous recovery of vocal fold movement. It also allows for continual re-evaluation of the vocal folds with flexible laryngoscopy with an unobstructed view of the larynx, while the tracheostomy maintains a stable airway.

Following tracheostomy placement, a further challenge in management arises due to the variable time intervals for potential spontaneous. The otolaryngologist is left to decide how often re-evaluation should take place and how long these children should be followed before further surgical intervention. Neither of these questions have a consensus within the literature. Most physicians advocate waiting several years before more invasive or irreversible procedures (e.g., lateralization, cordotomy, etc.) are performed, with studies demonstrating return of vocal fold movement up to 11 years after diagnosis [13, 28, 30]. In addition, normal laryngeal growth may allow for an increase in glottal aperture, which could decrease the need for any further intervention [30, 37]. Overall, it is shown that roughly 50% of children who have a tracheostomy placed for VFP require the tracheostomy tube to stay in place for greater than 3 years before decannulation is attempted [5, 36].

Once the airway is stable but prior to any irreversible laryngeal procedures in a child with bilateral VFP, dysphagia and the risk of aspiration should be addressed. This is especially true in children with a tracheostomy, as it has the potential to further exacerbate their dysphagia through impaired swallowing function due to decreased hyolaryngeal elevation. Speech therapy should be consulted on any child with bilateral VFP for swallowing evaluation. Studies have shown that roughly 50% of children with bilateral VFP need the assistance of a gastrostomy tube at initial diagnosis [7, 11, 38]. Children with developmental delay and bilateral VFP have been shown to require a gastrostomy tube at a much higher rate than developmentally normal children with bilateral VFP. Furthermore, children with developmental delay are less likely to regain or attain full feeds by mouth even with resolution of their vocal fold immobility [7].

Procedures Beyond Tracheostomy

Laryngeal surgeries and interventions following tracheostomy are most commonly performed to facilitate decannulation. Prior to committing to a surgery to enlarge the patency of the airway, there should be an active discussion with the parents so that they may understand the trade-offs involved, with the potential worsening of swallowing function and sacrifice of voice. This is also the case when performing procedures to widen the glottal aperture in children with bilateral VFP who do not have a tracheostomy. Surgical options fall into two categories: static vs. dynamic. Static procedures are further divided into tissue removal procedures or procedures that modify laryngeal framework. Dynamic procedures involve laryngeal reinnervation or functional electrical stimulation.

Surgeons who perform static procedures can often combine tissue removal techniques and laryngeal framework surgery simultaneously, such as the Woodman procedure or the arytenoid abduction laryngoplasty [39, 40]. Endoscopic techniques that can be used include posterior cordotomy, vocal process resection, arytenoidectomy, or posterior cricoid cartilage split and graft placement [41–43]. Due to the smaller dimensions of the pediatric glottis compared to the adult glottis, postsurgical scar tissue formation can have a large impact, both on the possibility of decannulation and phonation. Scar tissue formation has been noted to cause a higher rate of late failures in children than with adults [44].

The majority of studies involving static procedures have tracheostomy decannulation as the primary outcome. A meta-analysis found that a combination of anterior laryngofissure, arytenoidopexy, and vocal fold suture lateralization was the most reliable procedure to lead to tracheostomy decannulation in pediatric patients with bilateral VFP [4]. There is a paucity of literature that further examines these procedures and their specific effects on voice and/or swallowing in the pediatric population.

While static procedures widen the glottal diameter at the expense of swallowing, the dynamic procedure of selective laryngeal reinnervation by using the ansa cervicalis, phrenic nerve, or branches of the hypoglossal nerve shows some promise for bilateral VFP [45]. If successfully performed, abduction and adduction of the vocal folds may return, which can restore voice and protect airway during swallowing without disrupting the airway [45]. Another dynamic procedure option that can be employed is laryngeal chemodenervation, using injectable material such as botulinum toxin (Botox). Outcomes from a single-institution study demonstrated thyroarytenoid muscle injections to be more effective than cricothyroid muscle injections [46]. It was also more successful in maintaining decannulated status in children with a prior tracheotomy than preventing a tracheotomy in children without one

[46]. Similar to the static procedures, though, the majority of studies for dynamic procedures focus on primary outcome goal of tracheostomy decannulation and little to no focus on voicing and/or swallowing outcomes. Therefore, while success rates of procedures in relation to decannulation are fairly good, there have not been enough studies and adequate evidence to determine the impact of these procedures on dysphagia and dysphonia.

Unilateral Vocal Fold Paralysis

Unlike bilateral VFP, tracheostomy plays a much less prominent role in the treatment and management in children with unilateral VFP, as it usually only necessary if synchronous airway lesions are present [19]. Many of these patients (up to 80%) can be managed conservatively without surgical intervention. This is because the contralateral vocal fold can have effective compensation for glottal closure, which improves swallowing function and potentially dysphonia. Speech therapy can be used to help strengthen these compensatory methods and is often advocated as first line of therapy [18, 19, 47, 48]. The resolution rate of unilateral VFP varies within the literature and is quoted as high as 64%, but is thought to be much lower in iatrogenic cases [11, 29]. For those children who do have resolution of their unilateral VFP, roughly 80% of them will resolve within a year [11].

Surgical intervention is reserved for the 20–40% of patients who remain symptomatic after observation [49]. The challenge lies in deciding the length of the observation period prior to intervention. Most studies suggest waiting at least 1 year prior to intervention. Guiding these management decisions are symptom severity, effect of dysphonia and dysphagia on the child, and knowledge of the natural history of the unilateral VFP [11, 49, 50]. There are three primary surgical interventions that are employed for unilateral VFP: injection laryngoplasty, thyroplasty, and laryngeal reinnervation. There is a scarcity of data on these surgical interventions, and they are guided by level 4 evidence, which is somewhat expected given the low incidence of symptomatic unilateral VFP patients [49].

Injection laryngoplasty is considered a temporary intervention, as the materials used are designed to be eventually reabsorbed by the body (Fig. 16.3). A recent systematic review showed the most commonly used injectable materials include an absorbable gelatin sponge, sodium carboxymethyl cellulose gel, calcium hydroxylapatite, collagen, hyaluronic acid gels, and polytetrafluoroethylene [49]. However, most otolaryngologists who routinely address pediatric unilateral VFP are most likely to use carboxymethyl cellulose gel today, given the short-term nature of the injection material. Calcium hydroxylapatite is typically not used in the pediatric population, given the potential for an intense inflammatory response to the injection material [51]. Two of the studies in the review documented the injectable materials lasting longer in children than would expect in the adult population [49, 52, 53]. As more research is done to evaluate the resultant histologic changes to the tissue following injection, it is possible that further paradigm shifts may be seen in the future.

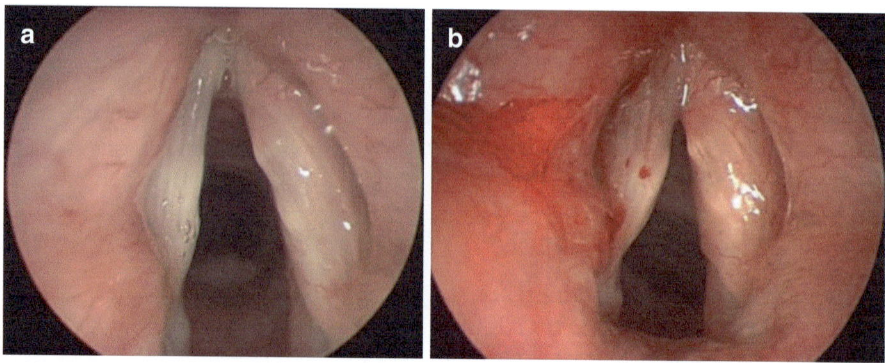

Fig. 16.3 Left injection laryngoplasty as seen on direct laryngoscopy. (**a**) Preinjection. The left vocal fold is paralyzed and demonstrates atrophy. (**b**) Postinjection. The left vocal fold is visibly fuller, with much significant decrease in the distance from the midline and contralateral vocal fold

With regard to outcomes following injection laryngoplasty, the majority of these studies documented that injection laryngoplasty was performed due to dysphonia symptoms with reported rates of objective or subjective improvement of 94–100% [30, 52–56]. These studies also consistently showed improvements in swallowing function on MBS, although the number of patients was limited [30, 52–56]. This surgical intervention is the only procedure for unilateral VFP that is considered temporary, so it is a good option in symptomatic children during the observation period. Recent studies have shown that patients may benefit from early injection as it may reduce the need for a more permanent procedure, such as thyroplasty or recurrent laryngeal nerve reinnervation [57, 58].

Medialization thyroplasty is a more permanent procedure and is commonly performed in the adult population, but is not often implemented in children. The largest case series by Link et al. [59] only involved eight patients treated with type I thyroplasty, most commonly for dysphonia or aspiration symptoms. A systematic review did find a high rate at 88% of aspiration recovery or swallowing function improvement after thyroplasty [49]. There are several reasons why this procedure has not been highly utilized in the pediatric population. First, in adults this is performed under local anesthesia and mild sedation, with the ability to adjust the position of the prosthesis based on real-time vocal feedback. However, with children, this is often difficult to carry out, although there are a few cases that report the use of intraoperative flexible laryngoscope through an LMA to adjust the position of the prosthesis [49, 60]. Another challenge with this laryngeal framework procedure is its effect on the size and continual growth of the pediatric larynx, particularly in very young children [19, 61].

Reinnervation of the paralyzed larynx with a direct neurorrhaphy of the recurrent laryngeal nerve and ansa cervicalis, or less commonly the phrenic nerve, is a much more popular permanent surgical intervention for children with unilateral VFP (Fig. 16.4). It is not performed for return of vocal fold movement but rather to restore tone, prevent atrophy, eliminate aspiration, improve dysphonia, and improve

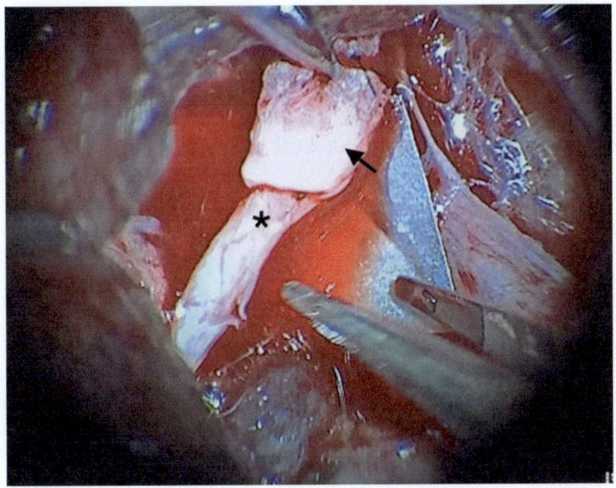

Fig. 16.4 Laryngeal reinnervation. The recurrent laryngeal nerve, depicted by the asterisk, has been anastomosed with the ansa cervicalis, depicted by the arrow

glottal closure [19]. It is recommended that the otolaryngologist perform laryngeal EMG prior to performing the procedure to ensure there is minimal chance of recovery of vocal fold movement [19]. Ansa cervicalis to recurrent laryngeal nerve (ansa-RLN) anastomosis is considered to have superior voice outcomes compared to thyroplasty in patients younger than 52 years of age according to a prospective surgical trial of 24 patients [62]. A single-institution case series of 13 children under the age of 10 who had ansa-RLN anastomosis performed and showed statistically significant improved voice outcomes using the parental global voice rating and GRBAS (grade, roughness, breathiness, asthenia, strain) scale [63]. Importantly, the study also showed statistically significant improvement in parental assessment of dysphagia with liquids [63]. Some authors argue that this procedure is superior to thyroplasty and injection laryngoplasty for several reasons, including no foreign body implant with risk of infection, reproducible results given the standardized technique, lack of a need for intraoperative adjustments, and durability of the procedure [63]. Long-term outcomes have yet to be published.

Conclusion

Some of the controversies and challenges surrounding the treatment of children with VFP include (1) poorly defined indications for surgical intervention, (2) a variety of treatment options without well-documented treatment outcomes, and (3) an inadequate understanding of the natural history of VFP in infants and young children regarding functional long-term effects on swallowing and voice [63]. Studies that focus on objective or subjective swallowing outcomes that include pre- and postsurgical MBS evaluations, FEES, and validated dysphagia surveys are lacking within the literature. Without these data, the choice of management and preferred surgical intervention are challenging, and the surgeon often relies on level 4 data [49]. Based on the present data, it appears that dysphagia due to VFP can often improve with conservative management, including time and feeding therapy. In those who do not improve, it is the job of the otolaryngologist to determine optimal timing for intervention, as well as the optimal surgical intervention on a patient-by-patient basis.

References

1. Crumley RL. Laryngeal synkinesis revisited. Ann Otol Rhinol Laryngol. 2000;109:365–71.
2. Bhattacharyya N. The prevalence of pediatric voice and swallowing problems in the United States. Laryngoscope. 2015;125:746–50.
3. Dedo DD. Pediatric vocal cord paralysis. Laryngoscope. 1979;89:1378–84.
4. Brigger MT, Hartnick CJ. Surgery for pediatric vocal cord paralysis: a meta-analysis. Otolaryngol Head Neck Surg. 2002;126:349–55.
5. Holinger LD, Holinger PC, Holinger PH. Etiology of bilateral abductor vocal cord paralysis. Ann Otol Rhinol Laryngol. 1976;85:428–36.
6. Parikh SR. Pediatric unilateral vocal fold immobility. Otolaryngol Clin N Am. 2004;37:203–15.
7. Hsu J, Tibbetts KM, Wu D, Nassar M, Tan M. Swallowing function in pediatric patients with bilateral vocal fold immobility. Int J Pediatr Otorhinolaryngol. 2017;93:37–41.
8. Sachdeva R, Hussain E, Moss MM, Schmitz ML, Ray RM, Imamura M, et al. Vocal cord dysfunction and feeding difficulties after pediatric cardiovascular surgery. J Pediatr. 2007;151(3):312–5, e1–e2
9. Truong MT, Messner AH, Kerschner JE, Scholes M, Wong-Dominguez J, Milczuk HA, et al. Pediatric vocal fold paralysis after cardiac surgery: rate of recovery and sequelae. Otolaryngol Head Neck Surg. 2007;137(5):780–4.
10. Benjamin JR, Smith PB, Cotton CM, Jaggers J, Goldstein RF, Malcolm WF. Long-term morbidities associated with vocal cord paralysis after surgical closure of a patent ductus arteriosis in extremely low birth weight infants. J Perinatol. 2010;30(6):408–13.
11. Jabbour J, Martin T, Beste D, Robey T. Pediatric vocal fold immobility natural history and the need for long-term follow-up. JAMA Otolaryngol Head Neck Surg. 2014;140(5):428–33.
12. Pemberton J, Frankfurter C, Bailey K, Jones L, Walton JM. Gastrostomy matters-the impact of pediatric surgery on caregiver quality of life. J Pediatr Surg. 2013;48(5):963–70.
13. Rosin DF, Handler SD, Potsic WP, Wetmore RF, Tom LWC. Vocal cord paralysis in children. Laryngoscope. 1990;100:1174–9.
14. Tibbetts KM, Wu D, Hsu JV, Burton WB, Nassar M, Tan M. Etiology and long-term functional swallow outcomes in pediatric unilateral vocal fold immobility. Int J Pediatr Otorhinolaryngol. 2016;88:179–83.
15. Randolph C, Lapey A, Shannon DC. Bilateral abductor paresis masquerading as asthma. J Allergy Clin Immunol. 1988;81:1122–5.
16. Chen EY, Inglis AF Jr. Bilateral vocal cord paralysis in children. Otolaryngol Clin N Am. 2008;41:889–901.
17. Raza SA, Mahendran S, Rahman N, Williams RG. Familial vocal fold paralysis. J Laryngol Otol. 2002;116:1047–9.
18. Grundfast KM, Harley E. Vocal cord paralysis. Otolaryngol Clin N Am. 1989;22:569–97.
19. Setlur J, Hartnick CJ. Management of unilateral true vocal cord paralysis in children. Curr Opin Otolaryngol Head Neck Surg. 2012;20:497–501.
20. Bogaard JM, Pauw KH, Versprille A, Stam H, Verbraak AF, Maas AJ. Maximal expiratory and inspiratory flow-volume curves in bilateral vocal-cord paralysis. Changes after surgical treat-

ment and comparison with glottis resistance characteristics. ORL J Otorhinolaryngol Relat Spec. 1987;49:35–41.
21. Vats A, Worley GA, de Bruyn R, Porter H, Albert DM, Bailey CM. Laryngeal ultrasound to assess vocal fold paralysis in children. J Laryngol Otol. 2004;118:429–31.
22. Carneiro-Pla D, Miller BS, Wilhelm SM, Milas M, Gauger PG, Cohen MS, et al. Feasibility of surgeon-performed transcutaneous vocal cord ultrasonography in identifying vocal cord mobility: a multi-institutional experience. Surgery. 2014;156(6):1597–602.
23. Parangi S. Editorial: Translaryngeal vocal cord ultrasound: ready for prime time. Surgery. 2016;159:67–9.
24. Berkowitz RG. Laryngeal electromyography findings in idiopathic congenital bilateral vocal cord paralysis. Ann Otol Rhinol Laryngol. 1996;105:207–12.
25. Wohl DL, Kilpatrick JK, Leshner RT, Shaia WT. Intraoperative pediatric laryngeal electromyography: experience and caveats with monopolar electrodes. Ann Otol Rhinol Laryngol. 2001;110:524–31.
26. Holinger PC, Holinger LD, Reichert TJ, Holinger PH. Respiratory obstruction and apnea in infants with bilateral abductor vocal cord paralysis, meningomyelocele, hydrocephalus, and Arnold Chiari malformation. J Pediatr. 1978;92:368–73.
27. Zbar RI, Chen AH, Behrendt DM, Bell EF, Smith RJ. Incidence of vocal fold paralysis in infants undergoing ligation of patent ductus arteriosus. Ann Thorac Surg. 1996;61:814–6.
28. Cohen SR, Geller KA, Birns JW, Thompson JW. Laryngeal paralysis in children: a long-term retrospective study. Ann Otol Rhinol Laryngol. 1982;91:417–24.
29. De Gaudemar I, Roudaire M, Francois M, Narcy P. Outcome of laryngeal paralysis in neonates: a long term retrospective study of 113 cases. Int J Pediatr Otorhinolaryngol. 1996;34:101–10.
30. Daya H, Hosni A, Bejar-Solar I, Evans JN, Bailey CM. Pediatric vocal fold paralysis. Arch Otolaryngol Head Neck Surg. 2000;126:21–5.
31. Andropoulos DG, Greene MF. Anesthesia and developing brains-implications of the FDA warning. N Engl J Med. 2017;376(10):905–7.
32. Nichols BG, Jabbour J, Hehir DA, Ghanayem NS, Beste D, Martin T, et al. Recovery of vocal fold immobility following isolated patent ductus arteriosus ligation. Int J Pediatr Otorhinolaryngol. 2014;78(8):1316–9.
33. Jang YY, Lee SJ, Lee SJ, Jeon JY, Lee SJ. Analysis of video fluoroscopic swallowing study in patients with vocal cord paralysis. Dysphagia. 2012;27(2):185–90.
34. Swift AC, Rogers J. Vocal cord paralysis in children. J Laryngol Otol. 1987;101:169–71.
35. Hollinger PH, Brown WT. Congenital webs, cysts, laryngoceles, and other anomalies of the larynx. Ann Otol Rhinol Laryngol. 1967;76:744–52.
36. Murty GE, Shinkwin C, Gibbin KP. Bilatearl vocal fold paralysis in infants: tracheostomy or not? J Laryngol Otol. 1994;108:329–31.
37. Berkowitz RG. Natural history of tracheostomy-dependent idiopathic congenital bilateral vocal fold paralysis. Otolaryngol Head Neck Surg. 2007;136:649–52.
38. Funk RT, Jabbour J, Robey T. Factors associated with tracheotomy and decannulation in pediatric bilateral vocal fold immobility. Int J Pediatr Otorhinolaryngol. 2015;79(6):895–9.
39. Woodman DG. A modification of the extralaryngeal approach to arytenoidectomy for bilateral abductor paralysis. Arch Otolaryngol. 1946;43:63–5.
40. Woodson G. Arytenoid abduction: indications and limitations. Ann Otol Rhinol Laryngol. 2010;119:742–8.
41. Thakkar K, Gerber ME. Endoscopic posterior costal cartilage graft placement for acute management of pediatric bilateral vocal fold paralysis without tracheostomy. Int J Pediatr Otorhinolaryngol. 2008;72:1555–8.
42. Bigenzahn W, Hoefler H. Minimally invasive laser surgery for the treatment of bilateral vocal cord paralysis. Laryngoscope. 1996;106:791–3.
43. Eckel HE, Thumfart M, Wassermann K, Vossing M, Thumfart WF. Cordectomy versus arytenoidectomy in the management of bilateral vocal cord paralysis. Ann Otol Rhinol Laryngol. 1994;103:852–7.

44. Ossoff RH, Duncavage JA, Shapshay SM, Krespi YP, Sisson GA. Endoscopic laser arytenoidectomy revisited. Ann Otol Rhinol Laryngol. 1990;99:764–71.
45. Marina MB, Marie JP, Birchall MA. Laryngeal reinnervation for bilateral vocal fold paralysis. Curr Opin Otolaryngol Head Neck Surg. 2011;19:434–8.
46. Smith ME, Park AH, Muntz HR, Gray SD. Airway augmentation and maintenance through laryngeal chemodenervation in children with impaired vocal fold mobility. Arch Otolaryngol Head Neck Surg. 2007;133:610–2.
47. Schindler A, Bottero A, Capaccio P, Ginocchio D, Adorni F, Ottaviani F. Vocal improvement after voice therapy in unilateral vocal fold paralysis. J Voice. 2008;22:113–8.
48. Tucker HM. Vocal cord paralysis in small children: principles of management. Ann Otol Rhinol Laryngol. 1986;95:618–21.
49. Butskiy O, Mistry B, Chadha NK. Surgical interventions for pediatric unilateral vocal cord paralysis: a systematic review. JAMA Otolaryngol Head Neck Surg. 2015;14(7):654–60.
50. Misono S, Merati AL. Evidence-based practice: evaluation and management of unilateral vocal fold paralysis. Otolaryngol Clin North Am. 2012;45(5):1083–108.
51. DeFatta RA, Chowdhury FR, Sataloff RT. Complications of injection laryngoplasty using calcium hydroxylapatite. J Voice. 2012;26(5):614–8.
52. Sipp JA, Kerschner JE, Braune N, Hartnick CJ. Vocal fold medicalization in children: injection laryngoplasty, thyroplasty, or nerve reinnervation? Arch Otolaryngol Head Neck Surg. 2007;133(8):767–71.
53. Tucker HM. Vocal cord paralysis in small children: principles in management. Ann Otol Rhinol Laryngol. 1986;95(6, pt 1):618–21.
54. Levine BA, Jacobs IN, Wetmore RF, Handler SD. Vocal cord injection in children with unilateral vocal cord paralysis. Arch Otolaryngol Head Neck Surg. 1995;121(1):116–9.
55. Patel NJ, Kerschner JE, Merati AL. The use of injectable collage in the management of pediatric vocal unilateral fold paralysis. Int J Pediatr Otorhinolaryngol. 2003;67(12):1355–60.
56. Cohen MS, Mehta DK, Maguire RC, Simons JP. Injection medicalization laryngoplasty in children. Arch Otolaryngol Head Neck Surg. 2011;137(3):264–8.
57. Yung KC, Likhterov I, Courey MS. Effect of temporary vocal fold injection medialization on the rate of permanent medialization laryngoplasty in unilateral vocal fold paralysis patients. Laryngoscope. 2011;121(10):2191–4.
58. Friedman AD, Burns JA, Heaton JT, Zeitels SM. Early versus late injection medialization for unilateral vocal cord paralysis. Laryngoscope. 2010;120(10):2042–6.
59. Link DT, Rutter MJ, Liu JH, Willging JP, Myer CM, Cotton RT. Pediatric type I thyroplasty: an evolving procedure. Ann Otol Rhinol Laryngol. 1999;108:1105–10.
60. Gardner GM, Altman JS, Balakrishnan G. Pediatric vocal fold medialization with silastic implant: intraoperative airway management. Int J Pediatr Otorhinolaryngol. 2000;52:37–44.
61. Isaacson G. Extraluminal arytenoid reconstruction: laryngeal framework surgery applied to a pediatric problem. Ann Otol Rhinol Laryngol. 1990;99(8):616–20.
62. Paniello RC, Edgar JD, Kallogjeri D, Piccirillo JF. Medialization versus reinnervation for unilateral vocal fold paralysis: a multicenter randomized clinical trial. Laryngoscope. 2011;121(10):2172–9.
63. Smith ME, Roy N, Houtz D. Laryngeal reinnervation for paralytic dysphonia in children younger than 10 years. Arch Otolaryngol Head Neck Surg. 2012;138:1161–9.

Chapter 17
Cricopharyngeal Dysfunction in Children

Joshua R. Bedwell

Introduction

The cricopharyngeus is the major functional component of the upper esophageal sphincter. Failure of this sphincter to relax in a coordinated fashion during swallowing is a rare cause of dysphagia in pediatric patients but can lead to significant morbidity. Diagnosis of cricopharyngeal achalasia is typically made with a video-fluoroscopic swallow study, with the potential support of other methods such as endoscopy and manometry. There are a number of described techniques for management ranging from dilation to open myotomy.

Anatomy and Physiology

The cricopharyngeus muscle (CPM) is a C-shaped striated muscle situated between the inferior pharyngeal constrictor and the esophagus. The CPM as well as the surrounding pharynx and proximal esophagus make up the pharyngoesophageal segment (PES). The CPM attaches to the lateral portions of the cricoid cartilage and has muscle fibers in both oblique and transverse orientations [1, 2]. Motor innervation is provided by both the pharyngeal plexus of the vagus nerve and the recurrent laryngeal nerve [3]. Sensory information is carried by the glossopharyngeal nerve.

At rest, the CPM is contracted. Such closure of the upper esophageal sphincter (UES) prevents aerophagia and protects the airway from refluxed gastric contents. The CPM reflexively relaxes during swallowing, coordinated with pharyngeal contraction and laryngeal elevation, thereby opening the UES and allowing the bolus to

J. R. Bedwell
Department of Otolaryngology, Baylor College of Medicine, Texas Children's Hospital, Houston, TX, USA
e-mail: jrbedwel@texaschildrens.org

J. Ongkasuwan, E. H. Chiou (eds.), *Pediatric Dysphagia*,
https://doi.org/10.1007/978-3-319-97025-7_17

move into the esophagus. Impaired or uncoordinated relaxation of the CPM during deglutition leads to symptoms of dysphagia, regurgitation, and potentially aspiration into the airway.

Pathophysiology

Swallowing problems arising in the PES may be due to a number of factors, including impaired CPM relaxation, weak pharyngeal constriction, and/or poor laryngeal elevation [1]. "Cricopharyngeal achalasia" (CPA) specifically refers to dysphagia due to failure of the CPM to adequately relax. Although this is a widely recognized entity in the adult population, CPA is a rare cause of dysphagia in children, often leading to delays in diagnosis [4].

The exact pathogenesis of CPA remains unclear. In adults, it is often associated with a neurologic process, but in children it is often an isolated finding. Gross and microscopic findings on specimens from open myotomy include muscle fiber hypertrophy as well as fibrosis [2]. Histologic findings at the time of autopsy of one of the earliest reported CPA cases demonstrated an absence of ganglion cells in the upper third of the esophagus, while the lower esophagus was normal [5]. It is possible that a variety of mechanisms may ultimately lead to the same outcome of CPM dysfunction.

Presentation and Workup

Patients with CPA tend to present in the perinatal period with feeding difficulties. Common symptoms include choking episodes, regurgitation, nasopharyngeal reflux of feeds, and aspiration into the lower airway. Patients may exhibit poor weight gain or failure to thrive. Frequent aspiration events can lead to recurrent respiratory infections. The differential diagnosis for such patients is broad and includes a number of congenital malformations such as esophageal atresia or stenosis, tracheoesophageal fistula, vascular rings, and laryngeal cleft, among others (Table 17.1). Because of the rarity of CPA in children, clinicians must maintain a high index of suspicion. While nearly 90% of reported cases are diagnosed in children under 12 months of age, only 15% are definitively diagnosed within the first month of life [6]. Brooks reported a series in which all patients had a significant delay in diagnosis, ranging from 11 to 138 months [4].

The initial workup includes a complete history and detailed head and neck and neurologic examination to rule out other causes for dysphagia. The videofluoroscopic swallow study (VFSS) is the gold standard for diagnosing CPA. The characteristic finding is the cricopharyngeal muscle bar narrowing or completely obstructing the PES. The pharynx above the CPM may be distended with contrast, and nasopharyngeal reflux and/or tracheal aspiration may be evident. Aside from the distinctive cricopharyngeal bar, VFSS allows an evaluation of other important components affecting the PES, including strength of the pharyngeal contraction and

Table 17.1 Differential diagnosis of dysphagia in the neonate

Anatomic	Choanal atresia
	Cleft palate
	Esophageal atresia/stenosis
	Tracheoesophageal fistula
	Laryngeal cleft
	Vascular rings/slings
Neurologic	Arnold-Chiari malformation
	Supranuclear palsy
	Spinal atrophy (Werdnig-Hoffman)
	Vocal fold immobility
	Cerebral palsy
	Hydrocephalus
Muscular	Myasthenia
	Muscular dystrophy
Other	Foreign body
	Prematurity
	Gastroesophageal reflux
	Idiopathic

hyolaryngeal elevation [1]. Evaluation of these other aspects of PES function is important, as patients with problems aside from poor CPM relaxation are less likely to benefit from the surgical techniques discussed below.

Flexible endoscopic evaluation of swallowing (FEES) is a frequently employed evaluation but is not able to specifically diagnose CPA. Findings on FEES may include pooled secretions and signs of laryngeal penetration or aspiration. It may be helpful in ruling out other causes for dysphagia or aspiration such as obstructive masses or vocal fold immobility.

Gross findings on esophagoscopy may include obvious CPM hypertrophy with a narrowed esophageal inlet, redundant mucosa at the inlet, or may be normal [6–9]. Therefore, endoscopy is primarily useful in ruling out other causes for dysphagia, such as severe reflux and eosinophilic esophagitis.

In theory, high-resolution impedance manometry would be very helpful in diagnosing CPA. Persistent high UES pressures following a swallow indicating failed relaxation of the CPM would be highly suggestive of CPA. Brooks demonstrated normalization of elevated mean UES pressures after myotomy in two pediatric cases [4]. There are challenges with the routine use of manometry in diagnosing CPA in children. First, there are no normative data on UES pressures for the pediatric population [10, 11]. Measurement techniques vary from institution to institution, and therefore "normal" pressure values will vary as well. In the absence of this data, studies in the literature present pre- and post-intervention measurements, demonstrating a change in UES pressure. Preoperative pressures reported range from 64 to 715 mmHg, and post-intervention pressures range from 19 to 32 mmHg [4, 12]. A second issue is that the probe itself will naturally move during a swallow, making it difficult to pinpoint the area of dysfunction, though pairing manometry with a videofluoroscopic evaluation has been suggested to improve accuracy [1].

Associated Conditions

While most cases are idiopathic, there are a number of conditions that have been associated with CPA. Neurologic and neuromuscular conditions have been associated with CPA, though the exact relationship remains unclear [4, 13–15]. An MRI to rule out an Arnold-Chiari malformation may be warranted.

The role of gastroesophageal reflux (GER) in pediatric CPA is not settled, with conflicting evidence in the literature. Adult studies have lent some support to the idea that GER may cause CPM spasm or uncoordinated relaxation during swallow, with subsequent elevated UES pressures seen on manometry [1]. However, comparisons of UES pressure via manometry in infants with and without GER show no difference in mean pressure or coordination of UES relaxation with swallowing [16]. On the other hand, Scholes found that of four infants with CPA who underwent endoscopy with biopsy, three were found to have esophagitis [8].

Treatment

Therapeutic options for children with CPA include watchful waiting with nasogastric or gastrostomy tube feeding, dilation, targeted botulinum toxin injections, and either endoscopic or open cricopharyngeal myotomy. Spontaneous resolution of CPA in infants has been reported, but there is not enough information available in the literature to define which patients are likely to resolve and how long one should observe. Given the potential for failure to thrive and complications from aspiration events, early intervention is the best option for most cases.

Medical Therapy

Medications such as nifedipine and nitrates that relax the smooth muscle of the esophagus have been reported on in the past, but significant side effects preclude their use in the pediatric population [13]. Although evidence on the contribution of GERD to CPA is lacking, several authors recommend treating empirically with proton-pump inhibitors [6, 17].

Dilation

Blank first reported on the use of bougienage dilation in a child with CPA in 1972 [18]. Several subsequent authors have reported on the successful use of bougies to dilate the UES [19, 20]. More recently, high-pressure balloons have been used successfully to dilate the CPM [13, 21]. There have been no adverse events or complications of dilation reported, and some advocate for an initial trial of dilation before progressing to more invasive techniques such as myotomy [9].

Botulinum Toxin

Botulinum toxin causes flaccid muscle paralysis by inhibiting presynaptic acetylcholine release at the neuromuscular junction. The effect is temporary, lasting weeks to months. Experience using targeted botulinum toxin injections in children with esophageal achalasia suggests it can be effective, though given the temporary nature of the toxin, most children will go on to need definitive procedures [22]. Bauman described her experience with a pediatric CPA patient in 2005, in which a 3.5-month infant improved after botulinum toxin injection into the CPM during a direct laryngoscopy [6]. The effect was short-lived (2 months), and after one repeat injection, he went on to have an open CPM myotomy. Several others have reported similar results, with mean interval between injections at about 3 months [7, 8, 23]. Doses reported have ranged from 10 to 100 units (1.4–7.9 U/kg) injected at 2–4 sites along the posterior aspect of the CPM. There has been only one reported complication with botulinum injection, namely, temporarily worsening aspiration in a patient who received a relatively high dose [23].

While most patients ultimately required myotomy, Scholes et al. have a series of six patients in which four resolved with only botulinum toxin injections [8]. Of those four, two resolved after one injection and two after two. This suggests that botulinum injection may be a reasonable first step in an infant with suspected CPA. Resolution of the symptoms after injection supports the diagnosis and suggests a positive outcome for the more invasive option of myotomy.

Cricopharyngeal Myotomy

Division of the transverse fibers of the CPM can be done to open the constricted UES and resolve dysphagia in CPA [24]. The open approach to CPM myotomy is well-described and effective. Briefly, the CPM is accessed via a transverse cervical incision (typically on the left to reduce the risk of recurrent laryngeal nerve injury). The sternocleidomastoid muscle and carotid sheath are retracted laterally, while the larynx is rotated to expose the transverse muscle fibers of the CPM. The muscle is sharply divided in the midline, taking care to preserve the pharyngeal and esophageal mucosa. Placement of a bougie or Foley catheter within the esophagus may prove useful in this regard. Reported results of open CPM myotomy with long-term follow-up are uniformly positive, with no major complications [2, 4, 25]. Theoretic risks abstracted from the adult literature include persistent symptoms due to inadequate myotomy, recurrent laryngeal nerve injury, mucosal perforation potentially leading to fistula formation, wound infection, or mediastinitis [13].

An endoscopic approach to CPM myotomy has gained favor more recently, after finding success in the adult population with CPM pathology [26–29]. Chun described the technique in an infant, using a carbon dioxide laser during direct suspension microlaryngoscopy [7]. CPM fibers are divided until the buccopharyngeal fascia is identified (and left intact). The endoscopic approach removes the risk of recurrent laryngeal nerve damage, though potentially increases the risk of salivary leak and mediastinitis from inadvertent entry into the retropharyngeal space.

Conclusion

Cricopharyngeal achalasia is a rare but serious cause of dysphagia in the pediatric population characterized by failed relaxation of the cricopharyngeal muscle during deglutition. Symptoms typically present early in life and include failure to thrive, regurgitation, nasopharyngeal reflux, and aspiration. Diagnosis is best confirmed by visualizing a prominent cricopharyngeal bar on a videofluoroscopic swallow study, constricting the upper esophageal sphincter, and limiting passage of the bolus into the esophagus. Management options include dilation, botulinum toxin injection, and cricopharyngeal myotomy. The literature in the pediatric population is limited; therefore, no one technique can be shown to be superior.

References

1. Kuhn MA, Belafsky PC. Management of cricopharyngeus muscle dysfunction. Otolaryngol Clin N Am. 2013;46(6):1087–99.
2. Muraji T, Takamizawa S, Satoh S, et al. Congenital cricopharyngeal achalasia: diagnosis and surgical management. J Pediatr Surg. 2002;37(5):E12.
3. Sasaki CT, Kim YH, Sims HS, Czibulka A. Motor innervation of the human cricopharyngeus muscle. Ann Otol Rhinol Laryngol. 1999;108(12):1132–9.
4. Brooks A, Millar AJ, Rode H. The surgical management of cricopharyngeal achalasia in children. Int J Pediatr Otorhinolaryngol. 2000;56(1):1–7.
5. Utian HL, Thomas RG. Cricopharyngeal incoordination in infancy. Pediatrics. 1969;43(3):402–6.
6. Sewell RK, Bauman NM. Congenital cricopharyngeal achalasia: management with botulinum toxin before myotomy. Arch Otolaryngol Head Neck Surg. 2005;131(5):451–3.
7. Chun R, Sitton M, Tipnis NA, et al. Endoscopic cricopharyngeal myotomy for management of cricopharyngeal achalasia (CA) in an 18-month-old child. Laryngoscope. 2013;123(3):797–800.
8. Scholes MA, McEvoy T, Mousa H, Wiet GJ. Cricopharyngeal achalasia in children: botulinum toxin injection as a tool for diagnosis and treatment. Laryngoscope. 2014;124(6):1475–80.
9. Skinner MA, Shorter NA. Primary neonatal cricopharyngeal achalasia: a case report and review of the literature. J Pediatr Surg. 1992;27(12):1509–11.

10. Goldani HA, Staiano A, Borrelli O, Thapar N, Lindley KJ. Pediatric esophageal high-resolution manometry: utility of a standardized protocol and size-adjusted pressure topography parameters. Am J Gastroenterol. 2010;105(2):460–7.
11. Nikaki K, Ooi JL, Sifrim D. Chicago classification of esophageal motility disorders: applications and limits in adults and pediatric patients with esophageal symptoms. Curr Gastroenterol Rep. 2016;18(11):59.
12. Watanabe T, Shimizu T, Takahashi M, et al. Cricopharyngeal achalasia treated with myectomy and post-operative high-resolution manometry. Int J Pediatr Otorhinolaryngol. 2014;78(7):1182–5.
13. De Caluwe D, Nassogne MC, Reding R, de Ville de Goyet J, Clapuyt P, Otte JB. Cricopharyngeal achalasia: case reports and review of the literature. Eur J Pediatr Surg. 1999;9(2):109–12.
14. Kornblum C, Broicher R, Walther E, et al. Cricopharyngeal achalasia is a common cause of dysphagia in patients with mtDNA deletions. Neurology. 2001;56(10):1409–12.
15. Reichert TJ, Bluestone CD, Stool SE, Sieber WK, Sieber AM. Congenital cricopharyngeal achalasia. Ann Otol Rhinol Laryngol. 1977;86(5 Pt 1):603–10.
16. Sondheimer JM. Upper esophageal sphincter and pharyngoesophageal motor function in infants with and without gastroesophageal reflux. Gastroenterology. 1983;85(2):301–5.
17. Huoh KC, Messner AH. Cricopharyngeal achalasia in children: indications for treatment and management options. Curr Opin Otolaryngol Head Neck Surg. 2013;21(6):576–80.
18. Blank RH, Silbiger M. Cricopharyngeal achalasia as a cause of respiratory distress in infancy. J Pediatr. 1972;81(1):95–8.
19. Lernau OZ, Sherzer E, Mogle P, Nissan S. Congenital cricopharyngeal achalasia treatment by dilatations. J Pediatr Surg. 1984;19(2):202–3.
20. Dinari G, Danziger Y, Mimouni M, Rosenbach Y, Zahavi I, Grunebaum M. Cricopharyngeal dysfunction in childhood: treatment by dilatations. J Pediatr Gastroenterol Nutr. 1987;6(2): 212–6.
21. Erdeve O, Kologlu M, Saygili B, Atasay B, Arsan S. Primary cricopharyngeal achalasia in a newborn treated by balloon dilatation: a case report and review of the literature. Int J Pediatr Otorhinolaryngol. 2007;71(1):165–8.
22. Hurwitz M, Bahar RJ, Ament ME, et al. Evaluation of the use of botulinum toxin in children with achalasia. J Pediatr Gastroenterol Nutr. 2000;30(5):509–14.
23. Barnes MA, Ho AS, Malhotra PS, Koltai PJ, Messner A. The use of botulinum toxin for pediatric cricopharyngeal achalasia. Int J Pediatr Otorhinolaryngol. 2011;75(9):1210–4.
24. Kaplan S. Paralysis of deglutition, a post-poliomyelitis complication treated by section of the cricopharyngeus muscle. Ann Surg. 1951;133(4):572–3.
25. Martin N, Prince JM, Kane TD, Goyal A, Mehta D. Congenital cricopharyngeal achalasia in a 4.5-year-old managed by cervical myotomy: a case report. Int J Pediatr Otorhinolaryngol. 2011;75(2):289–92.
26. Halvorson DJ, Kuhn FA. Transmucosal cricopharyngeal myotomy with the potassium-titanyl-phosphate laser in the treatment of cricopharyngeal dysmotility. Ann Otol Rhinol Laryngol. 1994;103(3):173–7.
27. Brondbo K. Treatment of cricopharyngeal dysfunction by endoscopic laser myotomy. Acta Otolaryngol Suppl. 2000;543:222–4.
28. Dauer E, Salassa J, Iuga L, Kasperbauer J. Endoscopic laser vs open approach for cricopharyngeal myotomy. Otolaryngol Head Neck Surg. 2006;134(5):830–5.
29. Pitman M, Weissbrod P. Endoscopic CO_2 laser cricopharyngeal myotomy. Laryngoscope. 2009;119(1):45–53.

Chapter 18
Esophageal Dysphagia

Rinarani Sanghavi and Rachel Rosen

Abbreviations

CT	Computed tomography
EA	Esophageal atresia
EGD	Esophagogastroduodenoscopy
EoE	Eosinophilic esophagitis
GERD	Gastroesophageal reflux disease
HRM	High-resolution manometry
LES	Lower esophageal sphincter
MRI	Magnetic resonance imaging
TEF	Tracheoesophageal fistula

Introduction

Dysphagia refers to the sensation of difficulty swallowing or food getting stuck in the esophagus after it is swallowed and as it traverses the esophagus. There are two primary types of dysphagia encountered by gastroenterologists: oropharyngeal dysphagia and esophageal dysphagia. The focus of this chapter is on esophageal dysphagia. The causes for esophageal dysphagia can vary widely and range from conditions which cause chronic or subacute dysphagia to those who present with

R. Sanghavi (✉)
Department of Pediatrics, UT Southwestern Medical Center/Children's Health Dallas,
Dallas, TX, USA
e-mail: rinarani.sanghavi@utsouthwestern.edu

R. Rosen
Division of Gastroenterology and Nutrition, Boston Childrens Hospital, Boston, MA, USA
e-mail: Rachel.rosen@childrens.harvard.edu

© Springer International Publishing AG, part of Springer Nature 2018

J. Ongkasuwan, E. H. Chiou (eds.), *Pediatric Dysphagia*,
https://doi.org/10.1007/978-3-319-97025-7_18

acute-onset symptoms. In most cases, children who develop sudden inability or refusal of oral solids or liquids, odynophagia, drooling, or concomitant respiratory symptoms will require urgent evaluation for conditions such as foreign body or caustic ingestion or infectious complications, including epiglottitis or retropharyngeal abscess. The primary scope of this chapter, however, will emphasize the diagnosis and management of chronic esophageal dysphagia in the context of feeding and swallowing disorders.

Estimated reports of the incidence and prevalence of pediatric dysphagia vary widely, in part due to it being underreported [1, 2]. It has been reported that 25–45% of typically developing children demonstrate feeding and swallowing problems though how much of this is a result of esophageal disorders is not known [2–4]. Rates of feeding and swallowing difficulties are even higher in children with developmental delay; the prevalence is estimated to be 30–80% for children with developmental disorders [1–3], and it is increasing perhaps due to improved survival of very low birth weight babies and medically complex children [1, 2].

Severe consequences of feeding problems (e.g., growth failure, susceptibility to chronic illness) have been reported to occur in 3–10% of children, with an even higher prevalence found in children with physical disabilities (26–90%) and those with history of chronic medical illness and prematurity (10–49%) [1–3]. The percentage of all of feeding issues which result from esophageal etiologies, however, is not known. When considering esophageal dysphagia, three key factors need to be considered as potential causes: anatomic, inflammatory, or dysmotility problems (primary or secondary).

Tests for Dysphagia

When evaluating a child with dysphagia, obtaining a thorough clinical history and performing a physical examination remain the most important diagnostic tools to distinguish between the different causes of dysphagia. Depending on the differential generated through a thorough history and physical examination, subsequent tests can be ordered to confirm initial suspicion.

Clinical Examination

From a historical perspective, patients may have dysphagia with solids, liquids, or both. Patients with oropharyngeal dysphagia typically have more difficulty with liquids and present with coughing, choking, gagging, vomiting, a wet voice, or throat clearing. Esophageal dysphagia typically presents with either solid food dysphagia (as seen with esophageal strictures or stenosis, such as in children with eosinophilic esophagitis, early achalasia, or caustic ingestion injury) or with both solid and liquid dysphagia (as seen with children with advanced achalasia, connective tissue disorders, or other primary or secondary motility disorders). Patients with esophageal dysphagia typically complain of food getting stuck, chest pain with eating, vomiting of undigested food, a sensation of gradual filling up of food and/or liquid as a meal progresses, or post-prandial and/or nocturnal (supine) coughing. In younger or nonverbal children, symptoms may be less definitive and may present only with feeding difficulties, food restriction, and weight loss. Signs of respiratory distress with feeds and growth using growth charts should be ascertained.

Physical Exam

For the child who presents with acute-onset esophageal dysphagia, attention to the cardiopulmonary exam is especially important. Signs of respiratory distress, such as stridor, chest retractions, hot potato voice or aphonia (inability to speak), tachypnea, or hypoxia, should prompt an urgent evaluation of the airway and lungs, with stabilization as needed. For chronic or gradual-onset esophageal dysphagia, the physical examination should include close examination of the oral cavity, pharynx, and neck looking for a mass such as a cyst or other inflammatory processes. The neurologic exam may be useful to elicit cranial nerve deficits which can be associated with swallowing difficulties. Finally, abnormal muscle tone, strength, or reflexes may indicate an underlying neuromuscular cause for dysphagia.

Radiology Studies

A plain X-ray may be performed to evaluate for a foreign body in cases of acute-onset dysphagia. A barium swallow (also known as an esophagram or upper GI series) is used to assess anatomy and is a key diagnostic tool to evaluate for esophageal strictures. Barium studies may suggest an underlying motility disorder through the presence of tertiary contractions, a bird's beak appearance to the lower esophageal sphincter (suggesting achalasia), a dilated sigmoid esophagus (late achalasia), and a fluid level or persistent barium in the esophagus 10 min after the barium is ingested. This test is in contrast to a modified barium swallow (also known as a video swallow fluoroscopic study) which focuses on the oropharynx and upper esophagus (cricopharyngeus and upper 1/3 of the esophagus only) in order to diagnose oropharyngeal dysphagia and tracheoesophageal fistulae. This is performed in the presence of feeding therapists for the evaluation of the mechanics of swallowing and specifically for aspiration or penetration and to assess therapeutic response [5]. Children with dysphagia may be fearful or unable to swallow an adequate amount of barium, which may cause a false-positive result on esophagram for a stricture. In these children, a barium tablet is a useful tool [6]. A barium tablet (12.5 mm diameter) is swallowed with a small amount of water. If the tablet gets lodged at a particular location, then a more detailed assessment is indicated [7].

Computed Tomography (CT)

Cross-sectional CT imaging of the neck and chest may be useful if a mass effect is seen on prior radiological studies for the evaluation of vascular malformations or esophageal tumors. Since these are rare entities in children, this diagnostic modality is not commonly indicated in the evaluation of childhood dysphagia. The exception is in children with esophageal atresia, in whom vascular anomalies (e.g., rings and slings) are more commonly encountered and should be suspected and investigated using chest CT or magnetic resonance imaging (MRI) [8]. CT can also reveal a dilated esophagus in patients presenting with atypical symptoms which may lead providers to consider primary motility disorders. It is frequently used to monitor for radiographic evidence of chronic lung disease which can be found in up to 50% of patients with motility disorders felt to be related to recurrent aspiration of esophageal contents from stasis [9].

Esophageal Manometry

If the history or imaging raises concern for an esophageal motility disorder, then an esophageal manometry is the gold standard test to assess for esophageal motility. High-resolution manometry (HRM) is now used almost exclusively at all centers. This test entails placing a nasal catheter and advancing it to the stomach under manometric visualization in an awake child. Multiple liquid swallows with 5 ml of water each are performed to assess upper esophageal sphincter tone and relaxation, esophageal peristalsis, and lower esophageal tone and relaxation. This test also can detect a hiatal hernia as well as rumination disorder. Combined manometry with impedance testing is superior to manometry alone and is used commonly to detect both reflux as well as dysmotility. When impedance monitoring is combined with HRM, any liquids given during the test need to contain ions; patients are typically given ten salt water swallows, ten viscous swallows, and ten solid swallows. To reveal more subtle motility disorders, rapid sequence swallows can be elicited to test for deglutitive inhibition.

Endoscopy

An upper GI endoscopy or esophagogastroduodenoscopy (EGD) is helpful to make the diagnosis of inflammatory conditions of the mucosa (e.g., eosinophilic esophagitis, reflux disease) but may also serve a therapeutic role in patients with anatomic lesions contributing to dysphagia (e.g., balloon dilation of strictures, lower esophageal sphincter (LES), or fundoplication). Dysphagia due to infectious esophagitis from *Candida*, *Cytomegalovirus* (CMV), herpes simplex virus (HSV), etc. is also diagnosed using endoscopy with biopsies and mucosal brushings. More recently, endoscopic ultrasound (EUS) examination with a radial probe is used to help identify subtle strictures and may predict the response to dilation, which usually requires more sessions when the *muscularis propria* is involved [10].

Causes for Esophageal Dysphagia

Anatomic Obstruction

Strictures

The most common causes of esophageal strictures in children are anastomotic strictures after esophageal atresia/tracheoesophageal fistula (EA/TEF) repair surgery and strictures following caustic ingestion. Distal esophageal strictures are more commonly seen with peptic disease, with congenital strictures being rare cause in children. In recent times, an increased awareness and understanding of eosinophilic esophagitis (EoE) and the potential for EoE-related strictures should also be considered in the differential.

Caustic Strictures

Caustic ingestion and resulting esophageal injury remains a significant medical and social concern despite various efforts to minimize hazards of caustic household products, which can include both acids and alkaline products. Damage to the esophagus should be assessed endoscopically, ideally within 12–18 h after the ingestion, and is classified according to severity of injury to the esophageal mucosa, ranging from grade 0 (no damage) to grade IIIb (extensive necrosis) [11] (see Table 18.1).

In a 10-year retrospective study of caustic ingestions, it was noted that 98% were accidental in nature. Fifty percent of patients of grade II injury subsequently developed strictures requiring multiple dilations [12]. Following a grade IIb and a grade III esophageal burn, stricture incidence was noted to be 71% and 100%, respectively [13, 14]. Strictures usually develop within 8 weeks after the ingestion in 80% of

Table 18.1 Endoscopic grading of caustic injury

Grade	Description
0	Normal
I	Edema and hyperemia of the esophagus
IIa	Friability; hemorrhage; erosion, blisters, exudates, or whitish membranes; superficial ulcers
IIb	Grade IIa plus deep, discrete, or circumferential ulceration
IIIa	Small scattered areas of necrosis; areas of brownish black-gray discoloration
IIIb	Extensive necrosis

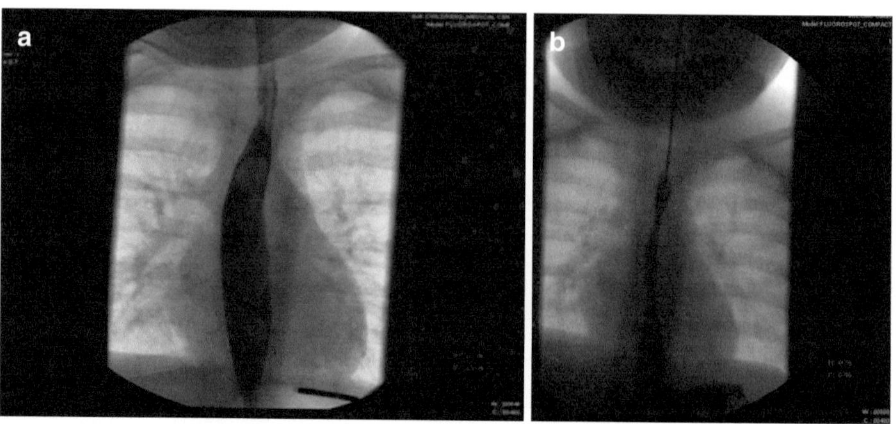

Fig. 18.1 Esophagram from a 2-year-old with caustic ingestion. (**a**) Initial (**b**) 5 weeks post-ingestion showing long stricture

patients, but can occur as early as 3 weeks after injury or as late as after 1 year. Ingestion of powerful caustic substances (e.g., sodium hydroxide) is followed by severe, long-standing strictures and dramatically altered esophageal motility leading to severe dysphagia [15]. The most common site of involvement was the upper third followed by the lower third of the esophagus [16].

Assessment for caustic strictures should be performed via esophagram done at 4–5 weeks after the initial injury (see Fig. 18.1). Management of caustic strictures is usually by dilation of the stricture [17]. Dilation can be carried out with balloons or bougies (usually Savary) without a clear advantage for either method [18]. Good nutrition has been linked to improved outcomes in caustic ingestions and management of sequelae, and therefore alternate methods of nutrition (e.g., gastrostomy tube) should be considered in patients if dysphagia is severe or in those with high-grade strictures [19, 20].

Esophageal Atresia

Esophageal atresia (EA) is a common foregut malformation, with an incidence of 1/3000–1/4000 live births, with a 0.5–2% risk of recurrence among siblings of the affected child. It is often associated with a tracheoesophageal fistula (TEF). In 2016, the European Society for Pediatric Gastroenterology, Hepatology, and Nutrition and the North American Society for Pediatric Gastroenterology, Hepatology, and Nutrition (ESGPHAN-NASPGHAN) published joint guidelines for the management of children with EA/TEF and specifically addressed dysphagia in these children [8].

The etiology of the dysphagia in EA/TEF is most likely multifactorial, with dysmotility, strictures, and reflux and/or eosinophilic esophagitis being implicated [21, 22]. Esophageal dysmotility is almost universally present in these patients even prior to surgical repair making it likely that there is a congenital etiology for the dysmotility [23]. A recent review reports a prevalence of more than 50% in patients with EA/TEF older than 10 years of age [24]. Abnormal motility of the esophagus is implicated in the pathophysiology of other complications associated with EA such as aspiration and gastroesophageal reflux disease (GERD) in addition to dysphagia [25]. In young children with EA/TEF who are unable to provide an accurate history, dysphagia in these children may be even more common than reported, especially since they are likely used to the sensation of dysphagia from an early age. The 2016 ESPGHAN/NASPGHAN guidelines recommend that dysphagia should be suspected in patients with EA who have food aversion, impaction, difficulty swallowing, cough, odynophagia, vomiting, or malnutrition [8]. An esophagram along with an upper endoscopy with biopsies are the recommended tests for these patients to rule out anatomic and inflammatory causes for symptoms. If the results of these tests are normal, esophageal manometry may be considered next in the diagnostic algorithm. (Fig. 18.2) In particular, when HRM is performed with simultaneous impedance, the degree of dysmotility can be further assessed via measurement of liquid bolus stasis associated with swallows. Three distinct motility patterns have been recognized in association with EA/TEF: pressurization, isolated distal contractions, and aperistalsis [23]. Management of dysphagia in EA should be tailored to the patient and include treatment of any underlying esophagitis with acid suppression, adaptation of feeding techniques, and management of strictures by dilation or endoscopic knife treatment [26].

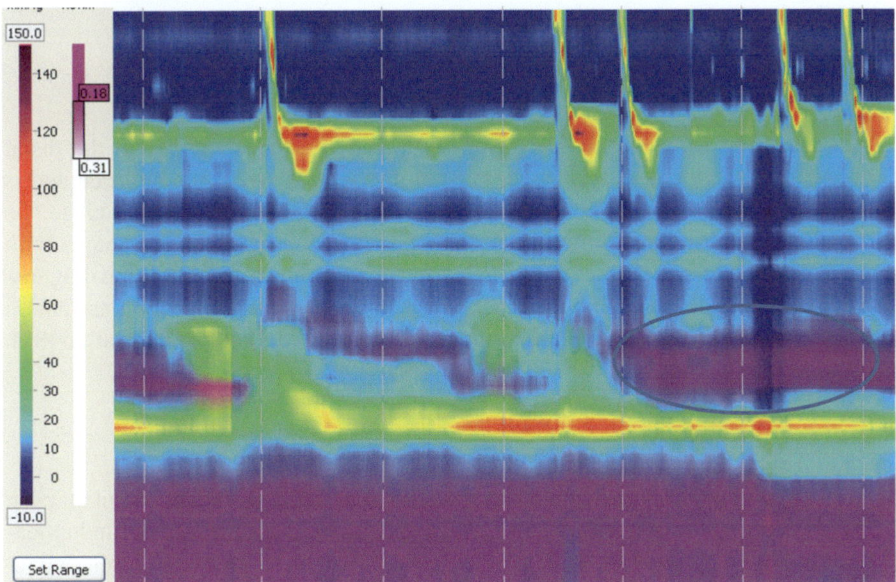

Fig. 18.2 Combined HRM with impedance tracing in a patient with esophageal atresia and a tight fundoplication. Absent peristalsis with incomplete relaxing LES and esophageal stasis of fluid just superior to LES (circled purple)

Vascular Rings and Slings

The term vascular ring refers to congenital vascular anomalies of the aortic arch system that compress the esophagus and trachea, causing symptoms related to those two structures. Double aortic arch is the most commonly reported vascular ring, followed by right aortic arch with left ligamentum arteriosum. Pulmonary artery sling is rare, and these patients need to be carefully evaluated for frequently associated tracheal stenosis. Another cause of tracheal compression occurring only in infants is the innominate artery compression syndrome. In the current era, the diagnosis of a vascular ring is best established by CT imaging that can accurately delineate the anatomy of the vascular ring and associated tracheal pathology. For patients with a right aortic arch, there recently has been an increased recognition of a structure called a Kommerell diverticulum which may require resection and transfer of the left subclavian artery to the left carotid artery though its role in producing symptoms of dysphagia is controversial. A very rare vascular ring is the circumflex aorta that is treated with the aortic uncrossing operation. Patients with vascular rings should all have an echocardiogram because of the incidence of associated congenital heart disease [27]. On occasion, esophageal manometry is needed to determine if these rings are causing a functional obstruction to help guide the cardiothoracic surgeon if a ring should be repaired or not. Persistent feeding difficulties and dysphagia have been reported in children with vascular rings and slings. While respiratory symptoms typically continue to persist over time, in a recent retrospective study, dysphagia almost always resolved [28].

Schatzki Ring

A Schatzki ring (or Schatzki-Gary ring) is a ring of mucosal tissue in the distal esophagus that can cause dysphagia. It is an uncommon finding in children and is usually associated with GER, hiatal hernia, or eosinophilic esophagitis [29]. The most frequent presenting symptom of these patients is progressive dysphagia with solid food and acute food impaction [30]. A barium esophagram is useful in diagnosing Schatzki rings. The goal in these patients is to treat any esophageal inflammation which may result in resolution of the ring or, when needed, esophageal dilation [31].

Post-fundoplication

Dysphagia is reported in up to 6.5% of patients post-fundoplication and in an even higher number in children with EA post-fundoplication [32]. The Nissen fundoplication is total (360°) and is the most common technique performed in children to treat GERD or a hiatal hernia. Dysphagia post-fundoplication is thought to be due to an overly tight wrap causing mechanical obstruction at the level of the wrap. Contrast esophagram, upper GI endoscopy, and esophageal HRM with impedance are useful diagnostic tests. An esophagram may reveal an air-fluid level or distal esophageal compression from a paraesophageal hernia secondary to slippage of a Nissen fundoplication over time. An upper endoscopy can also show evidence of fundoplication herniation, tightness at the lower esophageal sphincter, and/or a distal esophageal diverticulum, all of which could contribute to dysphagia. Finally, HRM with impedance can identify if there are elevated pressures in the gastroesophageal junction (suggesting a too-tight fundoplication), prolonged bolus stasis above the fundoplication (suggesting dysphagia or increased aspiration risk), or two separate distal esophageal high pressure zones (suggestive of a slipped fundoplication) (see Fig. 18.2). Treatment of dysphagia in this population should be tailored to individual patients but frequently includes a trial of botulinum toxin (Botox) injection to the LES (to see if dysphagia temporarily improves prior to considering dilation), esophageal balloon dilation, or, in extreme cases, takedown of the fundoplication.

Inflammatory conditions

EoE

Eosinophilic esophagitis (EoE) is a chronic inflammatory disease characterized by eosinophilic infiltration of the esophagus and clinical symptoms of dysphagia, feeding difficulties, vomiting, food impactions, or cough. The dysphagia associated with EoE may be multifactorial and result from inflammation, fibrosis, and/or the presence of a Schatzki ring [29]. The incidence of esophageal motor abnormalities is reported to be between 4% to 87% in patients with EoE [29, 33]. A range of manometric abnormalities have been reported in children with EoE, including aperistalsis, simultaneous contractions, diffuse esophageal spasm, nutcracker esophagus, and lower esophageal sphincter abnormalities. In adults, the prevalence of these abnormalities increases with longer disease duration [34]. It is not clear, however, if these nonspecific findings correlate with clinical symptoms. In children, abnormal peristalsis was seen in 41% of patients undergoing esophageal manometry [33]. When using prolonged esophageal manometry (24 h) with pH-monitoring, children with EoE showed an increase in the number of isolated and high-amplitude contractions and ineffective peristalsis both in the fasting and fed state [33]. The impact of therapies (steroids, acid suppression, and/or dietary interventions) on the restoration of esophageal motility in children is not known. An adult study comparing esophageal motility in EoE patients before and after therapy with topical budesonide was able to show that observed motility abnormalities resolved in 86% of patients after successful treatment [35].

GERD

Gastroesophageal reflux (GER) is a normal physiologic process in which there is an involuntary passage of gastric contents into the esophagus. Most reflux episodes are asymptomatic, short in duration, and limited to the distal esophagus and occur several times per day, particularly after meals. The most common trigger for a reflux episode is a transient relaxation of the LES [36]. Other causes for reflux include increased abdominal pressure not accompanied by an increase in the pressure of the LES or conditions where the LES pressure is reduced. In infancy, physiologic GER is associated with regurgitation or occasionally vomiting or may occur in the absence of symptoms. GER is frequently encountered in infancy and tends to self-resolve over time [37]. Gastroesophageal reflux disease (GERD) is diagnosed when reflux of gastric contents is the cause of troublesome symptoms and/or complications such as esophagitis, nutritional compromise, respiratory complications, or poor weight gain. Pathologic GERD may be primary or secondary. GERD is particularly common with a number of genetic syndromes such as Cornelia de Lange syndrome and trisomy 21; birth defects such as congenital diaphragmatic hernia, omphalocele, and gastroschisis; cystic fibrosis; and neurologic conditions such as hypotonia and myotonic dystrophy [38]. Dysphagia is not a typical presenting symptom of GERD unless there is esophagitis present which may have an impact on esophageal clearance. When adult patients with GERD and dysphagia were evaluated using high-resolution manometry combined with impedance, patients with pathologic acid exposure times were associated with decreased esophageal motility, reflected by a significantly lower mean distal contractile integral (DCI) associated with peristalsis. There was also a significant correlation between lower individual DCI and longer total bolus transit time. In these patients, proton-pump inhibitor (PPI) therapy decreased the frequency of dysphagia and improved the peristaltic force [39]. Chronic mucosal inflammation can also lead to a fibrotic stricture and in turn cause mechanical obstruction, worsening any symptoms of dysphagia. Therefore, in any patient with dysphagia and GERD, barium imaging should be performed prior to other testing. Chronic reflux is often associated with a hiatal hernia and is the most common etiology of dysphagia in patients with a hiatal hernia. The larger the hiatal hernia, the worse the dysphagia. Impaired contractile vigor due to repeated acid exposure of the hiatal pouch has also been associated with esophageal dysmotility and subsequent dysphagia [40].

Infection

Candida, herpes simplex virus (HSV), *Mycobacterium tuberculosis*, *Aspergillus*, histoplasmosis, and *Cytomegalovirus* (CMV) infections of the esophagus can all cause dysphagia in children.

Candida esophagitis is most commonly seen in children taking oral or inhaled steroids.

In a study of human immunodeficiency virus (HIV)-infected children, dysphagia was caused by abnormalities in both the oral and pharyngeal phase, likely related to underlying *Candida* esophagitis as well as HIV encephalopathy [41].

Neuromuscular/Motility disorders

Achalasia

Achalasia is a primary motility disorder of the esophagus defined as absence of peristalsis with a normal or hypertensive non-relaxing LES. The cause for achalasia is not known, but infectious, autoimmune, and inflammatory mechanisms have been proposed [42–44]. Histological analysis of achalasia has revealed an absence or degeneration of the Auerbach's plexus throughout the body of the esophagus. It is postulated that myenteric plexus damage leads to loss of the inhibitory ganglionic cells in the myenteric plexus. Thus, neurotransmitter inhibition is decreased with a relative deficiency in nitric oxide. This leads to an imbalance in the concentrations of inhibitory nitric oxide versus stimulatory acetylcholine, which in turn results in unchecked contraction of the LES mediated by acetylcholine. The most common cause of achalasia in children is idiopathic though it has been reported in paraneoplastic conditions and in the context of Chagas disease though the latter has only been reported in adults. In children, achalasia can be associated with Allgrove or triple A syndrome, an autosomal recessive syndrome characterized by a triad of achalasia, alacrima, and adrenal insufficiency/Addison's disease. It is also sometimes associated with autonomic instability [45]. Clinically, achalasia is an uncommon disorder in young children. In the pediatric population, the mean age of diagnosis is 10 years [46]. Classical presenting features include progressive dysphagia, more for solids initially but then eventually progressing to both liquids and solid food dysphagia. Regurgitation is common due to ingested food and liquid remaining in the esophagus for long periods. Sometimes these patients are mistakenly diagnosed with GERD, but in fact they are regurgitating esophageal rather than gastric contents. Because of the esophageal stasis, patients often have a cough that occurs especially when lying down. When esophageal contents are aspirated into the airways, this can develop into pneumonia. Up to 50% of adult achalasia patients have abnormalities seen on chest CT, and adult studies show that balloon dilation of the LES results in complete resolution of cough [45, 47]. Other presenting symptoms include weight loss and malnutrition because of the inability of food to pass into the esophagus, persistent vomiting of undigested esophageal contents, or progressive restriction of oral intake because of the severity of symptoms [48]. In addition, retrosternal discomfort and pain radiating to the interscapular area are other clinical features of achalasia.

As with all pediatric patients with dysphagia, a barium esophagram is the initial first step in diagnosis. Barium imaging may be normal or may show tertiary contractions, a dilated esophagus, an air-fluid level, and/or a slow trickle of barium through the LES creating a bird's beak appearance [49]. Over time, as the esophagus dilates, it develops the appearance of sigmoid colon. In adults, staging of the dilation of the esophagus exists. Stage 1 is proximal dilation <4 cm, stage II is dilation between 4 and 7 cm, and stage III is dilation greater than 7 cm. Stages II and III are more likely

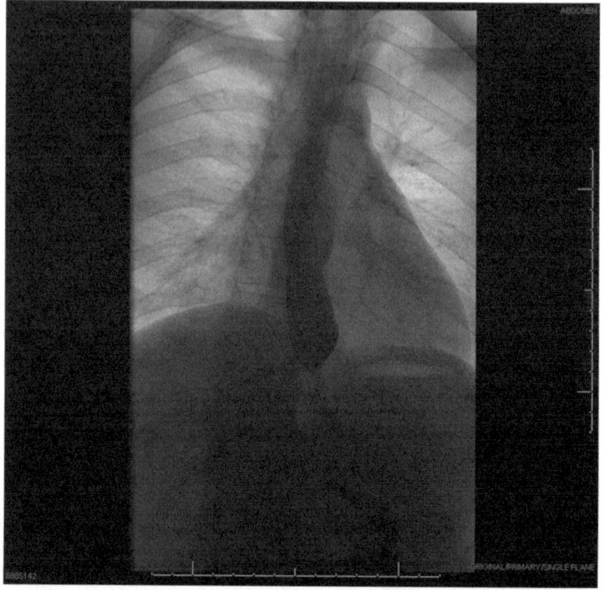

Fig. 18.3 Esophagram from a patient with achalasia showing the classical "bird's beak" appearance

to be type 3 achalasia on the Chicago classification [43] (Fig. 18.3). A plain chest X-ray may show a retro-cardiac air-fluid level on lateral views. On a plain abdominal X-ray, absence of the fundic air bubble is another clue that the patient may have achalasia [50].

Esophageal Manometry

Esophageal manometry remains the gold standard for diagnosing achalasia [50]. Manometry must document complete aperistalsis of the esophagus in association with liquid swallows as well as non-relaxation of the LES, as reflected by an elevated 4-s integrated relaxation pressure (IRP) >15 mmHg. The advent of high-resolution manometry (HRM) has allowed classification of achalasia into three major subtypes called the Chicago classification [51] (see Table 18.2). These subtypes are also seen in pediatrics but have not been clinically validated. The manometric criteria for diagnosis may differ as there are now studies in both adults and pediatrics showing that the IRP criteria may be lower for children. Apart from its value in diagnosis, esophageal manometry may predict prognosis with adult studies showing that patients with type 3 achalasia have a better therapeutic response than patients with types 1 and 2 [52]. Esophageal manometry also plays a critical role in the evaluation of children with persistent dysphagia after treatment with Heller myotomy or pneumatic dilation to assess if the persistent symptoms are related to esophageal body dysmotility or a persistent elevation in IRP requiring additional therapies directed at the LES (Figs. 18.4, 18.5, and 18.6).

Table 18.2 Chicago classification of achalasia

Disorder	Criteria
Type I achalasia (classic achalasia)	Elevated median IRP (>15 mmHg), 100% failed peristalsis (DCI <100 mmHg). *Premature contractions with DCI values less than 450 mmHg-s-cm meet criteria for failed peristalsis*
Type II achalasia (with esophageal compression)	Elevated median IRP (>15 mmHg), 100% failed peristalsis, pan-esophageal pressurization with ≥20% of swallows. *Contractions may be masked by esophageal pressurization, and DCI should not be calculated*
Type III achalasia (spastic achalasia)	Elevated median IRP (>15 mmHg), no normal peristalsis, premature (spastic) contractions with DCI >450 mmHg-s-cm with ≥20% of swallows. *May be mixed with pan-esophageal pressurization*

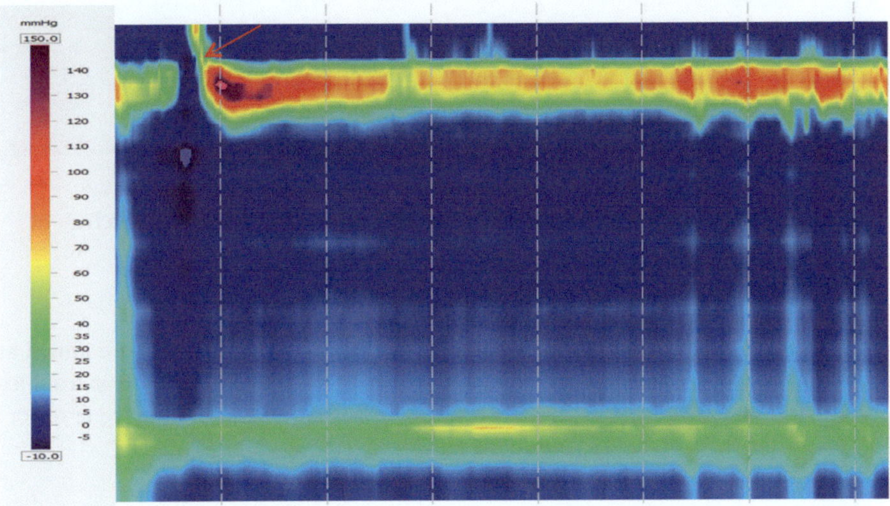

Fig. 18.4 Type I achalasia −100% failed contractions (arrow indicates swallow)

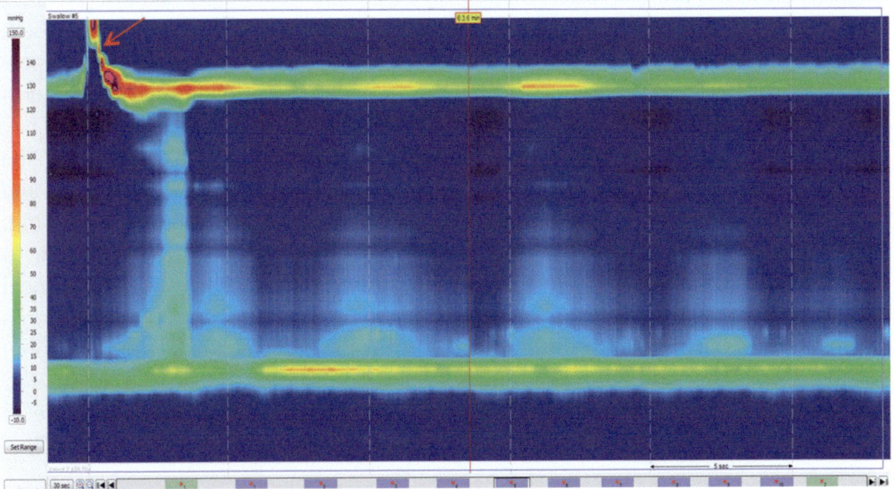

Fig. 18.5 Type II achalasia: pan-esophageal pressurization (arrow indicates swallow)

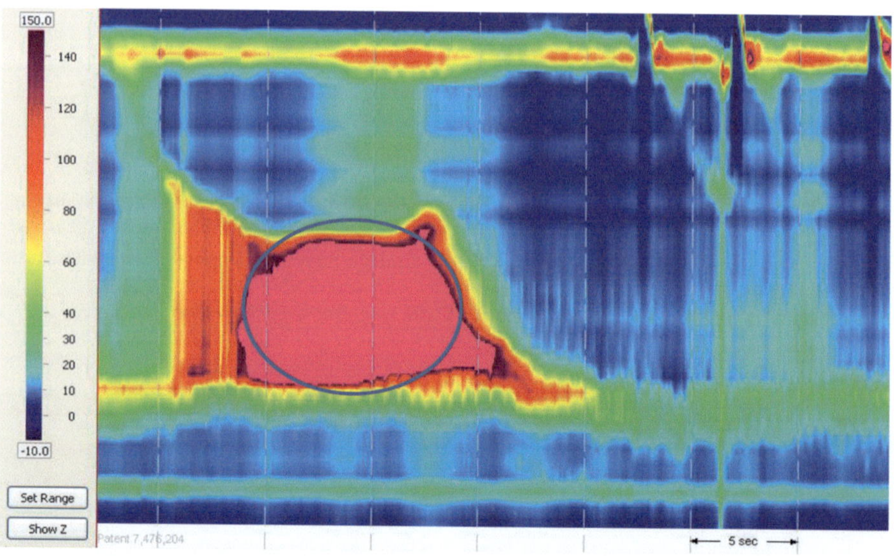

Fig. 18.6 Type III achalasia with spasticity of the distal esophagus (circled) and high IRP

Management

There are currently no therapeutic cures for achalasia. Most therapies are aimed at reducing the elevated LES pressure, hence palliating or alleviating the most troublesome symptoms of achalasia [53]. There are no effective therapies directed at restoring peristalsis or esophageal motility.

Pharmacological Therapy

Medications play a minor role in the treatment of achalasia. Nitrates or calcium channel blockers are the most commonly used pharmacologic agents. Nitrates inhibit normal LES contraction by increasing nitric oxide concentration in smooth muscle cells, which, in turn, increases cyclic adenosine monophosphate levels promoting muscle relaxation. Wen et al. in a recent review identified only two randomized studies assessing the success of nitrates in the treatment of achalasia. They concluded that no solid recommendations could be given on the use of nitrates in the treatment of achalasia [54]. Calcium channel antagonists block calcium entry and hence esophageal muscle contraction. Nifedipine, in sublingual doses of 10–20 mg, 15–30 min before meals, is the most commonly used oral drug for achalasia. It inhibits LES contraction and decreases LES resting pressure up to 60%. The clinical response is of short duration because drug tolerance develops rapidly. Symptom improvement is often incomplete, and side effects such as headache, hypotension, and leg edema are common limiting factors in their use.

Thus, these drugs are commonly reserved for patients who cannot or refuse to undergo other more invasive therapies and for those in whom Botox injection has failed.

Endoscopy

Endoscopy may reveal a dilated distal esophageal sac containing stagnant food and fluid with a concomitant *Candida* overgrowth and a closed LES with a rosette-like appearance. While endoscopy may be suggestive of an achalasia diagnosis, the primary role of endoscopy is for therapeutic intervention of the LES *after* manometric confirmation of the diagnosis has been obtained. In preparation for endoscopy and anesthesia, it is important to note that all patients with suspected achalasia are at high risk for aspiration during induction because of the retained esophageal contents and some institutions have a modified, longer NPO period for these patients. Most pediatric centers will perform a rapid sequence induction with intubation for all patients because of this risk [55, 56].

Botulinum Toxin

Botulinum toxin (Botox) is a neurotoxic protein produced by the bacterium *Clostridium botulinum* and related species, which prevents the release of acetylcholine from axon endings located in the neuromuscular junction, thus resulting in paralysis. Botox injection into the lower esophageal sphincter results in relaxation and may be considered in patients in whom the diagnosis is not clear and a less permanent therapy is needed to determine if symptoms improve or in patients that are too ill/unstable to undergo more definitive therapy such as pneumatic dilation or Heller myotomy. Botox is dosed on a per kilogram basis with a typical dose of 6 mg/kg/injection up to a maximum of 100 units in children. The Botox dose is usually divided into four aliquots and injected into the four quadrants of the lower esophageal sphincter under direct endoscopic vision. Efficacy, defined as improvement in global symptom scores and reduction in LES pressures, is 85% in the short term; however, this decreases to 50% at 6 months and 30% after 1 year [57]. It is generally a safe procedure, with rare adverse events including mucosal injury and very rarely bleeding, mediastinitis, or pneumothorax. In addition, repeat injections may be less effective [57]. Due to the poor long-term efficacy, this treatment is generally reserved for patients that are too unwell to undergo any of the other procedures.

Pneumatic Dilation

The aim of pneumatic dilation (PD) treatment is reduction of LES pressure which then alleviates symptoms related to the obstruction to the passage of food in the LES. This is one of the first-line treatments for pediatric achalasia with patients undergoing 1–6 dilations (median 2) to achieve symptom resolution [49]. Up to 87% of patients experience symptomatic improvement with PD [58, 59]. The procedure involves endoscopically placing a pneumatic balloon dilator across the LES and inflating the balloon with air to achieve disruption of the LES. In contrast to the hydrostatic balloons used for dilation of esophageal strictures, achalasia balloons are non-compliant and generate more radial force when inflated with air. Pneumatic dilation balloons are designed so that it can be inflated to a desired maximum diameter (typically 30, 35, or 40 mm). Because the balloon is rigid, further inflation can only result in the increase of the pressure at the stenotic zone, but not the diameter which in theory decreases the risk of perforation. A pediatric case series of 34 patients reported that 100% of PD patients experienced symptom recurrence, compared to 53% of Heller myotomy patients ($p < 0.01$) [60]. Large motility centers anecdotally experience higher response rates to both procedures. GERD is the most common adverse event seen with disruption of the LES. It occurs in 4% of patients treated with PD [53]. Other adverse effects include perforation (5%), chest pain, and rarely bleeding.

Laparoscopic Heller Myotomy

The goal of laparoscopic Heller myotomy (LHM) is to permanently disrupt the LES by extramucosal esophageal myotomy (cutting the muscle of the esophagus). The first report of surgical esophageal myotomy for achalasia was from Germany in 1914 by Ernest Heller [61]. The surgical myotomy slowly evolved over the next 80 years. LHM is now most commonly performed via 4–5 small abdominal incisions. Once the esophagus has been adequately freed up, approximately 6–8 cm of the esophageal muscle is cut with extension down 2–3 cm onto the stomach. Due to the disruption of the natural connections with the esophagus and surrounding structures, up to 4.7% of patients develop symptomatic reflux, and 2% have pathologic reflux by reflux testing after the procedure [62]. To restore the main antireflux barrier, a partial fundoplication is typically performed. A total 360° fundoplication is generally considered too great of an obstacle to esophagogastric transit for patients with an impaired esophageal peristalsis. Anterior 180° Dor and posterior 180° Toupet partial fundoplications are the two commonly performed antireflux procedures with LHM [63]. Adverse effects associated with LHM include tears to the mucosa during myotomy (12%, which are usually repaired without clinical consequences), GERD (highly variable, about 15%), rarely bleeding, and damage to the lung, spleen, stomach, esophagus, or liver [64]. In 2011, a randomized trial by Boeckxstaens and colleagues comparing PD to LHM was published in the *New England Journal of Medicine* [65]. Allowing for repeated PD to be performed if needed, the authors found that after 2 years of follow-up, there was no significant difference in success rates between the two treatments, with both modalities achieving therapeutic success of over 85%. A perforation rate of 4% for pneumatic dilation and 12% for Heller myotomy patients was also reported [65].

Per Oral Endoscopic Myotomy (POEM)

In 2008, Dr. Haruhiro Inoue performed the first human endoscopic myotomy, coined POEM (per oral endoscopic myotomy). Dr. Inoue subsequently published the first case series of POEM in 17 patients, reporting excellent clinical results for esophageal achalasia [66]. POEM appears to be emerging as a preferred modality for the treatment of achalasia in modern times. The POEM procedure starts with an endoscopic examination of the upper GI tract, and any residual debris is suctioned from the esophagus. After injection of a saline solution under the mucosa in the distal esophagus, a "submucosal tunnel" is created allowing for access to the diseased muscle. After completion of the tunnel, the inner circular muscle layer is cut along the length of the tunnel. An antibiotic solution is sprayed into the tunnel, and the entry site is closed with small clips. Adverse effects can include excessive gas in the abdominal cavity related to carbon dioxide insufflation, esophageal perforation, infection, bleeding, and aspiration pneumonia. Small pediatric case series suggest that symptom resolution occurs in 66–100% of patients, comparable to PD and LHM [67–69].

Emerging Therapies

Self-expanding metallic stents have recently been explored as a potential therapy for achalasia. There are very few studies available on this treatment. Stents are placed into the esophagus endoscopically. The stents gradually expand at body temperature over 24 h, resulting in more predictable tearing of the cardia muscle, less tissue scarring, and a lower rate of stenosis after the removal of the stent. A prospective randomized study evaluating the long-term efficacy of a partially covered removable metallic stent versus PD was reported from a group in China. Li et al. reported a clinical success rate of 83% for the 30 mm stent at 10 years, whereas the success rate for 20 mm stent and PD was 0%. However, the dilation protocol was less aggressive than the standard technique used in Europe with a maximal diameter of only 32 mm [70]. In another, single-center long-term prospective study, Zhao et al reported, using a 30 mm metallic stent, a clinical success rate of >80% [71]. No perforation or mortality was reported, but stent migration occurred in 5% of patients, GERD in 20%, and chest pain in 38.7%. Although these results appear promising, this technique needs to be evaluated more and tested in comparison with the therapeutic protocols of PD and LHM used in Europe and the USA.

Recently, there is limited data on the use of ethanolamine oleate (EO) to treat achalasia [72]. EO is a sclerosant agent and has been used in the treatment of bleeding esophageal varices, varicose veins, and reactive vascular lesions. Injection of EO into the LES has been theorized to induce an inflammatory response and fibrosis in the tissues, thus leading to damage of the excitatory neurons and decreased LES pressure. Moreto et al. performed injections every 2–4 weeks until dysphagia resolved in 103 patients over the last 20 years. The primary outcome was dysphagia relief. Secondary outcomes were LES pressure. They reported a 90% of cumulative expectancy of being free of recurrence at 50 months [72]. There is skepticism about this procedure because of the fibrotic nature of the narrowing.

Future Therapies

All the present approaches for the treatment of achalasia are targeting the disruption of the esophagus rather than trying to correct the underlying abnormality and restore the motility function. In view of the fact that the enteric neurons innervating the esophagus and the LES could disappear due to an autoimmune mechanism, theoretically immunosuppressive therapy could be considered to prevent disease progression. At the time of diagnosis, however, the number of neurons is already decreased, leading to significant dysfunction and symptoms. In an experimental study in mice, it was suggested that transplantation of neuronal stem cells might be a future therapeutic option [73]. The neurospheres, as they called the neural stem cells, can be isolated and cultured from mucosal biopsies as proven by Metzger et al. [74]. They generated neurosphere-like bodies capable of proliferating and generating multiple neuronal subtypes; when transplanted, they colonized cultured aganglionic human hindgut to generate ganglia-like structures comprised of enteric neurons and glia. Unfortunately, after in vivo transplantation into the mice intestine, these neurosphere-like bodies failed to adopt a neuronal phenotype. Similar findings were reported from other groups. Clearly, more research is required to develop optimized therapies and techniques of stem cell therapy to restore the functional anatomy of the LES.

Connective Tissue Disorders

Progressive systemic sclerosis (PSS) or scleroderma is a connective tissue disorder which causes smooth muscle atrophy and fibrosis of the distal esophagus. Clinically, patients typically report GI symptoms of gastroesophageal reflux and dysphagia. Manometry studies can show reduced amplitude or absent contractions and decreased LES pressure [75]. (Fig. 18.7) This complete loss of peristalsis causes food stasis in the esophagus, which can cause pulmonary symptoms from aspiration as well as primary pulmonary fibrosis [76]. Absent esophageal contractility on HRM was associated with increased skin disease severity and worse lung function [77].

While scleroderma is the most well-described connective tissue disorder causing esophageal motility abnormalities, very similar manometric patterns are seen in mixed connective tissue disorders, and in many cases, dysphagia is absent despite a complete lack of peristalsis. Strictures due to increasing fibrosis or uncontrolled reflux are also implicated in the dysphagia in these patients. Manometry is the gold standard for patients with PSS and dysphagia; however, there is poor correlation between manometric abnormalities and clinical presentation with many patients having an absence of symptoms despite severe disturbances of peristalsis. Treatment of these patients is largely supportive and includes acid suppression, aspiration precautions, and close monitoring for complications of GERD. The severity and extent of GERD in PSS is most closely related to the loss of distal esophageal peristalsis [78, 79].

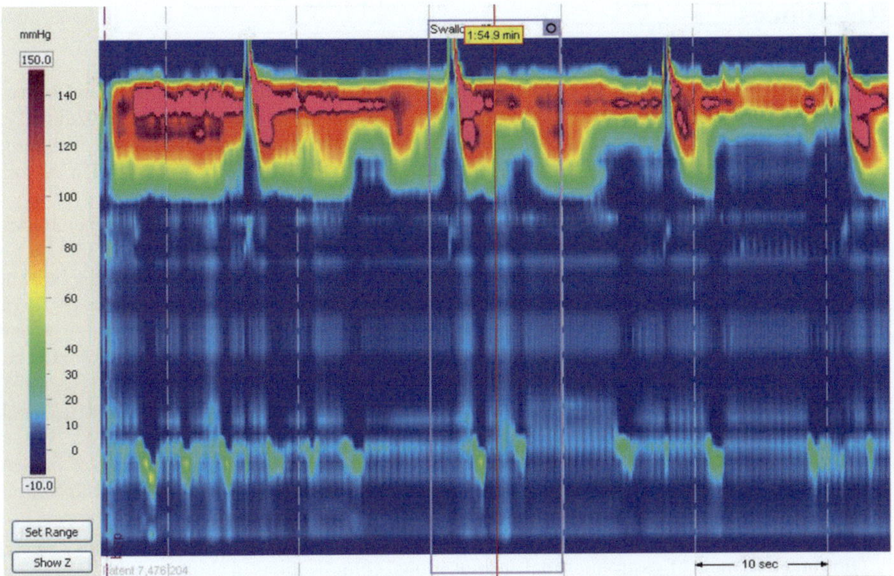

Fig. 18.7 Connective tissue disorder – HRM tracing showing absent peristalsis and low LES pressure

Esophageal Spasms

Diffuse esophageal spasm is a rare esophageal motility disorder in children. Clinically, it is characterized by dysphagia and chest pain. In 2011, the Chicago classification defined it by premature contractions in at least 20% of swallows with normal IRP (LES relaxation) [80]. In children, there are few case reports of DES [81]. In a retrospective review of 278 pediatric patients (aged 0–18 years) who underwent esophageal manometry, 13% had DES [81]. In patients diagnosed with DES, feeding refusal was the most common chief complaint followed by vomiting. Dysphagia was reported in three patients older than 5 years of age. Manometrically, all patients showed simultaneous contractions of the esophagus [81]. Use of Botox along with endoscopic ultrasound or peroral endoscopic myotomy is a promising approach [82], though there are no pediatric studies on efficacy of therapy.

Summary

Esophageal dysphagia in children can occur due to a variety of etiologies. A high level of suspicion, a thorough history, and clinical examination are helpful in distinguishing the different causes. After anatomic causes have been ruled out via radiographic studies, high-resolution esophageal manometry is a useful diagnostic tool to assist in the diagnosis and management of these children.

References

1. Arvedson JC. Assessment of pediatric dysphagia and feeding disorders: clinical and instrumental approaches. Dev Disabil Res Rev. 2008;14(2):118–27. https://doi.org/10.1002/ddrr.17.
2. Coyle J, Davis L, Easterling C, et al. Oropharyngeal dysphagia assessment and treatment efficacy: setting the record straight (response to Campbell-Taylor). J Am Med Dir Assoc. 2009;10(1):62–6. https://doi.org/10.1016/j.jamda.2008.10.003.
3. Manikam R, Perman JA. Pediatric feeding disorders. J Clin Gastroenterol. 2000;30(1):34–46. http://www.ncbi.nlm.nih.gov/pubmed/10636208. Accessed 15 Sept 2017.
4. Rudolph CD, Link DT. Feeding disorders in infants and children. Pediatr Clin N Am. 2002;49(1):97–112, iv. http://www.ncbi.nlm.nih.gov/pubmed/11826810. Accessed 15 Sept 2017.
5. Domenech E, Kelly J. Swallowing disorders. Med Clin North Am. 1999;83(1):97–113, ix. http://www.ncbi.nlm.nih.gov/pubmed/9927963. Accessed 15 Sept 2017.
6. Oh CH, Levine MS, Katzka DA, et al. Congenital esophageal stenosis in adults. Am J Roentgenol. 2001;176(5):1179–82. https://doi.org/10.2214/ajr.176.5.1761179.
7. Luedtke P, Levine MS, Rubesin SE, Weinstein DS, Laufer I. Radiologic diagnosis of benign esophageal strictures: a pattern approach. Radiographics. 2003;23(4):897–909. https://doi.org/10.1148/rg.234025717.
8. Krishnan U, Mousa H, Dall'Oglio L, et al. ESPGHAN-NASPGHAN guidelines for the evaluation and treatment of gastrointestinal and nutritional complications in children with esophageal atresia-tracheoesophageal fistula. J Pediatr Gastroenterol Nutr. 2016;63(5):550–70. https://doi.org/10.1097/MPG.0000000000001401.
9. Castor JM, Wood RK, Muir AJ, Palmer SM, Shimpi RA. Gastroesophageal reflux and altered motility in lung transplant rejection. Neurogastroenterol Motil. 2010;22(8):841–50. https://doi.org/10.1111/j.1365-2982.2010.01522.x.
10. Rana SS, Bhasin DK, Singh K. Role of endoscopic ultrasonography (EUS) in management of benign esophageal strictures. Ann Gastroenterol. 2011;24(4):280–4. http://www.ncbi.nlm.nih.gov/pubmed/24713797. Accessed 15 Sept 2017.
11. Cheng H-T, Cheng C-L, Lin C-H, et al. Caustic ingestion in adults: the role of endoscopic classification in predicting outcome. BMC Gastroenterol. 2008;8:31. https://doi.org/10.1186/1471-230X-8-31.
12. Riffat F, Cheng A. Pediatric caustic ingestion: 50 consecutive cases and a review of the literature. Dis Esophagus. 2009;22(1):89–94. https://doi.org/10.1111/j.1442-2050.2008.00867.x.
13. Baskın D, Urgancı N, Abbasoğlu L, et al. A standardised protocol for the acute management of corrosive ingestion in children. Pediatr Surg Int. 2004;20(11–12):824–8. https://doi.org/10.1007/s00383-004-1294-4.
14. Kay M, Wyllie R. Caustic ingestions in children. Curr Opin Pediatr. 2009;21(5):651–4. https://doi.org/10.1097/MOP.0b013e32832e2764.
15. Genç A, Mutaf O. Esophageal motility changes in acute and late periods of caustic esophageal burns and their relation to prognosis in children. J Pediatr Surg. 2002;37(11):1526–8. http://www.ncbi.nlm.nih.gov/pubmed/12407532. Accessed 15 Sept 2017.
16. Broor SL, Kumar A, Chari ST, et al. Corrosive oesophageal strictures following acid ingestion: clinical profile and results of endoscopic dilatation. J Gastroenterol Hepatol. 1989;4(1):55–61. http://www.ncbi.nlm.nih.gov/pubmed/2490943. Accessed 15 Sept 2017.
17. Doğan Y, Erkan T, Çokuğraş FÇ, Kutlu T. Caustic gastroesophageal lesions in childhood: an analysis of 473 cases. Clin Pediatr (Phila). 2006;45(5):435–8. https://doi.org/10.1177/0009922806289618.
18. Siersema PD, de Wijkerslooth LRH. Dilation of refractory benign esophageal strictures. Gastrointest Endosc. 2009;70(5):1000–12. https://doi.org/10.1016/j.gie.2009.07.004.
19. Contini S, Swarray-Deen A, Scarpignato C. Oesophageal corrosive injuries in children: a forgotten social and health challenge in developing countries. Bull World Health Organ. 2009;87(12):950–4. https://doi.org/10.2471/BLT.08.058065.

20. Sánchez-Ramírez CA, Larrosa-Haro A, Vásquez Garibay EM, Larios-Arceo F. Caustic ingestion and oesophageal damage in children: clinical spectrum and feeding practices. J Paediatr Child Health. 2011;47(6):378–80. https://doi.org/10.1111/j.1440-1754.2010.01984.x.
21. Sistonen SJ, Koivusalo A, Nieminen U, et al. Esophageal morbidity and function in adults with repaired esophageal atresia with tracheoesophageal fistula. Ann Surg. 2010;251(6):1167–73. https://doi.org/10.1097/SLA.0b013e3181c9b613.
22. Werlin SL, Dodds WJ, Hogan WJ, Glicklich M, Arndorfer R. Esophageal function in esophageal atresia. Dig Dis Sci. 1981;26(9):796–800. http://www.ncbi.nlm.nih.gov/pubmed/7285747. Accessed 15 Sept 2017.
23. Lemoine C, Aspirot A, Le Henaff G, Piloquet H, Lévesque D, Faure C. Characterization of esophageal motility following esophageal atresia repair using high-resolution esophageal manometry. J Pediatr Gastroenterol Nutr. 2013;56(6):609–14. https://doi.org/10.1097/MPG.0b013e3182868773.
24. Connor MJ, Springford LR, Kapetanakis VV, Giuliani S. Esophageal atresia and transitional care—step 1: a systematic review and meta-analysis of the literature to define the prevalence of chronic long-term problems. Am J Surg. 2015;209(4):747–59. https://doi.org/10.1016/j.amjsurg.2014.09.019.
25. Mahoney L, Rosen R. Feeding difficulties in children with esophageal atresia. Paediatr Respir Rev. 2016;19:21–7. https://doi.org/10.1016/j.prrv.2015.06.002.
26. Rodriguez-Baez N, Andersen JM. Management of esophageal strictures in children. Curr Treat Options Gastroenterol. 2003;6(5):417–25. http://www.ncbi.nlm.nih.gov/pubmed/12954148. Accessed 15 Sept 2017.
27. Backer CL, Mongé MC, Popescu AR, Eltayeb OM, Rastatter JC, Rigsby CK. Vascular rings. Semin Pediatr Surg. 2016;25(3):165–75. https://doi.org/10.1053/j.sempedsurg.2016.02.009.
28. François K, Panzer J, De Groote K, et al. Early and late outcomes after surgical management of congenital vascular rings. Eur J Pediatr. 2017;176(3):371–7. https://doi.org/10.1007/s00431-017-2850-y.
29. Towbin AJ, Diniz LO. Schatzki ring in pediatric and young adult patients. Pediatr Radiol. 2012;42(12):1437–40. https://doi.org/10.1007/s00247-012-2482-3.
30. Buckley K, Buonomo C, Husain K, Nurko S. Schatzki ring in children and young adults: clinical and radiologic findings. Pediatr Radiol. 1998;28(11):884–6. https://doi.org/10.1007/s002470050488.
31. Novak SH, Shortsleeve MJ, Kantrowitz PA. Effective treatment of symptomatic lower esophageal (Schatzki) rings with acid suppression therapy: confirmed on barium esophagography. Am J Roentgenol. 2015;205(6):1182–7. https://doi.org/10.2214/AJR.15.14704.
32. Holschneider P, Dübbers M, Engelskirchen R, Trompelt J, Holschneider A. Results of the operative treatment of gastroesophageal reflux in childhood with particular focus on patients with esophageal atresia. Eur J Pediatr Surg. 2007;17(3):163–75. https://doi.org/10.1055/s-2007-965087.
33. Nurko S, Rosen R, Furuta GT. Esophageal dysmotility in children with eosinophilic esophagitis: a study using prolonged esophageal manometry. Am J Gastroenterol. 2009;104(12):3050–7. https://doi.org/10.1038/ajg.2009.543.
34. van Rhijn BD, Smout AJPM, Bredenoord AJ. Disease duration determines health-related quality of life in adult eosinophilic esophagitis patients. Neurogastroenterol Motil. 2014;26(6):772–8. https://doi.org/10.1111/nmo.12323.
35. Nennstiel S, Bajbouj M, Becker V, et al. High-resolution manometry in patients with eosinophilic esophagitis under topical steroid therapy-a prospective observational study (HIMEOS-study). Neurogastroenterol Motil. 2016;28(4):599–607. https://doi.org/10.1111/nmo.12753.
36. Rybak A, Pesce M, Thapar N, Borrelli O. Gastro-esophageal reflux in children. Int J Mol Sci. 2017;18(8):pii: E1671. https://doi.org/10.3390/ijms18081671.
37. Chang AB, Cox NC, Faoagali J, et al. Cough and reflux esophagitis in children: their co-existence and airway cellularity. BMC Pediatr. 2006;6:4. https://doi.org/10.1186/1471-2431-6-4.

38. Henry SM. Discerning differences: gastroesophageal reflux and gastroesophageal reflux disease in infants. Adv Neonatal Care. 2004;4(4):235–47. http://www.ncbi.nlm.nih.gov/pubmed/15368216. Accessed 16 Sept 2017.

39. Ribolsi M, Biasutto D, Giordano A, Balestrieri P, Cicala M. Role of esophageal motility, acid reflux, and of acid suppression in nonobstructive dysphagia. J Clin Gastroenterol. 2017:1. https://doi.org/10.1097/MCG.0000000000000903.

40. DeLay K, Austin GL, Menard-Katcher P. Anatomic abnormalities are common potential explanations of manometric esophagogastric junction outflow obstruction. Neurogastroenterol Motil. 2016;28(8):1166–71. https://doi.org/10.1111/nmo.12814.

41. Nel ED, Ellis A. Swallowing abnormalities in HIV infected children: an important cause of morbidity. BMC Pediatr. 2012;12(1):615. https://doi.org/10.1186/1471-2431-12-68.

42. Goldblum JR, Whyte RI, Orringer MB, Appelman HD. Achalasia. A morphologic study of 42 resected specimens. Am J Surg Pathol. 1994;18(4):327–37. http://www.ncbi.nlm.nih.gov/pubmed/8141427. Accessed 16 Sept 2017.

43. Park W, Vaezi MF. Etiology and pathogenesis of achalasia: the current understanding. Am J Gastroenterol. 2005;100(6):1404–14. https://doi.org/10.1111/j.1572-0241.2005.41775.x.

44. Goldblum JR, Rice TW, Richter JE. Histopathologic features in esophagomyotomy specimens from patients with achalasia. Gastroenterology. 1996;111(3):648–54. http://www.ncbi.nlm.nih.gov/pubmed/8780569. Accessed 16 Sept 2017.

45. Hallal C, Kieling CO, Nunes DL, et al. Diagnosis, misdiagnosis, and associated diseases of achalasia in children and adolescents: a twelve-year single center experience. Pediatr Surg Int. 2012;28(12):1211–7. https://doi.org/10.1007/s00383-012-3214-3.

46. Hussain SZ, Thomas R, Tolia V. A review of achalasia in 33 children. Dig Dis Sci. 2002;47(11):2538–43. http://www.ncbi.nlm.nih.gov/pubmed/12452392. Accessed 16 Sept 2017.

47. Kwon HY, Lim JH, Shin YW, Kim C-W. A case of chronic cough caused by achalasia misconceived as gastroesophageal reflux disease. Allergy Asthma Immunol Res. 2014;6(6):573–6. https://doi.org/10.4168/aair.2014.6.6.573.

48. Morera C, Nurko S. Heterogeneity of lower esophageal sphincter function in children with achalasia. J Pediatr Gastroenterol Nutr. 2012;54(1):34–40. https://doi.org/10.1097/MPG.0b013e3182293d8c.

49. Franklin AL, Petrosyan M, Kane TD. Childhood achalasia: a comprehensive review of disease, diagnosis and therapeutic management. World J Gastrointest Endosc. 2014;6(4):105–11. https://doi.org/10.4253/wjge.v6.i4.105.

50. Vaezi MF, Pandolfino JE, Vela MF. ACG clinical guideline: diagnosis and management of achalasia. Am J Gastroenterol. 2013;108(8):1238–49. https://doi.org/10.1038/ajg.2013.196.

51. Bredenoord AJ, Fox M, Kahrilas PJ, et al. Chicago classification criteria of esophageal motility disorders defined in high resolution esophageal pressure topography1. Neurogastroenterol Motil. 2012;24:57–65. https://doi.org/10.1111/j.1365-2982.2011.01834.x.

52. Singendonk MMJ, Rosen R, Oors J, et al. Intra- and interrater reliability of the Chicago Classification of achalasia subtypes in pediatric high-resolution esophageal manometry (HRM) recordings. Neurogastroenterol Motil. 2017;29(11):e13113. https://doi.org/10.1111/nmo.13113.

53. Vela MF, Richter JE, Khandwala F, et al. The long-term efficacy of pneumatic dilatation and Heller myotomy for the treatment of achalasia. Clin Gastroenterol Hepatol. 2006;4(5):580–7. http://www.ncbi.nlm.nih.gov/pubmed/16630776. Accessed 16 Sept 2017.

54. Wen Z, Gardener E, Wang Y. Nitrates for achalasia. In: Cochrane database of systematic reviews. Chichester, UK: Wiley; 2002. https://doi.org/10.1002/14651858.CD002299.

55. Salem MR, Khorasani A, Saatee S, Crystal GJ, El-Orbany M. Gastric tubes and airway management in patients at risk of aspiration. Anesth Analg. 2014;118(3):569–79. https://doi.org/10.1213/ANE.0b013e3182917f11.

56. Iwakiri K, Hoshihara Y, Kawami N, et al. The appearance of rosette-like esophageal folds ("esophageal rosette") in the lower esophagus after a deep inspiration is a characteristic

endoscopic finding of primary achalasia. J Gastroenterol. 2010;45(4):422–5. https://doi.org/10.1007/s00535-009-0179-7.

57. Allescher HD, Storr M, Seige M, et al. Treatment of achalasia: botulinum toxin injection vs. pneumatic balloon dilation. A prospective study with long-term follow-up. Endoscopy. 2001;33(12):1007–17. https://doi.org/10.1055/s-2001-18935.

58. Di Nardo G, Rossi P, Oliva S, et al. Pneumatic balloon dilation in pediatric achalasia: efficacy and factors predicting outcome at a single tertiary pediatric gastroenterology center. Gastrointest Endosc. 2012;76(5):927–32. https://doi.org/10.1016/j.gie.2012.06.035.

59. Katz PO, Gilbert J, Castell DO. Pneumatic dilatation is effective long-term treatment for achalasia. Dig Dis Sci. 1998;43(9):1973–7. http://www.ncbi.nlm.nih.gov/pubmed/9753261. Accessed 16 Sept 2017.

60. Lee CW, Kays DW, Chen MK, Islam S. Outcomes of treatment of childhood achalasia. J Pediatr Surg. 2010;45(6):1173–7. https://doi.org/10.1016/j.jpedsurg.2010.02.086.

61. Heller E. Extramukose Cardiaplastik beim chronischen Cardiospasmus mit Dilatation des Oesophagus. Mitt Grenzgeb Med Chir. 1914;27:141–9.

62. Novais PA, Lemme EMO. 24-h pH monitoring patterns and clinical response after achalasia treatment with pneumatic dilation or laparoscopic Heller myotomy. Aliment Pharmacol Ther. 2010;32(10):1257–65. https://doi.org/10.1111/j.1365-2036.2010.04461.x.

63. Frantzides C, Moore RE, Carlson MA, et al. Minimally invasive surgery for achalasia: a 10-year experience. J Gastrointest Surg. 2004;8(1):18–23. https://doi.org/10.1016/j.gassur.2003.09.021.

64. Pandian TK, Naik ND, Fahy AS, et al. Laparoscopic esophagomyotomy for achalasia in children: a review. World J Gastrointest Endosc. 2016;8(2):56–66. https://doi.org/10.4253/wjge.v8.i2.56.

65. Boeckxstaens GE, Annese V, Des Varannes SB, et al. Pneumatic dilation versus laparoscopic Heller's myotomy for idiopathic achalasia. N Engl J Med. 2011;364(19):1807–16. https://doi.org/10.1056/NEJMoa1010502.

66. Inoue H, Minami H, Kobayashi Y, et al. Peroral endoscopic myotomy (POEM) for esophageal achalasia. Endoscopy. 2010;42(4):265–71. https://doi.org/10.1055/s-0029-1244080.

67. Phalanusitthepha C, Inoue H, Ikeda H, Sato H, Sato C, Hokierti C. Peroral endoscopic myotomy for esophageal achalasia. Ann Transl Med. 2014;2(3):31. https://doi.org/10.3978/j.issn.2305-5839.2014.02.04.

68. Tan Y, Zhu H, Li C, Chu Y, Huo J, Liu D. Comparison of peroral endoscopic myotomy and endoscopic balloon dilation for primary treatment of pediatric achalasia. J Pediatr Surg. 2016;51(10):1613–8. https://doi.org/10.1016/j.jpedsurg.2016.06.008.

69. Nabi Z, Ramchandani M, Reddy DN, et al. Per oral endoscopic myotomy in children with achalasia cardia. J Neurogastroenterol Motil. 2016;22(4):613–9. https://doi.org/10.5056/jnm15172.

70. Cheng Y-S, Li M-H, Chen W-X, Zhuang Q-X, Chen N-W, Shang K-Z. Follow-up evaluation for benign stricture of upper gastrointestinal tract with stent insertion. World J Gastroenterol. 2003;9(11):2609–11. http://www.ncbi.nlm.nih.gov/pubmed/14606108. Accessed 17 Sept 2017.

71. Zhao J-G, Li Y-D, Cheng Y-S, et al. Long-term safety and outcome of a temporary self-expanding metallic stent for achalasia: a prospective study with a 13-year single-center experience. Eur Radiol. 2009;19(8):1973–80. https://doi.org/10.1007/s00330-009-1373-y.

72. Moretó M, Ojembarrena E, Rodriguez M-L. Endoscopic injection of ethanolamine as a treatment for achalasia: a first report. Endoscopy. 1996;28(7):539–45. https://doi.org/10.1055/s-2007-1005551.

73. McCann CJ, Cooper JE, Natarajan D, et al. Transplantation of enteric nervous system stem cells rescues nitric oxide synthase deficient mouse colon. Nat Commun. 2017;8:15937. https://doi.org/10.1038/ncomms15937.

74. Metzger M, Caldwell C, Barlow AJ, Burns AJ, Thapar N. Enteric nervous system stem cells derived from human gut mucosa for the treatment of aganglionic gut disorders. Gastroenterology. 2009;136(7):2214–2225.e3. https://doi.org/10.1053/j.gastro.2009.02.048.
75. Crowell MD, Umar SB, Griffing WL, DiBaise JK, Lacy BE, Vela MF. Esophageal motor abnormalities in patients with scleroderma: heterogeneity, risk factors, and effects on quality of life. Clin Gastroenterol Hepatol. 2017;15(2):207–213.e1. https://doi.org/10.1016/j.cgh.2016.08.034.
76. Marie I, Dominique S, Levesque H, et al. Esophageal involvement and pulmonary manifestations in systemic sclerosis. Arthritis Rheum. 2001;45(4):346–54. https://doi.org/10.1002/1529-0131(200108)45:4<346::AID-ART347>3.0.CO;2-L.
77. Kimmel JN, Carlson DA, Hinchcliff M, et al. The association between systemic sclerosis disease manifestations and esophageal high-resolution manometry parameters. Neurogastroenterol Motil. 2016;28(8):1157–65. https://doi.org/10.1111/nmo.12813.
78. Yarze JC, Varga J, Stampfl D, Castell DO, Jimenez SA. Esophageal function in systemic sclerosis: a prospective evaluation of motility and acid reflux in 36 patients. Am J Gastroenterol. 1993;88(6):870–6. http://www.ncbi.nlm.nih.gov/pubmed/8503383. Accessed 17 Sept 2017.
79. Ebert EC. Esophageal disease in progressive systemic sclerosis. Curr Treat Options Gastroenterol. 2008;11(1):64–9. https://doi.org/10.1007/s11938-008-0008-8.
80. Singendonk MMJ, Kritas S, Cock C, et al. Applying the Chicago classification criteria of esophageal motility to a pediatric cohort: effects of patient age and size. Neurogastroenterol Motil. 2014;26(9):1333–41. https://doi.org/10.1111/nmo.12397.
81. Rosen JM, Lavenbarg T, Cocjin J, Hyman PE. Diffuse esophageal spasm in children referred for manometry. J Pediatr Gastroenterol Nutr. 2013;56(4):436–8. https://doi.org/10.1097/MPG.0b013e31827a7883.
82. Vanuytsel T, Bisschops R, Farré R, et al. Botulinum toxin reduces dysphagia in patients with nonachalasia primary esophageal motility disorders. Clin Gastroenterol Hepatol. 2013;11(9):1115–1121.e2. https://doi.org/10.1016/j.cgh.2013.03.021.

Chapter 19
Impact of Non-oral Feeding Methods on Feeding Development

Priya Raj

Introduction

The act of swallowing is a complex integrated series of neurological and physiological events which results first in the recognition of food in the mouth along with its taste and viscosity, followed by the breakdown of food to a consistency able to be swallowed, and ultimately safe and efficient propulsion of the food through the oral cavity, pharynx, and cervical esophagus. Dysphagia, or difficulty swallowing, is commonly encountered in children suffering from an underlying neurological, muscular, physiological, or structural disease or disorder. Problems may occur in the mouth, in the pharynx, in the larynx, or in the esophagus. The signs and symptoms of dysphagia can include coughing or choking with food or drink, difficulty triggering a swallow, or complete absence of a swallow, leading to complications such as frequent respiratory tract infections, weight loss, dehydration, malnutrition, aversion to food, and changes in behavior at mealtimes [1].

Non-oral tube feeding (NOTF) is useful for providing digestible nutrients in children suffering from short-term or long-term dysphagia who are unable to meet their nutritional requirements by mouth but continue to have a functional gastrointestinal tract. While the practice of NOTF dates back nearly 3500 years ago to the ancient Greeks and Egyptians, technical advances in the last few decades have made the process more acceptable for patients and a more cost-effective alternative to parenteral nutrition [2]. In general, the process of enteral feeding may be categorized into three stages. During the initial stage, the principal objective is to meet the defined nutritional and anthropometric targets. This is followed by the second stage during which these targets are maintained, while medical management is pursued to address the underlying issues causing dysphagia. If successfully addressed, the third and

P. Raj
Department of Pediatric Gastroenterology, Hepatology and Nutrition, Texas Children's Hospital, Houston, TX, USA
e-mail: praj@bcm.edu

© Springer International Publishing AG, part of Springer Nature 2018

J. Ongkasuwan, E. H. Chiou (eds.), *Pediatric Dysphagia*,
https://doi.org/10.1007/978-3-319-97025-7_19

final stage is aimed at weaning off the tube feeding and transitioning to complete oral alimentation [3].

The current chapter addresses the indications and considerations for non-oral feeding in children with dysphagia, the potential short-term and long-term complications, the implications of anti-reflux or fundoplication surgery, the challenges that may be encountered while attempting to transition to oral feeding and its overall impact on feeding development.

Indications for Non-oral Enteral Nutrition

Nonsupportive anatomy, impaired cardiorespiratory, neurologic and medical status, postural instability, gastrointestinal dysfunction, abnormal hunger and satiation cues, developmental delays, impaired oral-motor skills, oral/pharyngeal reflexes, poor airway protection, and secretion management can create barriers to successful oral feeding [4]. Enteral tube feedings are usually recommended in children with underlying dysphagia who demonstrate an impairment in at least one area of feeding that affects, (1) safety, (2) coordination, or (3) efficiency, and are unable to sustain normal growth patterns.

Safety The patient fails to demonstrate the necessary physiological function of oral, oropharyngeal, pharyngoesophageal, and esophageal phases to safely swallow oral feeds despite corrective postural techniques or modifications to the texture and consistency of their food. These children may clinically present with chronic choking or coughing, apneic spells, or recurrent respiratory infections.

Coordination This usually stems from underlying dysfunctional oral-motor skills which leads the patient to gag, vomit, have increased oral secretions, or display refusal behavior in association with oral feeds.

Efficiency When oral-motor integrity is compromised such as in children suffering from hypoxic brain damage or in those with acute or chronic cardiopulmonary disorders, they may lack the endurance and energy to sustain normal feeding behavior. This may lead to prolonged feeding time and decreased oral intake.

Enteral tube feedings may be used as a primary source of nutrition when deficits are severe (e.g., anoxic encephalopathy, head or spinal trauma, cerebral palsy, craniofacial abnormalities, neurodegenerative conditions, etc. that pose a high risk for pulmonary aspiration) or as a source of supplemental or supportive nutrition when the dysphagia is expected to be temporary (e.g., postoperative, trauma or burns, caustic ingestion, oral aversive behavior, etc.).

Table 19.1 summarizes the common indications for enteral tube feeding in children with underlying dysphagia. Early initiation of enteral nutrition is a consideration when rapid malnutrition is anticipated secondary to acute dysphagia, such as in premature infants with poor oral-motor skills; children suffering from dysphagia secondary to oral-esophageal mucosa injury from caustic ingestion, chemotherapy, or burns; children born with significant craniofacial or digestive tract malformations; or critically ill children suffering from acute respiratory failure and surgical or traumatic stress.

The Collaborative Approach and Considerations Prior to Initiating NOTF

The decision to initiate NOTF is a complex one which requires an integrated approach taking into account the medical, socioeconomic, and emotional standing of the patient and their family. It must not be forgotten that while dysphagia may present in isolation, it is often just one of the clinical impairments in a child with other complex medical or surgical issues. It can also include difficulties with child-caregiver interactions, social learning, developmental characteristics, and nutrition status. This calls for a multidisciplinary approach to tube feedings which involves a collaborative effort between the patient, their family, and various healthcare professionals [5].

Depending on the individual patient's underlying medical condition and management needs, this multidisciplinary team may involve the primary care provider, speech-language pathologist, feeding therapist, physical therapist, dietitian, nurse, gastroenterologist, otolaryngologist, neurologist, psychiatrist or psychologist, surgeon, pulmonologist, and pharmacist who help the family in their decision-making process prior to initiating NOTF and provide continued care and support thereafter. There is a growing consensus that this approach should be the standard of care for treating tube-fed children [6].

Table 19.1 Indications for enteral tube feeding in children with dysphagia

Structural/functional	Cleft lip/palate, choanal atresia, Pierre Robin sequence, craniofacial malformations, severe laryngomalacia, tracheoesophageal fistula, esophageal atresia, esophageal stricture (postsurgical, eosinophilic esophagitis, caustic ingestion, neoplastic), achalasia, and other gastrointestinal dysmotility disorders
Neurological	Anoxic encephalopathy, head or spinal trauma, meningitis, Chiari malformations, cerebral palsy, Möbius syndrome, muscular dystrophy, other neurodegenerative conditions
Inflammatory	Esophagitis secondary to chronic gastroesophageal reflux, inflammatory bowel disease, infectious, eosinophilic esophagitis, caustic ingestion, drug-induced
Behavioral/sensorial	Primary: oral aversion, textural issues, food refusal, pervasive developmental disorders, extreme food selectivity Secondary: abuse or neglect, forced feeding
Miscellaneous conditions affecting neuromuscular coordination	Prematurity, chronic lung disease, cystic fibrosis, congenital heart defects, post-organ transplant, status asthmaticus, recurrent pneumonia, burns, inborn errors of metabolism, genetic syndromes like trisomy 21, Prader-Willi and Rett syndromes, Treacher Collins syndrome, 22q11 deletion, etc.

Each member of the multidisciplinary team plays an integral role to help achieve the primary goal in children with dysphagia which is to provide optimal nutrition, hydration, and airway protection while working toward alleviating their underlying acute or chronic medical condition, attempting to restore normal swallowing function, and improving or maintaining the quality of life of patients and their caregivers. This collaboration of expert opinions within a developmental framework is crucial for building a comprehensive picture and achieving optimal outcomes in the pediatric dysphagia patient requiring NOTF.

Medical It is important to begin with a thorough, reliable, and valid evaluation of the patient's baseline clinical and nutritional status. The gastrointestinal function (digestive and absorptive) and the potential for continued or eventual transition to oral intake should also be estimated prior to committing to enteral tube feedings. The fact that many children experience improvement in swallow function over time should be a strong consideration while deciding on whether to place an enteral tube or not. Laboratory tests investigating micronutrient deficiency, food allergy testing, swallow function study, pulmonary function study, or sleep study may be useful before initiating NOTF.

Psychosocial and Cultural The process leading up to tube placement, nutrition education, equipment procurement, formula prescriptions and delivery, and ongoing care can be an overwhelming experience for the patient and their caregivers. It is important to investigate the patient's and their family's attitudes and belief systems (e.g., halal/kosher) before recommending non-oral feedings. This will help facilitate family-centered care and consequently improve outcomes after enteral tube placement.

This collaborative approach prior to initiating NOTF will help set the expectations for the family up front and will also enable the medical team to formulate a more concrete and favourable plan.

Routes of Delivery

Once the decision has been made to initiate enteral nutrition in a child with dysphagia, it is important to determine whether the patient will require it for a short-term or extended period of time. Other factors to take into consideration would be the functional status of the patient's gastrointestinal tract and their risk for aspiration [7, 8]. Possible routes of nutrient administration include (1) gastric (nasogastric or gastrostomy) and (2) post-transpyloric or transpyloric (nasoduodenal, naso-jejunal, gastrojejunostomy, or jejunostomy).

Nutrition can be delivered intravenously with total parenteral nutrition (TPN) or administered directly to the gastrointestinal (GI) tract through enteral tubes. TPN, although useful in a subgroup of children, has the well-known disadvantage of bypassing the GI tract, which may lead to bacteremia, sepsis, cholestatic liver disease, and, in rare circumstances, liver failure requiring liver transplantation [9].

Enteral feeding on the other hand is beneficial in maintaining gut function and reducing the risk of infections while promoting mucosal integrity. If short-term (less than 6–8 weeks) nutritional support is anticipated, the use of a naso-oral (NO), nasogastric (NG), nasoduodenal (ND), or naso-jejunal (NJ) tube is preferred. Silicone or polyurethane-based transnasal tubes are efficient and well tolerated for this purpose. When longer enteral nutrition is necessary, a more permanent means of providing nutritional supplementation, such as percutaneous gastrostomy or gastrojejunostomy (GJ) tube placement, may be considered. A retrospective review of enteral nutrition support practices at a tertiary pediatric hospital noted that food refusal was significantly associated with NG tube exposure >3 months (RR 3.3, $p < 0.001$, NNT = 3), and anthropometric outcomes were superior in gastrostomy-fed patients. Rates of aspiration pneumonia were similar in both groups. Despite more initial opposition to gastrostomy and a higher complication rate, gastrostomy users appeared more satisfied with their experience, as demonstrated by a much lower discontinuation rate than observed in the NG group [10].

Post-pyloric feeding beyond the stomach may be indicated in children with congenital upper gastrointestinal abnormalities, gastric dysmotility, severe vomiting resulting in growth failure, recent gastric surgery and those at increased risk of aspiration. Disadvantages of post-pyloric feeds include a requirement for longer feeding times, since continuous rather than bolus feeds must be used, and a tendency for accidental displacement (except with permanent, surgically placed primary jejunal tubes). A retrospective study in a group of children with neurological impairment found that the rates of aspiration pneumonia and mortality were similar among those treated with jejunal feeding as compared with those treated with fundoplication [11]. Gastrostomy feeds afford the benefit of tolerating large osmotic loads while retaining the stomach microbial properties during the feeding process. If ongoing need for non-oral feedings is anticipated in a child with underlying dysphagia, the gastrostomy tube may be better tolerated physically, socially, and functionally than NG or NJ tubes. The various routes and other salient features of NOTF methods are reviewed in Table 19.2.

Concurrent Anti-reflux Surgery

Children with dysphagia who qualify for percutaneous enteral tube placement may also have concomitant gastroesophageal reflux disease (GERD). GERD is especially common in children with neurodevelopmental disorders with a reported incidence as high as 70% [12]. In such patients in whom pharmacologic and/or dietary interventions have been suboptimal, anti-reflux surgery (ARS) or fundoplication is often a consideration around the time of gastrostomy tube placement. The gastric fundus is wrapped or plicated around the lower end of the esophagus and sutured in place to help reduce gastroesophageal reflux by reinforcing the lower esophageal sphincter and increasing basal lower esophageal sphincter pressure. It can also be useful to alleviate symptoms from hiatal hernia by restoring the angle of His. The

Table 19.2 Non-oral tube feedings

Tube	Duration	Placement	Delivery	Indications	Benefits	Considerations
Orogastric	Short term	Bedside. Transoral catheter to the stomach	Bolus, continuous/cyclical infusion via pump	Impaired nasal access, premature infant	Inexpensive, easy placement and removal	Impediment for suck/swallowing, risk for pulmonary aspiration from GERD or if dislodged
Nasogastric	Short term	Bedside. Transnasal catheter to the stomach	Bolus, continuous/cyclical infusion via pump	Useful in patients without active GERD/vomiting who have short-term dysphagia, supplemental feeding	Inexpensive, easy placement and removal	Nasopharyngeal/esophageal irritation, aesthetically unpleasing, impediment for suck/swallowing, risk for sinusitis/otitis media
Nasoenteric (N-D, N-J)	Short term	Fluoroscopy. Transnasal catheter beyond pylorus	Continuous infusion via pump	Useful in patients with short-term dysphagia/gastric dysmotility	Reduced risk for aspiration, decreased vomiting/GERD	Same as NG tube. Tube dislodgement, clogging or kinking of tube more prevalent
PEG/surgical gastrostomy	Long term	Endoscopic/radiological, surgical/laparoscopic. Tube inserted percutaneously into the stomach	Bolus, continuous/cyclical infusion via pump	Useful in patients with long-term dysphagia/impaired gastric dysmotility	Can continue oral feeding therapy, aesthetically more acceptable, improved mobility and patient comfort	Risks for pneumoperitoneum or colonic perforation with PEG placement, surgical placement more invasive. Stoma care for leakage/granulation tissue or ulceration. Entero-enteric fistula, buried bumper syndrome
Gastrojejunostomy (GJ)/jejunostomy	Long term	Radiological, surgical/laparoscopic. Tube inserted percutaneously into the stomach	Continuous infusion via pump	Useful in patients with severe GERD or gastroparesis and aspiration risk	Reduced risk for aspiration, decreased vomiting/GERD. With G-J can decompress gastric content with enteral feeding	Same as gastrostomy, tube migration, intestinal obstruction/volvulus. Continuous feeds can be cumbersome. Direct jejunostomy less likely to dislodge

Nissen fundoplication is total (360°), but partial fundoplications known as Thal (270° anterior), Belsey (270° anterior transthoracic), Dor (anterior 180–200°), Lind (300° posterior), and Toupet (posterior 270°) fundoplications are alternative procedures with somewhat different indications and outcomes [13].

The value of fundoplication surgery with or without gastrostomy tube placement has been and continues to be a hot topic of debate. Data from various evidence-based outcome studies related to fundoplication surgery fail to provide clarity on the issue. Hament et al. suggested that ARS together with gastrostomy tube placement was successful in treating GERD in their study group of mainly neurodevelopmentally challenged pediatric patients, but did not necessarily eliminate preexistent vomiting. If significant clinical symptoms of reflux were absent prior to tube placement, they recommended against combining ARS with it. Only if symptoms progress after PEG, ARS should be considered [14]. Patients with primary neurodevelopmental disorders however are often unable to express their discomfort due to communication deficits. This cohort of patients may exhibit nonspecific signs of GERD like increased seizures or spasticity and are also at a higher risk of resulting GERD complications like aspiration and worsening swallowing difficulties. Careful evaluation may be warranted before surgery to confirm GERD and to rule out differential diagnosis like eosinophilic esophagitis. That said, a study by Barnhart and group showed that infants with neurodevelopmental delays who underwent fundoplication at the time of gastrostomy placement did not have a reduced rate of reflux-related hospitalizations (including asthma, inhalation, GERD, pneumopathies) when compared with those who underwent gastrostomy placement alone [15].

Although Nissen fundoplication has been deemed as a generally safe and efficacious surgical procedure, over time a proportion of patients develop new or recurrent foregut symptoms. It can have a negative impact on gastric compliance and tone and sensory function leading to symptoms like recurrent retching, early satiety, accelerated gastric emptying or "dumping syndrome," "gas bloating syndrome" (inability to belch and vomit, abdominal pain after eating, and/or dysphagia), and delayed gastric emptying. These postoperative symptoms have been hypothesized to stem from visceral afferent hypersensitivity, impaired gastric accommodation, and possible vagal nerve injury. Mousa et al. prospectively evaluated the effect of Nissen fundoplication on gastric sensory and motor functions in 13 children with gastroesophageal reflux. Gastric barostat and mixed meal gastric-emptying studies were performed before surgery in all patients and were repeated after surgery in 8 and 9 children, respectively. After Nissen fundoplication, children with gastroesophageal reflux had significantly higher minimal gastric distending pressure, decreased gastric compliance, and significantly higher pain scores with no effect on gastric emptying [16].

Current literature is lacking in high levels of evidence either to support or refute fundoplication at the time of percutaneous enteral tube placement. Thus the decision may boil down to a case-by-case consideration or personal preferences of the family and dysphagia team [17].

Caregivers' Perceptions and Impact on Quality of Life

Primary caregivers are often burdened down by the stress and anxiety associated with their child's nutritional status and health. While many studies have elucidated the advantages of tube feedings to help overcome the clinically detrimental sequelae of oral-motor dysfunction, it also has a sizeable impact on quality of life and various psychosocial factors [18]. The literature presents many conflicting opinions on parental perceptions surrounding non-oral enteral nutrition modalities. The concept of NOTF has a multitude of meanings for caregivers. It is an intervention that deviates from the expected normal feeding patterns of children, and it can have a significant impact upon family routines and social dynamics. Caregiver's decisions about gastrostomy feeding are complex and difficult and must be taken into account in making therapeutic recommendations [19].

Healthcare professionals have traditionally advised earlier percutaneous enteral tube placement in children with severe neurologic disabilities, marked feeding disorders, and high risk of malnutrition in order to improve their medical and social outcomes. Potential benefits of early GT placement may include reduction of facial irritation, nasal adhesions, and oral and nasal irritation associated with an indwelling NG tube. Risks of chronic infection and aspiration due to migration of the NG tube may also be decreased. However, a delay in acceptance of the procedure by parents/guardians is often the main issue of concern [20, 21]. When families are broached with the recommendation of initiating tube feedings, it is not uncommon for them to react with a sense of "giving up hope," "relinquishing normality," or "maternal or care-giver failure," while others welcome the "end of a struggle." On the other hand, there is also evidence that ultimately the social and psychological impact of gastrostomy feeding is positive, and many parents report that they wish the intervention had taken place earlier [22]. In a study by Smith et al., 90% of the 45 families evaluated using a semi-structured interview reported satisfaction with the effects of tube feeding on their child and family life. Negative reports in this study were associated with increased stress related to feeding prior to enteral access. In addition to the clinical benefits it affords, tube feeding is also valuable for the primary care takers who feel more confident and relaxed with respect to their child's medical and nutritional status [23].

Children with complex medical and developmental disorders are often faced with significant feeding difficulties, which consequently predispose them to suboptimal growth, and poor developmental outcomes. Gastrostomy feeding has been found to improve weight z-scores and mid-arm circumference, reduce feeding time, and improve the quality of life of caregivers and children with complex neurodevelopmental disorders [24, 25]. Studies have also shown that malnourishment during the critical periods of rapid neurological development can lead to neurochemical changes within brain cells influencing cell function and structure. This could possibly result in long-lasting deficits in intelligence and school performance [26].

Poor growth not only acts as an impediment to the child's clinical well-being but also negatively impacts their integration into normal society. In a population-based study of children with moderate or severe cerebral palsy by Samson-Fang et al., they explored the relationships between nutritional status and health and functional outcomes. They noted that poor nutritional status correlated with increased health-care utilization (hospitalizations, doctor visits) and decreased participation in usual activities by the child and parent [27]. Studies have also demonstrated improved parental satisfaction in children with major feeding problems along with better parent-child communication during meals after insertion of a gastrostomy tube in the child. Heine et al. reported reduced family and child distress during feeding after gastrostomy tube insertion and that parents were happier with the gastrostomy tube than with the nasogastric tube [28]. NOTF have also been shown to reduce cumulative time spent on meals in children who had difficulties with regular oral feeding [29]. Some studies have shown an actual increase in oral intake after gastrostomy tube insertion. They postulated that improved satisfaction during meals, removal of the nasogastric tube, and improvement in the child's physical and psychological well-being may have all contributed to increased oral intake [30].

In some children with severe neurodevelopmental disabilities resulting in oropharyngeal incoordination, their families may choose to pursue some "pleasure feeding" in tandem with tube feedings despite the known risks of aspiration and potential pulmonary injury. These considerations require a clear and detailed discussion of goals and risks between the family and medical care providers [4].

Other Outcomes Related to Non-oral Tube Feeding

Approximately 4 in 100,000 children require enteral tube feeding, the rate being higher among children with complex clinical disorders [31]. It is estimated that anywhere between 40% and 70% of children with chronic medical conditions experience significant feeding difficulties. Their need for enteral tube feeding may span over months or years, which may result in chronic oral food refusal [32, 33]. Actual measurable outcomes of NOTF are dependent on whether the need is short term or long term. The duration is in turn related to factors like severity of the underlying dysphagia, age of the child at commencement of tube feedings, and complexity of the child's medical or surgical issues. Depending on the route of delivery, outcomes could be based on the attainment of specific nutrition or hydration goals, survival rates, hospitalization time, complications, overall clinical progress, and status of aspiration risk, cost, or quality of life parameters.

Although early percutaneous enteral tube placement may be beneficial in some cohorts of patients with dysphagia, the benefits need to be balanced with the risks such as infection or postoperative complications. The medical literature is conflicted with some studies suggesting improved respiratory outcomes, including decreased antibiotic use and respiratory-related hospitalizations in children at high risk for aspiration who received enteral nutrition via gastrostomy tube [34–36]. On the other hand, in a retrospective study by McSweeney et al., children who underwent gastrostomy tube placement for the treatment of aspiration had two times as many admissions as compared with aspirating patients who were fed orally. They recommended a trial of oral feeding in all children cleared to take nectar- or honey-thickened liquids prior to gastrostomy tube placement [37].

Additional studies have shown that once placed, GTs can be often fraught with complications, ranging from minor (tube leakage, skin irritation, or granulation tissue formation) to severe (worsened gastroesophageal reflux disease, cellulitis, or tube dislodgement) or prolonged oral aversions [38]. Cellulitis requiring hospitalization for antibiotics and wound care has been found to be the most common percutaneous enteral tube-related major adverse event [39]. Some studies have suggested that children with gastrostomy tubes require double the home care costs of those allocated to medically complex children without gastrostomy tubes and were more likely to have higher rates of hospital readmission. More studies are required to examine the financial implications of enteral tube feeding-associated long-term complications [40, 41].

It is therefore essential to provide close monitoring and preventative care for children with enteral tubes to help mitigate the associated risks. With the emergence of multidisciplinary team-based care for children with dysphagia, there has been an effort to encourage early oral feedings (when indicated) in order to avoid the potential comorbidities of tube feedings like tube dislodgement, mechanical obstruction, infections, potential worsening of gastroesophageal reflux, or development of prolonged oral aversions preventing patients from weaning off their enteral tube feeds [38].

Prolonged Tube Feedings and Transitioning to Oral Feeds

Though much discussion and research have focused on which patients will require feeding tubes, there is limited data available focused on who qualifies for transition to oral feeding. The need for initiating non-oral feeding mechanisms is typically determined by the nature of the underlying disease causing the dysphagia and the general health status of the child. The question of how long any individual patient will require or benefit from tube feedings is difficult to answer. Comprehensive feeding and swallowing evaluations by trained speech-language pathologists play a central role in the placement of feeding tubes and, for some patients, in the removal of feeding tubes. Close multidisciplinary follow-up and clinical reevaluation of tube-fed children are critical to identify positive changes in swallowing ability that may permit transition from tube to oral feeding.

The decision to transition back to complete oral feeds is usually driven when the following parameters are met: (1) the child demonstrates efficient and coordinated oral feeding that is safe and adequately meets their nutritional goals, and (2) enteral nutrition modalities have led to improvement in the quality of life and survival rates in many children who otherwise would have been at a high risk for malnourishment and cardiopulmonary compromise along with other morbidities. However, prolonged tube feeding may have some unintended deleterious consequences [42].

While premature infants in neonatal intensive care units often require tube feeding support owing to their immature sucking skills, as the infant matures, the need for continued tube feeding is more likely to be related to underlying medical and neurodevelopmental problems or complications. Infants requiring tube feeding in the first 6 months of life and preterm infants have been found to have a higher risk for developing long-term severe feeding disorders. Several studies of premature infants without medical complications showed that frequent non-nutritive sucking exercises during NG tube feeding can accelerate the transition to complete oral feeding and consequently decrease length of hospital stay [43]. In a retrospective study by Bazyk, 100 infants who had commenced NG tube feeding in the first 6 months of life but who were reintroduced to oral feeds before the end of the first year were evaluated. The study suggested that while prematurity in itself did not significantly impact the transition from tube to oral feeding, multiple medical complications associated with respiratory, digestive, or cardiac systems were significantly related to the length of transition. The study also pointed out that although these complications were identified as predictors of length of transition, they did not necessarily imply causation [44].

Challenges with Tube Weaning

As the prevalence of NOTF has increased, so have the challenges associated with transitioning a child from tube to oral feeding. Parental anxiety, age at which oral feeding commences, and aversive experiences along with underlying medical complications are the most common obstacles that may impede successful tube weaning.

Parental Anxiety It is important for the dysphagia team to predetermine the family's ability to cope with the stresses associated with transitioning to oral feedings. A cohesive approach with the help of a psychologist will help to build up parental confidence in their child's capacity to feed by mouth and improve the chances of positive long-term outcomes [45].

Age Later age at the time of tube feeding withdrawal has been found to be strongly associated with failure or protracted weaning course. It has been suggested that tube feeding may disrupt the establishment of physiological pathways allowing integration of sensory information. This is especially true in the case of children with complex clinical needs who have had long intensive care stays or repeated hospitalizations and may have missed out on critical periods for feeding skills development [46]. Illingworth and Lister identified that readiness for chewing occurred at around 6 months for most normal children [47]. They presented a number of case studies of children who were introduced to solid foods at a late stage, having either had previous tube feeding or a liquid or pureed diet. These children exhibited aversive or refusal behavior, including vomiting, and failure to chew. This hypothesis of a sensitive period or window for development of chewing skills has not been tested experimentally however.

Aversive Stimuli Primary feeding difficulties related to neurologic and respiratory status may also be compounded by repeated aversive oral experiences such as endotracheal and nasogastric tube placement, force feeding, and delayed establishment of normal feeding patterns, leading patients to associate oral feeding with pain or discomfort. Chronic nausea and vomiting have a particularly strong effect on human dislike of food [48]. Poorly controlled gastroesophageal reflux disease can lead to nausea, vomiting, and esophagitis, all of which may link feeding with aversive experiences. In a matched sample study, Mathisen et al. reported how children of 6 months of age with GERD had significantly more feeding difficulties and food refusal [49]. Hence in symptomatic children, it may be prudent to use modalities like combined pH-impedance monitoring or esophagogastroduodenoscopy to determine the presence of GERD and proactively address it medically or surgically.

Tube Dependency

"Tube dependency" can either be medically necessary or preventable. Permanent or unavoidable tube feeding may be deemed medically necessary for some children. This may include but is not limited to children with severe underlying metabolic disorders, those dependent on bad-tasting specific diets, patients who experience recurrent episodes of aspiration pneumonias or anyone too ill to be stressed with oral feedings [50]. Preventable tube dependency is characterized by the active refusal to eat (or drink), lack of motivation or inability to learn, or failure to demonstrate precursors of feeding skills after long-term enteral feeding, despite being medically stable to safely transition to normal oral nutrition [3]. The intensity of the avoidant/restrictive behavior can manifest as an attitude of opposition or avoidance to food, an aversion to certain foods or all food in general, a phobia of introducing food into the mouth, a textural issue, a prominent gag reflex as well as effortless vomiting, a general disinterest in food, or a hypersensitivity affecting the whole body. These unintended consequences often lead to significant psychological problems that can fracture their personal and social relationships [51].

Weaning Strategies for Tube-Dependent Children

Manikam and Perman noted that tube-fed children experienced difficulty with identifying and experiencing hunger [52]. The concept of "hunger" is a key stimulus that drives the acquisition of oral feeding skills, and it helps infants and children to precisely regulate their energy intake. When energy intake completely meets or exceeds the patients' needs, hunger can be suppressed in the short term by gastric distension and in the longer term by leptin produced by fat stores [53]. Long-term enteral feeds have been shown to suppress this hunger drive, hence making the weaning process challenging. The age at which weaning of tube feeding is attempted is also key. One study assessing the impact of tube feed reduction on growth and identification of factors associated with its successful cessation found that majority of children on tube feeds for more than 6 months eventually ceased feeds successfully, but slow and failed weaning was more likely after age 5 years [54]. Although it is difficult to evaluate the hunger and appetite levels of pediatric patients, one of the strategies proposed to enable tube feed weaning in dependent children is to reduce the amount of energy intake derived from tube feeding in order to stimulate hunger. This method when carried out in close conjunction with a multidisciplinary medical team has been used successfully in numerous studies [55, 56].

Mason et al. suggested that stimulating appetite by simply reducing tube feedings does not lead to increased oral intake. A major determinant of successful weaning from tube feeding was the child's existing acceptance of any food into the mouth. They stressed the importance of creating a link between eating orally and satisfying hunger with the help of behavioral therapy and proactive caregiver involvement [57]. Other studies have demonstrated effective weaning off tube feeding with in-patient or home-based multidisciplinary hunger provocation programs that used standardized protocols. One home-based weaning program outlined five phases to treat tube dependency, assessment, preparation, hunger induction, intensive treatment, and follow-up, with an overall success rate of 90% in those enrolled [58, 59]. A Japanese study encouraged self-feeding/finger feeding in addition to the reduction in or discontinuation of tube feeding and suggested that excessive control by parents and clinicians reduces the child's interest in food and self-feeding [60]. Majority of the tube-dependent children are capable of transferring items from one hand to the other. In order to develop the child's interest in food, activities such as cooking, messy play activities, and activities involving actions such as touching food can be used. Force feeding should be avoided in order to create a healthy and positive environment that would encourage children to eat orally [61]. Many specialized tube-weaning clinical programs exist worldwide, predominantly dedicated to short-term stays. Some favor rapid weans, while others outline a more protracted transition course. While rapid withdrawal regimes are widely publicized and are highly appealing in terms of apparent cost-effectiveness, there is limited data available with regard to long-term patient outcomes.

Conclusion

Infants and children with dysphagia requiring non-oral enteral feedings often belong to a medically fragile group with many comorbidities. It is estimated that approximately half of all children who undergo percutaneous enteral tube placement are likely to still have it 10 years later. While it affords many medical and social advantages, prospective longitudinal studies are needed to fully understand the outcomes of tube feedings on infants and children with dysphagia suffering from chronic health conditions. There is a dearth of well-structured strategies assessing the long-term efficacy and safety of weaning regimens. Future randomized controlled trials will be useful to address this. It is pivotal for this population of children to be managed with a multidisciplinary approach in order to identify risk factors for complications early and, when indicated, to proactively encourage oral intake skills to promote a shorter duration of tube feeding.

References

1. Logemann JA. The evaluation and treatment of swallowing disorders. Curr Opin Otolaryngol Head Neck Surg. 1998;6(6):395–400.
2. Chernoff R. An overview of tube feeding: from ancient times to the future. Nutr Clin Pract. 2006;21(4):408–10.
3. Dunitz-Scheer M, Marinschek S, Beckenbach H, Kratky E, Hauer A, Scheer P. Tube dependence: a reactive eating behavior disorder. Infant Child Adolesc Nutr. 2011;3(4):209–15.
4. Duffy KL. Dysphagia in children. Curr Probl Pediatr Adolesc Health Care. 2018;48(3):71–3.
5. Dusick A. Investigation and management of dysphagia. Semin Pediatr Neurol. 2003;10(4): 255–64. Elsevier.
6. Byars KC, Burklow KA, Ferguson K, et al. A multicomponent behavioral program for oral aversion in children dependent on gastrostomy feedings. J Pediatr Gastroenterol Nutr. 2003;37(4):473–80.
7. Agostoni C, Axelson I, Colomb V, et al. The need for nutrition support teams in pediatric units: a commentary by the ESPGHAN committee on nutrition. J Pediatr Gastroenterol Nutr. 2005;41:8–11.
8. Adams RC, Elias ER, Council on Children with Disabilities. Nonoral feeding for children and youth with developmental or acquired disabilities. Pediatrics. 2014;134:e1745.
9. Lewis EC, Connolly B, Temple M, John P, Chait PG, Vaughan J, Amaral JG. Growth outcomes and complications after radiologic gastrostomy in 120 children. Pediatr Radiol. 2008;38(9):963.
10. Ricciuto A, Baird R, Sant'Anna A. A retrospective review of enteral nutrition support practices at a tertiary pediatric hospital: a comparison of prolonged nasogastric and gastrostomy tube feeding. Clin Nutr. 2015;34(4):652–8.
11. Srivastava R, Downey EC, O'Gorman M, et al. Impact of fundoplication versus gastrojejunal feeding tubes on mortality and in preventing aspiration pneumonia in young children with neurologic impairment who have gastroesophageal reflux disease. Pediatrics. 2009;123:338.
12. Gangil A, Patwari AK, Bajaj P, Kashyap R, Anand VK. Gastroesophageal reflux disease in children with cerebral palsy. Indian Pediatr. 2001;38(7):766–70.
13. Minjarez RC, Jobe BA. Surgical therapy for gastroesophageal reflux disease. GI Motility online. 2006 May 16.
14. Hament JM, Bax NM, Van der Zee DC, De Schryver JE, Nesselaar C. Complications of percutaneous endoscopic gastrostomy with or without concomitant antireflux surgery in 96 children. J Pediatr Surg. 2001;36(9):1412–5.
15. Barnhart DC, Hall M, Mahant S, Goldin AB, Berry JG, Faix RG, Dean JM, Srivastava R. Effectiveness of fundoplication at the time of gastrostomy in infants with neurological impairment. JAMA Pediatr. 2013;167(10):911–8.
16. Mousa H, Caniano DA, Alhajj M, Gibson L, Di Lorenzo C, Binkowitz L. Effect of Nissen fundoplication on gastric motor and sensory functions. J Pediatr Gastroenterol Nutr. 2006;43(2):185–9.

17. Gilger MA, Yeh C, Chiang J, Dietrich C, Brandt ML, El-Serag HB. Outcomes of surgical fundoplication in children. Clin Gastroenterol Hepatol. 2004;2(11):978–84.
18. Sullivan PB, Juszczak E, Bachlet AM, Thomas AG, Lambert B, Vernon-Roberts A, Grant HW, Eltumi M, Alder N, Jenkinson C. Impact of gastrostomy tube feeding on the quality of life of carers of children with cerebral palsy. Dev Med Child Neurol. 2004;46:796–800.
19. Thorne SE, Radford MJ, McCormick J. The multiple meanings of long-term gastrostomy in children with severe disability. J Pediatr Nurs. 1997b;12:89–99.
20. Martinez-Costa C, Borraz S, Benlloch C, et al. Early decision of gastrostomy tube insertion in children with severe developmental disability: a current dilemma. J Hum Nutr Diet. 2011;24:115–21.
21. Fortunato JE, Troy AL, Cuffari C, et al. Outcome after percutaneous endoscopic gastrostomy in children and young adults. J Pediatr Gastroenterol Nutr. 2010;50:390–3.
22. Tawfik R, Dickson A, Clarke M, Thomas AG. Caregivers' perceptions following gastrostomy in severely disabled children with feeding problems. Dev Med Child Neurol. 1997;39:746–51.
23. Smith SW, Camfield C, Camfield P. Living with cerebral palsy and tube feeding: a population-based follow-up study. J Pediatr. 1999;135:307–10.
24. Sullivan PB, Lambert B, Rose M, et al. Prevalence and severity of feeding and nutritional problems in children with neurological impairment: Oxford feeding study. Dev Med Child Neurol. 2000;42:674–80.
25. Marchand V, Motil KJ. Nutrition support for neurologically impaired children: a clinical report of the North American Society for Pediatric Gastroenterology, Hepatology, and Nutrition. J Pediatr Gastroenterol Nutr. 2006;43:123–35.
26. Engle PL, Black MM, Behrman JR, De Mello MC, Gertler PJ, Kapiriri L, Martorell R, Young ME, International Child Development Steering Group. Strategies to avoid the loss of developmental potential in more than 200 million children in the developing world. Lancet. 2007;369(9557):229–42.
27. Samson-Fang L, Fung E, Stallings VA, et al. Relationship of nutritional status to health and societal participation in children with cerebral palsy. J Pediatr. 2002;141:637–43.
28. Heine RG, Reddihough DS, Catto-Smith AG. Gastro-oesophageal reflux and feeding problems after gastrostomy in children with severe neurological impairment. Dev Med Child Neurol. 1995;37:320–9.
29. Srinivasan R, O'Neill C, Blumenow W, Dalzell AM. Perceptions of care-givers following percutaneous endoscopic gastrostomy in children with congenitally malformed hearts. Cardiol Young. 2009;19:507–10.
30. Avitsland TL, Kristensen C, Emblem R, Veenstra M, Mala T, Bjornland K. Percutaneous endoscopic gastrostomy in children: a safe technique with major symptom relief and high parental satisfaction. J Pediatr Gastroenterol Nutr. 2006;43:624–8.
31. Diamanti A, Di Ciommo VM, Tentolini A, et al. Home enteral nutrition in children: a 14-year multicenter survey. Eur J Clin Nutr. 2013;67(1):53–7.
32. Rudolph CD, Link DT. Feeding disorders in infants and children. Pediatr Clin. 2002;49(1):97–112.
33. Staiano A. Food refusal in toddlers with chronic diseases. J Pediatr Gastroenterol Nutr. 2003;37:225–7.
34. Sullivan PB, Morrice JS, Vernon-Roberts A, Grant H, Eltumi M, Thomas AG. Does gastrostomy tube feeding in children with cerebral palsy increase the risk of respiratory morbidity? Arch Dis Child. 2006;91:478–82.
35. Mahant S, Friedman JN, Connolly B, et al. Tube feeding and quality of life in children with severe neurological impairment. Arch Dis Child. 2009;94:668–73.
36. Lemale J, Martin SR, Gervais F, et al. Outcome of percutaneous endoscopic gastrostomy in children: a 10 year review. Gastroenterology. 2009;236:0016–5085.
37. McSweeney ME, Kerr J, Amirault J, Mitchell PD, Larson K, Rosen R. Oral feeding reduces hospitalizations compared with gastrostomy feeding in infants and children who aspirate. J Pediatr. 2016;170:79–84.

38. van der Merwe WG, Brown RA, Ireland JD, Goddard E. Percutaneous endoscopic gastrostomy in children—a 5-year experience. S Afr Med J. 2003;93:781–5.
39. Fox VL, Abel SD, Malas S, et al. Complications following percutaneous endoscopic gastrostomy and subsequent catheter replacement in children and young adults. Gastrointest Endosc. 1997;45:64–71.
40. Berry JG, Hall DE, Kuo DZ, et al. Hospital utilization and characteristics of patients experiencing recurrent readmissions within children's hospitals. JAMA. 2011;305:682–90.
41. Heyman MB, Harmatz P, Acree M, et al. Economic and psychologic costs for maternal caregivers of gastrostomy-dependent children. J Pediatr. 2004;511–6(30):145.
42. Senez C, Guys JM, Mancini J, Paz Paredes A, Lena G, Choux M. Weaning children from tube to oral feeding. Childs Nerv Syst. 1996;12:590–4.
43. Burklow KA, McGrath AM, Valerius KS, Rudolph C. Relationship between feeding difficulties, medical complexity, and gestational age. Nutr Clin Pract. 2002;17(6):373–8.
44. Bazyk S. Factors associated with the transition to oral feeding in infants fed by nasogastric tubes. Am J Occup Ther. 1990;44(12):1070–8.
45. Blackman JA, Nelson CL. Reinstituting oral feedings in children fed by gastrostomy tube. Clin Pediatr. 1985;24(8):434–8.
46. Zangen T, Ciarla C, Zangen S, DiLorenzo C, Flores AF, Cocjin J, et al. Gastrointestinal motility and sensory abnormalities may contribute to food refusal in medically fragile toddlers. J Pediatr Gastroenterol Nutr. 2003;37:287–93.
47. Illingworth RS, Lister J. The critical or sensitive period, with special reference to certain feeding problems in infants and children. J Pediatr. 1964;65:839–48.
48. Pelchat ML, Rozin P. The special role of nausea in the acquisition of food dislikes by humans. Appetite. 1982;3(4):341–51.
49. Mathisen B, Worrall L, Masel J, Wall C, Shepherd RW. Feeding problems in infants with gastro-oesophageal reflux disease: a controlled study. J Paediatr Child Health. 1999;35(2):163–9.
50. Krom H, de Winter JP, Kindermann A. Development, prevention, and treatment of feeding tube dependency. Eur J Pediatr. 2017;176(6):683–8.
51. Mirete J, Thouvenin B, Malecot G, Le Gouez M, Chalouhi C, du Fraysseix C, Royer A, Leon A, Vachey C, Abadie V. A program for weaning children from enteral feeding in a general pediatric unit: how, for whom, and with what results? Front Pediatr. 2018;6:10.
52. Manikam R, Perman JA. Pediatric feeding disorders. J Clin Gastroenterol. 2000;30:34–46.
53. Druce M, Bloom SR. The regulation of appetite. Arch Dis Child. 2006;91:183–7.
54. Wright CM, Smith KH, Morrison J. Withdrawing feeds from children on long term enteral feeding: factors associated with success and failure. Arch Dis Child. 2011;96(5):433–9.
55. Benoit D, Wang EE, Zlotkin SH. Discontinuation of enterostomy tube feeding by behavioral treatment in early childhood: a randomized controlled trial. J Pediatr. 2000;137:498–503.
56. Kindermann A, Kneepkens CM, Stok A, van Dijk EM, Engels M, Douwes AC. Discontinuation of tube feeding in young children by hunger provocation. J Pediatr Gastroenterol Nutr. 2008;47:87–91.
57. Mason SJ, Harris G, Blissett J. Tube feeding in infancy: implications for the development of normal eating and drinking skills. Dysphagia. 2005;20:46–61.
58. Trabi T, Dunitz-Scheer M, Kratky E, Beckenbach H, Scheer PJ. Inpatient tube weaning in children with long-term feeding tube dependency: a retrospective analysis. Infant Ment Health J. 2010;31(6):664–81.
59. Wilken M, Cremer V, Echtermeyer S. Home-based feeding tube weaning: outline of a new treatment modality for children with long-term feeding tube dependency. ICAN: Infant Child Adolesc Nutr. 2015;7(5):270–7.
60. Ishizaki A, Hironaka S, Tatsuno M, Mukai Y. Characteristics of and weaning strategies in tube-dependent children. Pediatr Int. 2013;55(2):208–13.
61. Harding C, Faiman A, Wright J. Evaluation of an intensive desensitisation, oral tolerance therapy and hunger provocation program for children who have had prolonged periods of tube feeds. Int J Evid Based Healthc. 2010;8(4):268–76.

Chapter 20
Secretion Management

Elton Lambert

Introduction

Secretions within the upper aerodigestive tract assist with functions of deglutition, breathing, and immune protection among others. Secretions including mucous from the nasal cavity, oral cavity, pharynx, and lower respiratory tract and saliva from the salivary glands assist in the humidification and warming of air during respiration, the lubrication of food and liquid during deglutition, and the trapping and neutralization of pathogens as a part of adaptive and innate immune systems.

Nasal Cavity

2 Liters of nasal mucous is produced every day. This mucous is composed of water, electrolytes, immunoglobulins, and various serum and glycoproteins. Submucosal, seromucous glands, goblet cells, blood plasma transudate, mucosal tissue fluid, and tear fluid form nasal mucous [1]. Parasympathetic stimulation within the nasal cavity leads to increased nasal secretions [2].

Mucociliary clearance of nasal mucous proceeds in a coordinated manner from the paranasal sinuses through their respective outflow tracts to the nasal cavity, while secretions within the nasal cavity are transported toward the nasopharynx and the pharynx and eventually swallowed.

A variety of insults can cause increased nasal secretions. Rhinitis is inflammation of the nasal lining. A discussion of all possible etiologies of acute and chronic rhinitis is beyond the scope of this chapter. Allergies, nasal irritants, temperature/

E. Lambert
Pediatric Otolaryngology, Texas Children's Hospital/Baylor College of Medicine,
Houston, TX, USA
e-mail: emashela@texaschildrens.org

© Springer International Publishing AG, part of Springer Nature 2018
J. Ongkasuwan, E. H. Chiou (eds.), *Pediatric Dysphagia*,
https://doi.org/10.1007/978-3-319-97025-7_20

humidity changes, exposure to drugs, and infections by bacteria, viruses, parasites, or fungi causing an inflammatory process in the nasal mucosa lead to increased vascularity and transudation of water and serum proteins [1]. Increased nasal secretions with anterior rhinorrhea can be caused by nasal obstruction. Patients with deficient swallowing mechanisms can have a build of nasal secretions within the pharynx. A buildup of nasal secretions can occur due to conditions that impair mucociliary clearance.

Respiratory Epithelium

Tracheobronchial glands produce mucin-rich secretions. The mucous blanket forms a barrier between particles inhaled and the respiratory epithelium. Functions of humidification and immunity are similar to those discussed earlier in the nasal cavity. Mucous production within the tracheobronchial tree is not well known, but estimates range from 30 to 300 ml/day [3].

Ciliated epithelium extends from the larynx to the terminal bronchioles. Parasympathetic innervation stimulates secretion production and as with the nasal epithelium is modulated by inflammatory, irritants, pathogens, and agents that affect the autonomic nervous system. Mucociliary clearance, which ascends from the terminal bronchioles to the larynx, is assisted by expiratory airflow and augmented by the cough reflex [4].

Impaired mucociliary clearance can be due to primary disorders like primary ciliary dyskinesia and cystic fibrosis, secondarily due to pathogens and irritants such as cigarette smoke, or due to anatomic causes like tracheobronchomalacia. Impaired clearance of secretions may lead to chronic cough and chronic/recurrent lower respiratory infections. Mucous plugging and bronchiectasis can occur impairing ventilation. In children with impaired swallowing, aspiration can lead to increased tracheobronchial secretions taxing the tracheobronchial mucociliary system. Impaired swallowing also decreases clearance of tracheobronchial secretions transported through the glottis to the pharynx, thus increasing pharyngeal secretions.

Salivary Glands

There are three pairs of major salivary glands – the parotid, submandibular, and sublingual – and hundreds of minor salivary glands located submucosally in the oral cavity and pharynx. The parotid gland is located anterior to the external auditory canal with saliva secreted through Stensen's duct that pierces the buccal mucosa at the level of maxillary second molar. The submandibular gland lies within the submandibular triangle inferior to the mandible. Saliva secreted from the submandibular gland enters Wharton's duct and exits into the anterior floor of the mouth. The sublingual gland is located at the posterior floor of the mouth. Its associated duct of Bartholin empties into the submandibular duct.

Afferents from cranial nerves V, VII, IX, and X travel toward the solitary tract and salivary nucleus in the medulla. Parasympathetic innervation reaches the submandibular and sublingual glands via the seventh cranial nerve, and the parotid via the ninth cranial nerve. Preganglionic fibers travel along the chorda tympani to the main facial nerve trunk, and synapse in the submandibular ganglion within the submandibular space. The postganglionic fibers then innervate the submandibular and sublingual gland. Preganglionic fibers destined for the parotid gland synapse at the otic ganglion from cranial nerve IX, and continue onto the parotid via branches of cranial nerve V. Sympathetic innervation originates from the thoracic segments with preganglionic fibers synapsing in the superior cervical ganglion. Postganglionic fibers travel along the external carotid artery system [5].

1 to 1.5 L of saliva flow is produced every day. Unstimulated saliva flows at about 0.3 ml/min, while stimulated flow can be up to 7 ml/min. The submandibular glands contribute about 71% of the unstimulated flow, while the parotid gland produces 25% and sublingual gland about 3%. The parotid gland produces two thirds of stimulated saliva [6]. The minor salivary glands contribute a small percentage to overall salivary flow.

Saliva consists of many electrolytes including sodium, potassium, calcium, magnesium, bicarbonates, phosphates, urea, and ammonia. Saliva also contains proteins including immunoglobulins, enzymes, and mucin. The parotid produces mucinous saliva, while the submandibular gland produces more serous saliva. The sublingual gland produces a mixed seromucinous secretion. Saliva lubricates and protects the mucosal lining of the oral cavity and pharynx, acts as a buffering solution, maintains tooth integrity, has antibacterial properties, and assists taste function [7].

Intact swallowing mechanisms are necessary for clearance of saliva. Just as with swallowing of food, propulsion of saliva from the oral cavity into the pharynx, coordination of oropharyngeal structures and laryngeal elevation, cricopharyngeal relaxation, and esophageal propulsion are necessary for transfer of saliva to the digestive system. The causes of swallowing dysfunction described in earlier chapters can lead to the accumulation of saliva in oral cavity and pharynx, termed sialorrhea. While we will describe later some states where there can be an overproduction of saliva, most children with sialorrhea have impairment of swallowing with resultant issues with saliva clearance.

Gastroesophageal Reflux

Gastroesophageal reflux leads to the reflux of gastric and esophageal contents into the pharynx. In children, there can be some physiologic reflux, but pathologic reflux may affect the upper aerodigestive tract and tracheobronchial tree. Refluxed contents can add to the volume of secretions within the pharynx and oral cavity. Gastrointestinal reflux is an important consideration in secretion management. Pediatric patients who present with aerodigestive and swallowing complains will often have associated gastroesophageal reflux (GER) disease. A more focused review of the management of GER can be found in Chap. 19.

Secretion Management and Pediatric Dysphagia

Why is secretion management so important in children who have dysphagia? Poorly handled secretions can be associated with significant morbidity in patients with dysphagia. In discussions about dysphagia, the focus is typically on feeding and nutrition. However, while the safe transfer of food and liquid from the oral cavity is important, the transfer of secretions occurs volitionally and reflexively throughout a patient's day. Therefore, modalities such as diet modification that seek to decrease aspiration of food do not necessarily help with a patient's oropharyngeal secretions.

As established earlier, nasal, pharyngeal, and tracheobronchial mucous, saliva, and GER can contribute to 3 L or more of oropharyngeal secretions in adults. Normal values in children are difficult to establish, but we can still recognize the significant amount of secretions that needs to be cleared from the oropharynx each day. One of our fears in pediatric patients with dysphagia is the risk of aspiration, but it is not only the presence of aspiration that is important but also what is being aspirated.

During an aspiration event, a chemical tracheobronchitis/pneumonitis can occur when fluids toxic to the airway such as organic solvents and milk are aspirated. Inert fluids such as water, barium, and gastric contents with a pH greater than 2.5 typically do not cause much reaction. Oropharyngeal secretions in addition to the presence of various proteins and enzymes, with or without gastric contents, can cause bacterial infections and/colonization by commensal organisms of the upper aerodigestive tract [8]. Karim et al. showed that in patients admitted for aspiration sequelae, those who had aspiration of oropharyngeal flora had increased need for ventilatory support, increased hospital length of stay, and increased mortality, when compared to aspiration of inert and reactive fluids [8]. This is clearly an issue in cases of known aspiration events and aspiration pneumonia, but also in patients with chronic poor handling of secretions. The presence of amylase in the tracheobronchial tree and positive 99 m technetium sulfur colloid sialograms illustrating the presence of saliva in the lower respiratory system is associated with chronic respiratory complaints and reactive airway disease [9].

Primer in the Management of Secretions

Chronic rhinitis and rhinosinusitis can lead to increased nasal secretions. Antihistamines and intranasal corticosteroids can be used in cases of allergic and non-allergic causes of chronic rhinitis to decrease nasal secretions. Environmental controls of increased nasal secretions including cigarette smoke should also be considered.

Patients with impaired tracheobronchial clearance should be followed by a pulmonologist. Considerations should be given for etiologies of primary mucociliary dysfunction. Pulmonary consultation can assist in choosing modalities used for airway clearance including inhaled mucolytics, bronchodilators, corticosteroids, cough assist devices, and chest physiotherapy. The measures can also help clearance of aspirated oropharyngeal secretion. A discussion of anticholinergic agents to manage tracheobronchial secretions will follow in the section on sialorrhea.

Acute increases in secretions as evidenced by increased rhinorrhea, oropharyngeal secretions, sputum production, or tracheal secretions in intubated patients or patients with tracheostomy tubes can be worrisome. These increases when accompanied by fever and changes in the color and smell of secretions point to an infectious etiology. Viral panels, watchful waiting, and bacterial and fungal cultures with or without empiric therapy can be employed based on the clinical assessment. Infections including acute sinusitis, tracheobronchitis, and pneumonia should be considered.

Management of chronic secretions is difficult. It is important to remember that poor handling of secretions is often the result of poor swallowing. Therefore, all measures described in this text to improve swallow function can also improve handling of secretions. Alternately, most of our interventions on secretion management seek to decrease the production of secretions. Beside the control of nasal and tracheobronchial secretions briefly described above and GER control described elsewhere in this text, saliva control is a cornerstone in secretion management for children with dysphagia.

Management of Sialorrhea

Pathophysiology and Significance of Sialorrhea

Control within oral preparatory stage is paramount to adequate swallowing. Efficient oral control requires that food, liquid, and saliva introduced into the oral cavity remain in the oral cavity until it is ready to be passed on to the oropharynx. Sialorrhea is the involuntary loss or spillage of saliva/secretions from the oral cavity. Anterior sialorrhea refers to the loss of saliva pass the lips and out of the mouth, while posterior sialorrhea occurs when saliva enters the oropharynx involuntarily. Posterior drooling carries an aspiration risk. These can occur concurrently, and often the presence of anterior sialorrhea may be the only historical feature that points to the presence of posterior drooling [9].

Drooling can be normal in infants, but typically subsides between ages of 15 and 36 months when control of saliva is established. Sialorrhea is typically considered abnormal after age 4 [10]. Sialorrhea is not generally due to hypersalivation. Psychotropic drugs such as clozapine can cause hypersalivation [11]. Caregivers of children with neurologic conditions often endorse a change in drooling severity with changes in their anticonvulsant medication neuromodulators. There may be some role for dysregulation of the autonomic system in patients with cerebral palsy with respect to the development of drooling. Despite this, the presence of sialorrhea is generally considered to be due to ineffective swallowing as opposed to factors that may cause hypersalivation [5]. Contributions to sialorrhea include dysfunction in the oral phase of swallowing, deficient lip closure, open mouth position, poor cervical posture, reduced intraoral sensitivity, emotional state, degree of concentration, disorganized tongue movement, and reduced frequency of swallowing. Disturbances in the coordination of orofacial, palate, and lingual musculature lead to pooling anteriorly, while deficiencies in the swallow reflex lead to spilling posteriorly.

In the pediatric population, children with neurologic diseases are most likely to have sialorrhea. The prevalence of sialorrhea is 10% to 58% in patients with cerebral palsy [5] but is common in patients with other neuromuscular diseases and intellectual disabilities. Patients with acquired neurological conditions including those with brain masses, hypoxic ischemic encephalopathy, and meningoencephalitis may also develop sialorrhea. Over 50% of children who are at risks of aspiration and penetration and who have swallowing issues will also have neurologic condition [12].

Patients with sialorrhea may face social rejection and teasing because of drooling. Clothing may be constantly damp or soiled, and patients often need bibs or diapers to prevent exposing clothing to saliva. Saliva may damage books, keyboards, and other communication devices. An unpleasant odor may be present. Facial skin may be irritated. Oral and perioral infections including angular cheilitis and other fungal infections can develop. Loss of saliva from the mouth can lead to dehydration. Although one may view the problem as excess saliva, it is important to recognize that saliva loss from the oral cavity impedes the normal function of saliva in the mouth. Patients with sialorrhea have decreased masticatory function due to lack of lubrication, and dental issues may be compounded as saliva remineralizes teeth [13]. Sialorrhea also places additional demands on caregivers in them having to remind individuals to swallow saliva and to clean excess saliva from the chin and other areas and the increased workload of washing towels and clothes [14].

With posterior drooling comes the risk of aspiration. Caregivers of patients with posterior drooling additionally have concerns with having to suction oropharyngeal secretions very regularly. Patients with posterior sialorrhea, who also have aspiration, have increased respiratory complaints. These include chronic cough and recurrent respiratory infections including aspiration pneumonia with sequelae such as frequent hospitalizations and need for antibiotics and bronchodilators.

There is not much known about the relationship between GER and saliva. There is not enough evidence to suggest that GER can be so severe that it can unilaterally account for excess posterior sialorrhea. Saliva may play a role in protecting esophageal mucosa from GER, so loss of saliva anteriorly may impair this protective effect. This may be only of significance in patients who are already at risks for esophagitis [15]. Chemical irritation of esophageal and pharyngeal mucosa by GER may lead to increased saliva production through parasympathetic vasovagal reflexes, but this remains unproven [16].

Evaluation of Patients with Sialorrhea and Increased Secretions

The history of a patient with increased secretions focuses on factors such as underlying etiologies, social and medical effects, and previous interventions. Duration and severity of secretions should be investigated. Many patients with cerebral palsy may have a prolonged history of poor handling of secretions. However, changes can occur with neuromodulatory medications or in neurological function.

It can be difficult to quantify the amount of secretions/sialorrhea. Subjective evaluations include the number of times sialorrhea must be wiped from the chin and lips, number of bibs and diapers used a day to collect saliva, and number of times oropharyngeal secretions have to be suctioned. Frequency of tracheostomy tube suctioning in patients who have a tracheostomy should also be noted. Dental health, destruction of books, clothing and other communication devices, and presence of teasing will give the examiner an assessment of the psychosocial impact of sialorrhea on the patient. There have been objective measurements developed to quantify secretions. These include the Drooling Quotient (DQ) that quantifies the number of sialorrhea episodes every 15 s in 1 h; Sochaniwskyj's technique where the amount of saliva that escapes through the mouth is quantified (Table 20.1); a scale developed by Thomas-Stonell and Greenberg, a qualitative assessment sialorrhea as assessed by the examiner; and various other assessments including weighing collection units, diapers, and towels [5].

Features of secretions should be noted. Smell and color of secretions are not necessarily reliable attributes; however, during respiratory infections, changes in the amount, smell, and color of oral, oropharyngeal, and tracheal secretions can be evident. The thickness of secretions can also be important. Thicker secretions, especially in the presence of glycopyrrolate, may be harder to swallow or more difficult for caregivers to remove.

Patient attributes should be noted including physical and cognitive impairments. Cognitive impairments may lead to sialorrhea due to lack of motor control or due to lack of attention. Cognitive ability also determines how effective behavioral modifications and oral motor therapy may be. Specific neurological signs and symptoms including state of alertness, cranial nerve function, motor skills, posture, and tone are important factors. Deficits in language including dysarthria and dyspraxia may point to issues with oral motor control.

Table 20.1 Thomas-Stonell and Greenberg examiner graded sialorrhea severity scale [17]

Grade	Observation
1	Dry lips (no sialorrhea)
2	Wet lips (mild sialorrhea)
3	Wet lips and chin (moderate sialorrhea)
4	Wet clothing around the neck (severe sialorrhea)
5	Wet clothing, hands, and objects (profuse sialorrhea)

As a part of an aerodigestive evaluation, the presence and absence of GER, dysphagia, and routes of nourishment are important to note. Of greatest importance is the presence of respiratory symptoms. The presence of increased respiratory symptoms, choking and gasping on secretions, reactive airway disease, recurrent infections such as aspiration pneumonia, need for bronchodilators, and number of hospitalizations should be assessed. The social impacts of sialorrhea are clear, but associated respiratory symptoms can be associated with increased morbidity and mortality. Patients who have respiratory compromise may warrant more aggressive interventions.

A medication and therapeutic history should be obtained. Anticonvulsants, benzodiazepines, and neuroleptics can increase sialorrhea. Prior treatments for secretion management should be known. Examiners should be aware of any history of behavioral and speech therapy and their associated responses. Responses and side effects associated with previously used medical therapy, like glycopyrrolate, may give insight to future responses and the willingness of parents to undertake these therapies. Reponses to previous botulinum toxin injection, including techniques used (with anesthesia or ultrasound), should also be known. Variable technique and dosing can affect efficacy. Previous salivary gland surgeries and tracheostomy placement may influence treatment plans.

Treatment of Sialorrhea

Behavioral Modifications

Pharmacologic agents and surgeries to manage sialorrhea can be effective but decrease the production of saliva or change the flow of secretion instead of tackling dysfunctional swallowing. Children who can follow prompts and directions should have a trial of oral, swallowing, and physical therapy. Oral stimulation can increase sensory awareness and improve physical constraints like lip sealing and tongue control. Redirection can help with patients who have open mouth positions, although orthodontic treatment may be necessary. One must also recognize potential weaknesses in jaw and cervical musculature that may lead to posturing that can contribute to spillage of saliva. Physiotherapeutic strategies can help patients with hypotonia in these groups and thus decrease sialorrhea. These modalities can be very successful but are dependent on the cognitive abilities of the child, are time intensive often requiring many hours per week of therapy, and require the help of a trained experienced professional versed in these techniques. Despite these disadvantages – in children who can benefit – they should form the foundation of any secretion control treatment plan.

Medical Therapy

Systemic anticholinergic therapy can be very affective. Glycopyrrolate is the only FDA-approved medication for pediatric patients in the management of drooling in neurologically impaired patients. It is an antimuscarinic anticholinergic medication. Up to 75% of children with cerebral palsy will notice a decrease in drooling with glycopyrrolate [18]. It can decrease saliva, but may also have some activity against mucosal secretions from the nasal cavity, pharynx, and trachea. Glycopyrrolate can be used as a first line for secretion management, based on parental preference or as an alternative/adjunct to surgical management. It is available as an oral solution and thus can be titrated based on a patient's weight and tolerance.

Significant side effects can occur because of the glycopyrrolate and other anticholinergics. Side effects include xerostomia and thick oral secretions. Although these are a result of the desired effect, one must recognize that dental hygiene can be negatively impacted by xerostomia, and thicker oral secretions can be harder to handle. Anticholinergic effects including urinary retention, skin flushing, irritability and other behavioral effects, gastrointestinal effects like constipation, blurred vision, and facial flushing may occur. When prescribing glycopyrrolate, these side effects must be monitored and may limit therapy. Many of the patients who require glycopyrrolate are at high risks for these symptoms [13].

Transdermal scopolamine can also be used for control of drooling. Advantages include constant dosing and ease of administration. Usage is limited by the anticholinergic side effects outlined above [19]. Scopolamine patches are difficult to dose in pediatric patients due to its constant release. Many prescribers will modify patches to use small portions of them, but clinical judgment in this practice is necessary. There are also concerns for withdrawal symptoms, when patches are discontinued [20].

Benzatropine, trihexyphenidyl, and atropine are other anticholinergic agents that have been used. Oral, intramuscular, intravenous, and nebulized preparations have been tried. Sublingual atropine drops have variable effects on sialorrhea. Onset of action can be as little as 15 min, and can last up to 6 h. Systemic absorption appears to be low, with decreased systemic cholinergic effects. Tachycardia can be noted, so care must be taken in those with cardiac conditions and arrhythmias [21].

Some patients with sialorrhea and poor handling of secretions may have very thick secretions. Secretions can be innately thickened and be dried due to ambient air and open mouth posturing or as a side effect of concurrent anticholinergic therapy. In these patients, a trial of mucous thinning agent or mucolytic may be useful. Guaifenesin and acetylcysteine may be used in this regard. In patients with respiratory symptoms, these medications may not affect the amount of secretions (although patients may complain of dry mouth indicating some antisialagogue effect). However, the ability of these medications to mobilize secretions out of the respiratory tract may be beneficial. Guaifenesin and acetylcysteine may also improve mucociliary transport in the respiratory tract [22].

Botulinum Toxin

Botulinum toxin is an anticholinergic agent that can be used in the management of sialorrhea and oral secretions. Botulinum toxin blocks the presynaptic release of acetylcholine. It has the advantage of expressing its anticholinergic effects locally without side effects typically associated with systemic anticholinergic therapies. Due to its anticholinergic properties, botulinum toxin has found applications in cosmetics in the management of rhytids, muscle contractures, blepharospasm, excessive sweating, and overactive bladder [23].

Botulinum toxin is injected into the parotid and submandibular glands for management of sialorrhea. Dosing strategies vary. 0.5–1 units/kg per gland is often used, while doses of 20–30 units may be most efficacious [24–27]. In the author's experience, a dose of 1 U/kg per gland is injected, with a max of 20 U. If desired effect is not obtained with 20 U, then 30 U may be used [27]. Botulinum toxin can be injected in the clinic setting using palpation and landmarks to localize the parotid and submandibular glands [28]. Ultrasound guidance leads to real-time, precise localization of the salivary glands and injections. Although it requires specialized equipment, training, and increased cost, it does improve efficacy and decrease adverse events [29].

Botulinum toxin does not have an immediate effect, and this must be expressed when counselling families. Salivary flow decreases through anticholinergic effects about 3–5 days postinjection with noticeable effects by the end of the first week. The anticholinergic activity continues to increase up until the third week. Botulinum toxin's effects reverse after 3–4 months [30]. The need for repeat injections should be assessed and may not require an exact interval of every 3–4 months. The interval for repeat injection can range from 7 to 65 weeks [30]. This variability may be related to parental preference and issues with follow-up. However, there is much that we don't know about response of patients with differing neuromuscular diseases to botulinum toxin. Some patients with reduced salivary flow may develop improved techniques to handle saliva after the botulinum toxin's effect has expired. There is also some controversy in the permanent effect that the toxin has on the structure of the gland that may lead to a long-lasting decrease in salivary flow [31].

Salivary gland botulinum toxin injection is an effective treatment for salivary control in children. Success rates vary between 60% and 83% based on visual analog scales, saliva collection, number of wet towels a day, qualitative assessments of sialorrhea, and frequency of suctioning oral/oropharyngeal secretions [24–30]. In patients with dysphagia and respiratory complaints who have sialorrhea, botulinum toxin can decrease admissions, hospital days, ICU days, need for antibiotics, and episodes of aspiration pneumonia [30, 32]. Adverse effects can be present in 16% of cases but may be less than 1% when using ultrasound guidance [29]. Local effects like bruising, flushing, and pain at the injection site are common. Xerostomia, increased saliva thickness, and paradoxical increased saliva production have been reported. The most worrisome effects occur when botulinum toxin is injected or spreads outside of the salivary glands. Muscle weakness, causing jaw weakness, dysphagia, and speech problems can occur but are rare. Families should be instructed not to massage the injection site to prevent potential spread [33].

Surgery

Surgical treatments used in secretion management can be categorized as (1) salivary gland and duct surgery that decreased or changed the flow of saliva, (2) procedures that allow of improved clearance of respiratory secretions, and (3) procedures that decrease the chance of secretions entering the airway.

Salivary Gland Surgery

Salivary duct surgeries are a class of procedures used for secretion management. These procedures can be performed on the submandibular duct and/or the parotid duct and can encompass rerouting or ligating the duct. Parotid duct and submandibular gland rerouting involve changing the direction of salivary flow. The submandibular and parotid ducts are oriented anteriorly with the opening of the submandibular duct located in the anterior floor of the mouth just posterior to the mandibular incisors and that of the parotid gland occurring within the buccal mucosa adjacent to second maxillary mucosa. Procedures involve releasing the respective ducts from the mucosa, surrounding musculature and connective tissue, and then transposing the opening more posteriorly, typically at the level of the tonsillar pillars. These procedures work well for anterior sialorrhea. Rates of control range from 74% to 91% [34]. However, care should be taken in children with posterior sialorrhea with or without dysphagia, as these procedures can increase oropharyngeal secretions and thus aspiration risk. Bleeding and infection are additional risks. Bleeding within the floor of the mouth can cause airway obstruction. Lingual nerve injury can occur with submandibular gland duct rerouting [35].

The ducts of the submandibular and parotid gland can be ligated. This involves dissection of a mucosal cuff of tissue around the respective ducts, microdissection and mobilization of the openings, and suture ligation. This ceases the flow of saliva from the ducts ligated. Concurrent submandibular and parotid ligation is a common method for salivary control in patients who aspirate with rates of control ranging from 27% to 100% [34]. Complications can arise from the backup of salivary flow. Transient salivary gland swelling and sialadenitis are common, and up to 23% can have a persistent facial swelling [36]. Sialoceles and fistulas can also occur. Despite these issues, duct ligation is a simple, effective, and minimal invasive approach for sialorrhea management.

Bilateral submandibular gland excision is effective for decreasing saliva and addresses the gland that is most important for resting salivary flow. Although transoral submandibular gland excision is described, a transcervical approach is classically used. The submandibular space is bordered by the inferior border of the mandible and the digastric muscle. After exposure of the space, the submandibular gland is dissected from the facial vessels, marginal mandibular nerve, submandibular lymph nodes, and mylohyoid muscle. Dissection deep to the mylohyoid leads to the submandibular duct, submandibular ganglion, and lingual and hypoglossal nerves. Transection of the submandibular ganglion and duct releases the submandibular gland with care to preserve the lingual and hypoglossal nerve. Success rates for submandibular gland resection range from 78% to 91% especially when paired with parotid duct ligation or rerouting [34]. Risks include wound complications, bleeding, infection, and weakness of the marginal mandibular, lingual, and hypoglossal nerves.

Sublingual gland excision is performed transorally after exposure within the floor of the mouth. Typically, it is combined with other procedures such as duct rerouting [35]. One should recognize that any intervention of the submandibular duct will decrease output from the sublingual gland as the gland empties into this duct. Transection of the nerve to the submandibular ganglion may also interrupt parasympathetic (secretory) function to the sublingual gland.

Due to the risk of facial nerve injury and questionable efficacy, parotidectomy whether partial or total is not recommended for saliva management.

Airway Surgery

Pulmonary toilet and clearance of airway secretions are common indications for the placement of a tracheostomy. However, care should be taken when recommending tracheostomy tube placement for the sole reason of clearing secretions. Patients with poor handling of secretions also have swallowing dysfunction. Secretion handling and aspiration may worsen with tracheostomy placement as tracheostomy tubes: tether and inhibit laryngeal elevation during swallow, reduce anterior rotation of the larynx, desensitize the larynx, and cause atrophy of laryngeal muscles. Cuffed tracheostomy tubes may compress the esophagus, and the cough reflex may lose its effectiveness due to loss of subglottic pressure. Placement of a speaking valve in appropriate patients can combat these downsides in patients who have a tracheostomy by improving swallowing function [37]. Patients with poor handling of secretions may have concurrent comorbidities like respiratory failure and severe obstructive sleep apnea in which a tracheostomy tube may be needed. Frequent suctioning of the tracheostomy tubes may be needed to maintain pulmonary clearance, but long-term medical and secretion management is often necessary.

There are many airway procedures that have been developed to manage secretions in those that have recurrent aspiration pneumonia. These should only be considered in children who have chronic life-threatening aspiration of secretions after exhausting other options for secretion management. These procedures do not affect secretion production but prevent aspiration of the said secretions. Irreversible procedures include narrow field laryngectomy where the laryngeal complex is removed and a tracheostoma is brought to the skin so that all oral and pharyngeal secretions can only be passed to the esophagus. Glottic closure involves obliterating the laryngeal outlet by stitching the true and false vocal cords together preventing secretions from entering the airway. In a subperichondrial cricoidectomy, the cricoid cartilage is resected with closure of the infraglottic airway. Glottic closure and subperichondrial cricoidectomy are also irreversible and require tracheostomy placement, and a patient cannot be intubated from above after these procedures.

Reversible airway procedures to manage aspiration include the epiglottic flap closure and partial cricoidectomy. In epiglottic flap closure, the epiglottis and aryepiglottic folds are used to close the glottis aperture. It requires a tracheostomy, and the patient cannot be intubated from above. Partial cricoidectomy involves removal of the posterior portion of the cricoid. This is thought to increase the caliber of the cervical esophagus while narrowing the subglottic airway. This allows secretions to preferentially enter the esophagus.

Laryngotracheal separation and diversion are two of the most common reversible airway procedures used in the management of chronic aspiration in children. Both procedures involved transection of the cervical trachea and creation of a tracheostoma by bringing the distal transected end to the skin. With a laryngotracheal resection, the proximal trachea is closed, thus creating a blind pouch. The proximal trachea is anastomosed to the cervical esophagus during a laryngotracheal diversion allowing for the passage of aspirated secretions into the esophagus. Laryngotracheal separation and diversion have been shown to decrease hospitalizations and respiratory infections in neurologically impaired children [38]. Wound complications, fistulas, and airway obstruction can complicate these surgeries. Wound complications may be more common in laryngotracheal diversion due to issues with the tracheoesophageal anastomosis.

References

1. Beule AG. Physiology and pathophysiology of respiratory mucosa of the nose and the paranasal sinuses. GMS Curr Top Otorhinolaryngol Head Neck Surg. 2010;9:Doc07.
2. Malcomson KG. The vasomotor activities of the nasal mucous membrane. J Laryngol Otol. 1959;73(2):73–98.
3. Clarke SW, Pavia D. Lung mucus production and mucociliary clearance: methods of assessment. Br J Clin Pharmacol. 1980;9(6):537–46.
4. Brand-Saberi BE, Schafer T. Trachea: anatomy and physiology. Thorac Surg Clin. 2014;24(1):1–5.
5. Dias BL, Fernandes AR, Maia Filho HS. Sialorrhea in children with cerebral palsy. J Pediatr. 2016;92(6):549–58.
6. Edgar WM. Saliva: its secretion, composition and functions. Br Dent J. 1992;172(8):305–12.
7. Flint PW, Haughey BH, Lund VJ, Niparko JK, Thomas Robbins K, Regan Thomas J, Lesperance MM. Cummings otolaryngology: head and neck surgery, 6e – 3-volume set. 6th ed. Philadelphia: Sauders Elsevier; 2014.
8. Karim RM, et al. Aspiration pneumonia in pediatric age group: etiology, predisposing factors and clinical outcome. J Pak Med Assoc. 1999;49(4):105–8.
9. Rajaei A, et al. The association between saliva control, silent saliva penetration, aspiration, and videofluoroscopic findings in Parkinson's disease patients. Adv Biomed Res. 2015;4:108.
10. Garnock-Jones KP. Glycopyrrolate oral solution: for chronic, severe drooling in pediatric patients with neurologic conditions. Paediatr Drugs. 2012;14(4):263–9.

11. Hung CC, et al. Treatment effects of traditional Chinese medicines Suoquan Pill and Wuling Powder on clozapine-induced hypersalivation in patients with schizophrenia: study protocol of a randomized, placebo-controlled trial. Zhong Xi Yi Jie He Xue Bao. 2011;9(5):495–502.
12. Bae SO, et al. Clinical characteristics associated with aspiration or penetration in children with swallowing problem. Ann Rehabil Med. 2014;38(6):734–41.
13. Walshe M, Smith M, Pennington L. Interventions for drooling in children with cerebral palsy. Cochrane Database Syst Rev. 2012;11:CD008624.
14. van der Burg J, et al. Drooling in children with cerebral palsy: a qualitative method to evaluate parental perceptions of its impact on daily life, social interaction, and self-esteem. Int J Rehabil Res. 2006;29(2):179–82.
15. Heine RG, Catto-Smith AG, Reddihough DS. Effect of antireflux medication on salivary drooling in children with cerebral palsy. Dev Med Child Neurol. 1996;38(11):1030–6.
16. Erasmus CE, et al. Clinical practice: swallowing problems in cerebral palsy. Eur J Pediatr. 2012;171(3):409–14.
17. Thomas-Stonell N, Greenberg J. Three treatment approaches and clinical factors in the reduction of drooling. Dysphagia. 1988;3(2):73–8.
18. Mier RJ, et al. Treatment of sialorrhea with glycopyrrolate: a double-blind, dose-ranging study. Arch Pediatr Adolesc Med. 2000;154(12):1214–8.
19. Lewis DW, et al. Transdermal scopolamine for reduction of drooling in developmentally delayed children. Dev Med Child Neurol. 1994;36(6):484–6.
20. Chowdhury NA, Sewatsky ML, Kim H. Transdermal scopolamine withdrawal syndrome case report in the pediatric cerebral palsy population. Am J Phys Med Rehabil. 2017;96:e151.
21. Rapoport A. Sublingual atropine drops for the treatment of pediatric sialorrhea. J Pain Symptom Manag. 2010;40(5):783–8.
22. Seagrave J, et al. Effects of guaifenesin, N-acetylcysteine, and ambroxol on MUC5AC and mucociliary transport in primary differentiated human tracheal-bronchial cells. Respir Res. 2012;13:98.
23. Esquenazi A, et al. International consensus statement for the use of botulinum toxin treatment in adults and children with neurological impairments – introduction. Eur J Neurol. 2010;17(Suppl 2):1–8.
24. Schroeder AS, et al. Botulinum toxin type A and B for the reduction of hypersalivation in children with neurological disorders: a focus on effectiveness and therapy adherence. Neuropediatrics. 2012;43(1):27–36.
25. Wu KP, et al. Botulinum toxin type A on oral health in treating sialorrhea in children with cerebral palsy: a randomized, double-blind, placebo-controlled study. J Child Neurol. 2011;26(7):838–43.
26. Alrefai AH, Aburahma SK, Khader YS. Treatment of sialorrhea in children with cerebral palsy: a double-blind placebo controlled trial. Clin Neurol Neurosurg. 2009;111(1):79–82.
27. Moller E, et al. Onabotulinumtoxin a treatment of drooling in children with cerebral palsy: a prospective, longitudinal open-label study. Toxins (Basel). 2015;7(7):2481–93.
28. Raval TH, Elliott CA. Botulinum toxin injection to the salivary glands for the treatment of sialorrhea with chronic aspiration. Ann Otol Rhinol Laryngol. 2008;117(2):118–22.
29. Shariat-Madar B, et al. Safety of ultrasound-guided botulinum toxin injections for sialorrhea as performed by pediatric otolaryngologists. Otolaryngol Head Neck Surg. 2016;154(5):924–7.
30. Pena AH, et al. Botulinum toxin a injection of salivary glands in children with drooling and chronic aspiration. J Vasc Interv Radiol. 2009;20(3):368–73.
31. Oliveira JB, Evencio-Neto J, Baratella-Evencio L. Histological and immunohistochemical findings of the action of botulinum toxin in salivary gland: systematic review. Braz J Biol. 2016;77(2):251–9.
32. Faria J, et al. Salivary botulinum toxin injection may reduce aspiration pneumonia in neurologically impaired children. Int J Pediatr Otorhinolaryngol. 2015;79(12):2124–8.
33. Vashishta R, et al. Botulinum toxin for the treatment of sialorrhea: a meta-analysis. Otolaryngol Head Neck Surg. 2013;148(2):191–6.

34. Reed J, Mans CK, Brietzke SE. Surgical management of drooling: a meta-analysis. Arch Otolaryngol Head Neck Surg. 2009;135(9):924–31.
35. Kok SE, et al. The impact of submandibular duct relocation on drooling and the well-being of children with neurodevelopmental disabilities. Int J Pediatr Otorhinolaryngol. 2016;88:173–8.
36. Khan WU, et al. Four-duct ligation for the treatment of sialorrhea in children. JAMA Otolaryngol Head Neck Surg. 2016;142(3):278–83.
37. Ongkasuwan J, et al. The effect of a speaking valve on laryngeal aspiration and penetration in children with tracheotomies. Laryngoscope. 2014;124(6):1469–74.
38. Chida I, et al. Clinical outcomes of tracheoesophageal diversion and laryngotracheal separation in neurologically impaired children. Auris Nasus Larynx. 2013;40(4):383–7.

Chapter 21
Dysphagia in Patients with Craniofacial Anomalies

Ellen E. Moore and Tara L. Rosenberg

Introduction

Patients with various craniofacial anomalies and related genetic disorders are at high risk for feeding/swallowing dysfunction and dysphagia. They may have a wide range of abnormalities causing these issues, such as functional and anatomical factors. Many have associated anomalies, such as congenital heart disease, that may worsen their overall feeding abilities. These patients benefit from early feeding assessment in the neonatal period, and they require close monitoring of weight gain and growth. A multidisciplinary approach with experienced practitioners in the specialty care of these patients is key to their management. This team approach allows for assessment from various perspectives and permits multiple problems to be addressed for each patient, leading to a comprehensive assessment and management plan.

History and Physical Exam

Performing a thorough history and physical exam is important in the identification of craniofacial anomalies and associated findings that may indicate the presence of a syndrome. Genetics team evaluation is paramount in patients with craniofacial anomalies. During the initial patient assessment, general appearance of the patient,

E. E. Moore
Speech, Language and Learning, Texas Children's Hospital, Houston, TX, USA
e-mail: eemoore@texaschildrens.org

T. L. Rosenberg (✉)
Department of Otolaryngology/Head and Neck Surgery, Baylor College of Medicine/Texas Children's Hospital, Houston, TX, USA
e-mail: tlrosenb@texaschildrens.org

© Springer International Publishing AG, part of Springer Nature 2018
J. Ongkasuwan, E. H. Chiou (eds.), *Pediatric Dysphagia*,
https://doi.org/10.1007/978-3-319-97025-7_21

including any signs of respiratory distress or airway obstruction, should be noted and managed accordingly. Once medically stable, a clinical swallow assessment by an experienced speech pathologist is important to identify any initial signs of feeding/swallowing problems or dysphagia in the neonate.

Cleft Lip and/or Cleft Palate

Unrepaired cleft lip and palate often present challenges to oral feeding. In general, the primary impact is on suction, which reduces efficiency of feeding. Significant pharyngeal phase disorders and tracheal aspiration are uncommon in children with orofacial clefts without syndromic involvement. There are general considerations for feeding based on the type and location of cleft, but the importance of individualized assessment and treatment should not be overlooked [1].

Cleft Lip

Typically, infants with isolated cleft lip are able to breastfeed or use a standard bottle without compromising efficiency. The ability to generate suction remains adequate given the intact soft palate. Although a cleft lip may have a slight impact on the labial seal around a nipple, either breast tissue or the base of an artificial nipple generally occludes the area of the cleft.

Cleft Lip and Alveolus

Cleft lip and alveolus, with or without extension into the anterior portion of the hard palate, may have a slightly increased impact on feeding skills than isolated cleft lip. The uneven surface of the alveolar ridge further reduces lip seal and may cause the nipple to shift within the oral cavity. Nutritive breastfeeding or the use of a standard bottle system is generally still successful, but modifications to positioning or cheek support may be helpful in assisting the infant maintain a consistent latch (see [2]). Rarely, the use of a modified cleft palate bottle system is necessary to improve efficiency.

Cleft Palate

Clefts involving the soft palate impact the infant's ability to generate negative pressure, or suction, due to inability to close the velopharyngeal port. This leads to limited expression of milk from the breast or a standard bottle and reduced efficiency of feeding. Poor weight gain, fatigue during feeds, and difficulty with caregiver-infant bonding may result. Although a subset of infants with clefts affecting the soft palate may be able to generate a degree of suction, this may not be maintained for the duration of the feed [3]. The ability to generate positive pressure (compression) via movement of the jaw and tongue is unaffected. Masarei et al. reported that infants with cleft palate (with or without cleft lip) typically use compression as the primary method of expressing milk. Their rate of sucking and ratio of sucks to swallows were found to be higher than in infants without clefts, possibly due to the slower rate of expression from the bottle [4]. The majority of infants with cleft palate will require the use of a modified bottle system (Fig. 21.1). These most frequently use a one-way flow valve at the base of the nipple, allowing for compression of the nipple between the anterior hard palate and tongue/mandible to express fluid. Squeeze-bottle systems are also available, through which the feeder compresses the bottle to express liquid. There is limited evidence supporting one adapted bottle type over another [5, 6], but appropriate parent education on system use and feeding strategies is essential.

Given the communication between the oral and nasal cavities, infants with cleft palate may have nasal regurgitation and increased ingestion of air while feeding. Upright positioning during feeds and appropriate pacing/flow rate generally minimize nasal regurgitation (Fig. 21.2) (see [7]). Frequent burping is recommended, at least once per 0.5–1 ounce of milk. In most cases, efficient oral feeding is achieved once appropriate modifications to bottles and positioning are implemented [8]. Children with cleft palate associated with an underlying genetic syndrome may have additional challenges to oral feeding related to neurological or respiratory complications. Adapted bottle systems are appropriate for this population to compensate for the cleft palate, while feeding therapy is often required targeting additional oral and pharyngeal deficits.

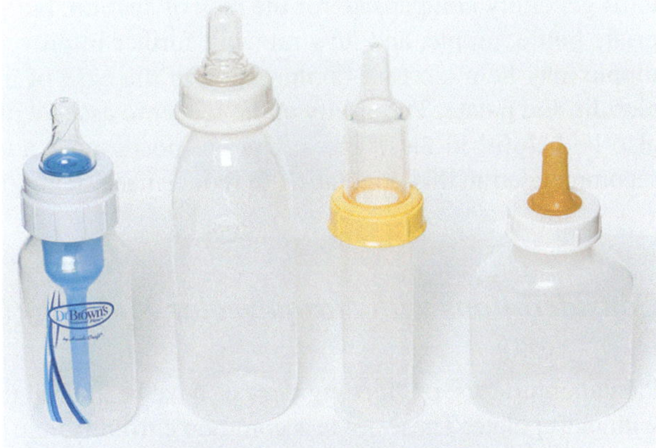

Fig. 21.1 Common modified bottle systems for cleft patients

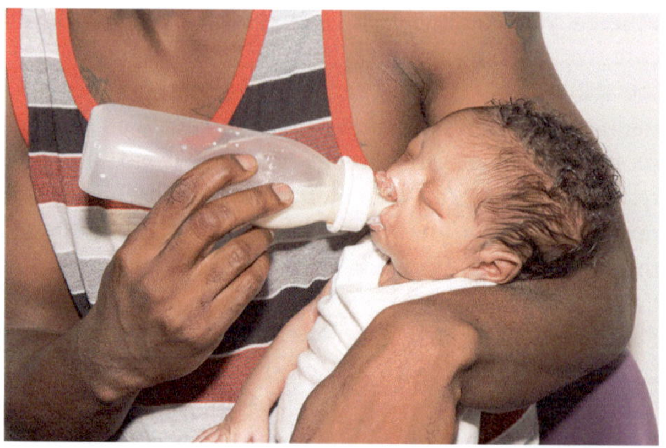

Fig. 21.2 Appropriate position for feeding cleft patient

Submucous Cleft Palate

Effects of a submucous cleft palate on feeding vary widely. While many children are able to feed effectively from the breast or standard bottle, some may experience similar features to children with overt cleft palates (see [2]). Use of a modified bottle system or faster flow standard nipple may be indicated in cases when feeds are taking greater than 30 min or weight gain is poor. Standard recommendations for feeding with cleft palate including upright positioning and frequent burping are also used for this population.

Cleft Lip and Palate

A complete cleft lip and palate (unilateral or bilateral) eliminates ability to generate negative pressure and may reduce force of compression/positive pressure [3]. Depending on the width of the cleft, the defect in the hard palate may significantly reduce the surface for compression against the top of a nipple. Modified bottle systems generally compensate for the lack of suction, but selection of the most appropriate bottle, nipple, and flow rate will further improve feeding outcomes. A wider nipple may help increase compression in the case of a wide unilateral or bilateral cleft lip and palate. The ability of the feeder to assist with external compression may also be helpful in these cases. Upright positioning and frequent burping are also recommended in this population to reduce nasal regurgitation and gas.

Considerations with Nasoalveolar Molding (NAM)

Palatal obturators, or "feeding plates," have been used to improve feeding in infants with cleft palate. These are less common currently, and they have not been found to significantly improve feeding [9]. Even with an obturator in place, the infant remains unable to generate suction [10]. Modified bottle systems are sufficient to overcome this difficulty without the use of an appliance. However, the use of nasoalveolar molding (NAM) is a common practice in pre-surgical preparation for cleft lip repair [11]. Infants are fitted with the removable device within weeks after birth, and adjustments are made weekly. For infants with significant alveolar defects, this may provide a more consistent surface for compression of a nipple and slightly improve efficiency. The device should not be expected to significantly improve feeding skills in infants already experiencing difficulties in the neonatal period. Suction remains reduced and the use of a modified bottle system is still required. While most infants are able to feed with NAM in place after a brief period of adjustment, a small subset has ongoing difficulty. Frequent troubleshooting and collaboration between the orthodontist, feeding specialist, and primary care provider are recommended to monitor weight gain and feeding skills during NAM treatment.

Pierre Robin Sequence

The presence of micrognathia, glossoptosis, and airway obstruction in Pierre Robin sequence (PRS) has a significant impact on feeding skills (Fig. 21.3). When significant micrognathia is present, the discrepancy between the superior and inferior dental arches may impact the strength of compression and limit expression of milk. Posterior positioning of the tongue due to micrognathia limits the infant's ability to cup the tongue around the nipple. This impacts both expression of milk and bolus control, often leading to premature spillage of fluid into the pharynx. A cleft palate is reported in up to 90% of infants with PRS [12]. The presence of a cleft palate requires modifications similar to those used for infants with isolated cleft palate and is, in general, more easily compensated for than the other anatomical differences in PRS. Airway obstruction is the primary contributor to feeding difficulties in this population [13].

A stable airway is necessary for successful feeding. As the severity of airway obstruction varies greatly between patients, differing levels of intervention for feeding will be required. For infants who display only mild obstruction while in supine and improve with prone positioning, successful oral feeding may be possible without additional intervention. Feeding for this population is most successful in an elevated side-lying or a nearly prone position, which allows the tongue to move anteriorly, reducing obstruction by the tongue base in the pharynx. Anterior movement of the tongue also increases tongue cupping around the nipple and allows the tongue to contribute to compression. A longer nipple is often more successful in reaching the retracted tongue. Slow flow rate and frequent breaks for ventilation are typically required. These infants may fatigue quickly while feeding due to the increased effort required for respiration and may have difficulty coordinating the suck-swallow-breathe triad. If they are unable to complete the prescribed volume within an appropriate timeframe (about 20 min), supplemental feeding nasogastric (NG) or gastric (G) tube may be required. Infants receiving supplemental feeds

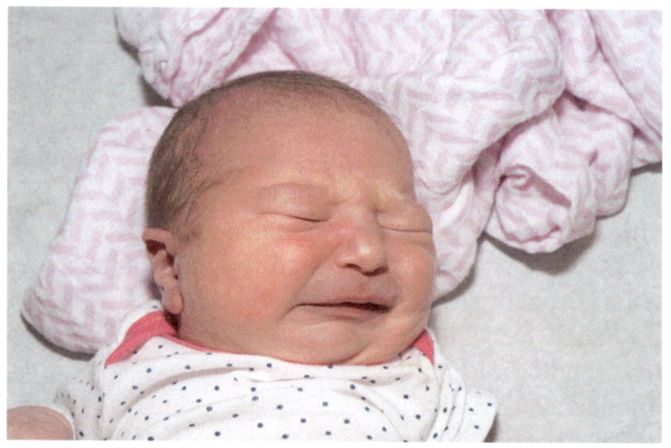

Fig. 21.3 Infant with Pierre Robin sequence. Note micrognathia on exam

should have opportunities to feed orally as often as is feasible to maintain skills and continue with progression of skills.

Difficulties with oral feeding increase along with the degree of airway obstruction. If the infant is unable to maintain the airway with side-lying or prone positioning, oral feeds are generally not appropriate until the obstruction is addressed. Nasopharyngeal airways have been used to improve respiratory status but may also place the infant at a higher risk for aspiration. The presence of the nasopharyngeal airway between the tongue base and posterior pharyngeal wall reduces contact between the two structures during the swallow, increasing the risk of aspiration. Surgical options for addressing the anatomical differences of PRS and reducing airway obstruction include tongue-lip adhesion and mandibular distraction osteogenesis (MDO). Tongue-lip adhesion reduces glossoptosis but may limit anterior tongue movement for feeding. Difficulties may persist in patients treated with tongue-lip adhesion [14], and more positive feeding outcomes have been reported for MDO, with faster progression to full oral feeding [15]. Following mandibular distraction, the mandible and tongue are placed more appropriately for efficient feeding, and numerous authors have reported positive outcomes for feeding. Following a learning period when supplemental gavage feeds may be required, most infants progress to full oral feeds. Monasterio et al. reported aspiration rates of 5.5% prior to MDO, which resolved after the procedure [16]. Complete avoidance of gastronomy tube placement after early MDO has also been reported [17].

Down Syndrome

The incidence of Down syndrome is about 1 in 700 live births. Patients with Down syndrome may have feeding/swallowing problems and/or dysphagia related to several factors: airway anomalies, relative macroglossia, poor oral skills, dental abnormalities, hypotonia, congenital heart disease, esophageal anomalies, and other gastrointestinal dysfunction [13]. Some airway anomalies found in Down syndrome patients at a higher incidence include laryngomalacia, laryngeal cleft, tracheal bronchus, and tracheal rings (Fig. 21.4) [18]. Since approximately half of patients with Down syndrome have associated congenital heart disease, this plays a large role in feeding/swallowing problems and/or dysphagia for many of them. The threshold for referral of a patient with Down syndrome for feeding evaluation should be low, since dysphagia is found in about half of this pediatric patient population, and frequently, the dysphagia is noted to be silent aspiration on video swallow studies [19, 20].

22q11 Deletion Syndrome

The incidence of 22q11 deletion syndrome is 1 in 4000 to 6000 births [21]. They have a wide range of phenotypic expression. Therefore, they may have feeding/swallowing difficulties and/or dysphagia caused by multiple different factors. Some of the common features in these patients that may affect feeding and swallowing are congenital heart disease, cleft palate/submucous cleft palate, velopharyngeal incompetence, airway anomalies, hypotonia, and gastrointestinal tract dysfunction [22, 23]. The suck-swallow-breathe sequence may be affected by some of these factors, leading to disorganized swallow and possible aspiration, prolonged feeding times, and fatigue. They may have insufficient caloric intake and subsequent failure to thrive [13, 24]. They may also have nasopharyngeal reflux, gagging or choking, and difficulty advancing textures later in childhood [21–23]. Multidisciplinary management of feeding and swallowing in this patient population is important, as is true in many genetic disorders. A feeding evaluation early in the neonatal period may also be helpful [22].

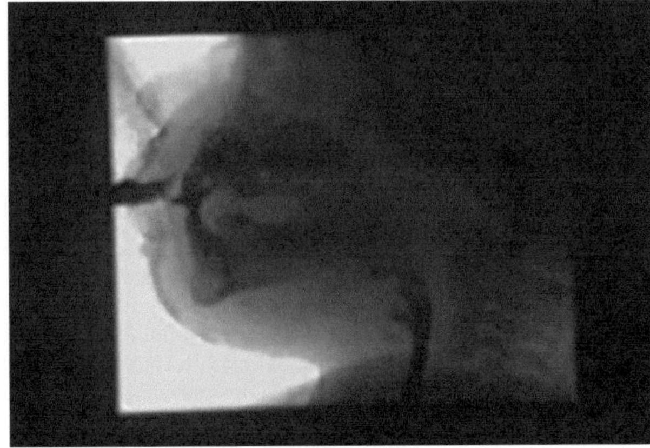

Fig. 21.4 Video swallow study of a patient with Down syndrome showing aspiration through type 1 laryngeal cleft

Hemifacial Microsomia

This broad group of first and second branchial arch malformations results in mandibular hypoplasia and facial weakness of varying degrees. Usually, only one side is affected, but both sides are. Feeding and swallowing difficulties may result from structural anomalies of the jaw, tongue, face, and pharynx or from neurologic dysfunction and/or congenital heart defects [24].

Summary

Feeding/swallowing dysfunction and dysphagia in various craniofacial anomalies and related genetic disorders are common. They have many factors contributing to this issue. These patients benefit from early feeding assessment and close monitoring of weight gain and growth. Experienced practitioners in the multidisciplinary care of these patients are essential to their management. The various perspectives of the team members permit multiple problems to be addressed for each patient. This allows for a comprehensive assessment and management plan to benefit the patient.

References

1. Clarren SK, Anderson B, Wolf LS. Feeding infants with cleft lip, cleft palate, or cleft lip and palate. Cleft Palate J. 1987;24(3):244–9.
2. Arvedson JC, Brodsky L, Arvedson JC, Brodsky LB. Feeding with craniofacial anomalies. In: Arvedson JC, Brodsky LB, editors. *Pediatric swallowing and feeding: assessment and management*. 2nd ed. Albany: Singular Publishing Group; 2002. p. 527–61.
3. Reid J, Reilly S, Kilpatrick N. Sucking performance of babies with cleft conditions. Cleft Palate Craniofac J. 2007;44(3):312–20.
4. Masarei AG, et al. The nature of feeding in infants with unrepaired cleft lip and/or palate compared with healthy noncleft infants. Cleft Palate Craniofac J. 2007;44(3):321–8.
5. Reid J. A review of feeding interventions for infants with cleft palate. Cleft Palate Craniofac J. 2004;41(3):268–78.
6. Bessell A, et al. Feeding interventions for growth and development in infants with cleft lip, cleft palate or cleft lip and palate. Cochrane Database Syst Rev. 2011;(2):CD003315.
7. Cooper-Brown L, Copeland S, Dailey S, Downey D, Petersen MC, Stimson C, Van Dyke DC. Feeding and swallowing dysfunction in genetic syndromes. Dev Disabil Res Rev. 2008;14(2):147–57.
8. Reid J, Kilpatrick N, Reilly S. A prospective, longitudinal study of feeding skills in a cohort of babies with cleft conditions. Cleft Palate Craniofac J. 2006;43(6):702–9.
9. Prahl C, et al. Infant orthopedics in UCLP: effect on feeding, weight, and length: a randomized clinical trial (Dutchcleft). Cleft Palate Craniofac J. 2005;42(2):171–7.
10. Choi BH, et al. Sucking efficiency of early orthopaedic plate and teats in infants with cleft lip and palate. Int J Oral Maxillofac Surg. 1991;20(3):167–9.
11. Sischo L, et al. Nasoalveolar molding: prevalence of cleft centers offering NAM and who seeks it. Cleft Palate Craniofac J. 2012;49(3):270–5.

12. Cohen SM, et al. Robin sequence: what the multidisciplinary approach can do. J Multidiscip Healthc. 2017;10:121–32.
13. Cooper-Brown L, et al. Feeding and swallowing dysfunction in genetic syndromes. Dev Disabil Res Rev. 2008;14(2):147–57.
14. Denny AD, Amm CA, Schaefer RB. Outcomes of tongue-lip adhesion for neonatal respiratory distress caused by Pierre Robin sequence. J Craniofac Surg. 2004;15(5):819–23.
15. Papoff P, et al. Outcomes after tongue-lip adhesion or mandibular distraction osteogenesis in infants with Pierre Robin sequence and severe airway obstruction. Int J Oral Maxillofac Surg. 2013;42(11):1418–23.
16. Monasterio FO, et al. Swallowing disorders in Pierre Robin sequence: its correction by distraction. J Craniofac Surg. 2004;15(6):934–41.
17. Lidsky ME, Lander TA, Sidman JD. Resolving feeding difficulties with early airway intervention in Pierre Robin Sequence. Laryngoscope. 2008;118(1):120–3.
18. McDowell KM, Craven DI. Pulmonary complications of Down syndrome during childhood. J Pediatr. 2011;158(2):319–25.
19. O'Neill AC, Richter GT. Pharyngeal dysphagia in children with Down syndrome. Otolaryngol Head Neck Surg. 2013;149(1):146–50.
20. Jackson A, et al. Clinical characteristics of dysphagia in children with Down syndrome. Dysphagia. 2016;31(5):663–71.
21. Goldmuntz E. DiGeorge syndrome: new insights. Clin Perinatol. 2005;32(4):963–78. ix–x
22. Eicher PS, et al. Dysphagia in children with a 22q11.2 deletion: unusual pattern found on modified barium swallow. J Pediatr. 2000;137(2):158–64.
23. Cuneo BF. 22q11.2 deletion syndrome: DiGeorge, velocardiofacial, and conotruncal anomaly face syndromes. Curr Opin Pediatr. 2001;13(5):465–72.
24. Merrow JM. Feeding management in infants with craniofacial anomalies. Facial Plast Surg Clin North Am. 2016;24(4):437–44.

Chapter 22
Psychological and Behavioral Disorders in Dysfunctional Feeding: Identification and Management

Alan H. Silverman and Andrea M. Begotka

Abbreviations

ARFID   Avoidant/restrictive food intake disorder
DSM-5   *Diagnostic and Statistical Manual* Version 5
FTT   Failure to thrive
ICD-10   *The International Classification of Diseases*, Tenth Edition

Introduction

Feeding a child is one of the most fundamental tasks of parenting. Successful feeding fosters secure attachments and supports appropriate growth and development for the child [1, 2]. Conversely, feeding problems can be upsetting to the family and may lead to insecure attachments and disruptive caregiver-child interactions [3, 4]. A pediatric feeding disorder is characterized by food refusal, disruptive mealtime behavior, rigid food preferences, suboptimal growth, and failure to master self-feeding skills commensurate with the child's developmental abilities [5]. In the United States, pediatric feeding disorders affect 3–20% of children (i.e., 720,000–5 million) and accounts for 3% of hospital admissions [6]. A chronic feeding disorder can negatively affect growth (final adult height), cognition (lower IQ and educational achievement), behavior (decreased attention and poorer social skills), and quality of life [7, 8]. Pediatric feeding disorders also negatively affect the financial and emotional well-being of affected families [3, 4]. This chapter focuses on psychological and behavioral aspects of feeding disorders. Psychological considerations along with a behavioral conceptualization will be reviewed

A. H. Silverman (✉)
Department of Pediatrics, Medical College of Wisconsin, Milwaukee, WI, USA
e-mail: asilverm@mcw.edu

A. M. Begotka
Psychiatry and Behavioral Medicine, Children's Hospital of Wisconsin, Milwaukee, WI, USA
e-mail: abegotka@chw.org

J. Ongkasuwan, E. H. Chiou (eds.), *Pediatric Dysphagia*,
https://doi.org/10.1007/978-3-319-97025-7_22

including diagnostic considerations, interdisciplinary team assessment, and methods of treatment.

Prevalence and Etiology

There is ongoing debate about how to best define a behavioral feeding disorder. In fact, there has been so much disagreement that several diagnostic systems have evolved to address this concern [6]. These various systems likely developed due to the heterogeneous nature of feeding problems with each discipline developing a system to meet the needs of their specific areas of concern with their own set of standards for diagnosis corresponding to their specific treatment codes. Historically, descriptions of feeding problems tended to define them in terms of organic disease versus behavioral etiologies [9, 10]. While this type of system was easily used by providers, it did little to describe the complexity with which most patients present. Over time systems evolved that did not exclusively assign a physiological or behavioral etiology but rather a blend of etiologies that captures the complexity and heterogeneity of these concerns [6]. Regrettably, there is still no one system that is widely accepted by the full composite of disciplines, and this remains an obstacle to the establishment of diagnostic standards and the development of treatment guidelines. Regardless, the existence of multiple systems has further complicated the question of what constitutes a feeding disorder.

Diagnosis

Presently, the two major diagnostic systems that are in greatest use are the (DSM-V) [11] and the (ICD-10) [12]. The DSM-V, published in 2013, is broadly used by mental health practitioners use to make psychiatric diagnoses, whereas the ICD-10 is a clinical cataloging system that went into effect for the US healthcare industry in 2015, primarily used by medical professionals, allied health providers, and interdisciplinary treatment centers. Each system has its relative strengths and weaknesses.

Avoidant/restrictive food intake disorder (ARFID) is the new DSM-V diagnosis taking the place of the diagnosis of feeding disorder of childhood. Changes made to the diagnosis in this edition are vastly superior to the diagnostic criteria from previous editions of the DSM as this edition allows for the presence of or history of physical ailments that contribute to the etiology. In the most recent edition, ARFID is defined by a clinically significant lack of or insufficient nutrition due to avoidance or restriction of oral intake. It must include one or more of the following: (1) weight loss or failure to meet growth expectations, (2) nutritional deficiencies, (3) dependence on enteral feeding or oral nutritional supplements, and (4) interference with psychosocial functioning. Exclusionary criteria include the presence of eating disorders such as anorexia or bulimia, lack of available food, and feeding behaviors associated with cultural practices. Food avoidance or restriction can often be a result for these children from a negative experience(s) they may have had in the past (e.g., vomiting, esophagitis, gagging, choking, forced feeding), where the child then develops a conditioned negative response to food and, therefore, avoids or restricts some or most foods. Children may also avoid or restrict foods based on the sensory characteristics of foods (e.g., smell, color, texture, taste, temperature of food).

The International Classification of Diseases, Tenth Edition (ICD-10) [12] system adopts a more descriptive framework for describing behavioral feeding concerns and does not attempt to determine whether the etiology is primarily biological or behavioral. The ICD-10 characterizes these feeding difficulties as specific to infancy or early childhood typically with the presence of adequate food supply, reasonably capable caregivers feeding the child, without current medical illnesses or conditions that are maintaining the feeding condition. This diagnostic system is typically used in a medical setting and is well suited to interdisciplinary team clinicians as the code may be used across disciplines, whereas ARFID is typically only diagnosed and used by mental health providers.

Other behaviorally oriented diagnostic systems exist but are less commonly used. Perhaps the best known of these is the psychodynamically oriented system developed by Chatoor and colleagues [13]. This method classifies feeding disorders into six subcategories according to various organic and nonorganic causes: (1) feeding disorder of state regulation, (2) feeding disorder of caregiver-infant reciprocity, (3) infantile anorexia, (4) sensory food aversions, (5) feeding disorder associated with concurrent medical condition, and (6) feeding disorder associated with insults to the gastrointestinal tract. While the use of the diagnostic system has been popular, little evidence has been provided to support its validity, and secondary payers have not recognized these diagnoses further limiting their use clinically.

Regardless of which system is used, a behavioral feeding disorder is generally characterized by disruptive feeding behaviors that are sufficiently divergent from age and/or culturally expected feeding behavior such that the well-being of the child is threatened. Disruptive feeding behaviors are often classified as active, such that the child physically resists caregiver efforts to feed (e.g., hits, spits), or passive, such that the child engages in nonphysical avoidance strategies (e.g., dawdling) [14]. Frequently, children will engage in a combination of active and passive forms of resistance when attempting to avoid feeding [15, 16]. These behaviors thus result in decreased intake of food and/or drink at mealtimes contributing to poor growth, limited nutrition, delayed advance of diet, picky eating, need for supplemental nutrition, and/or stressful mealtimes for the child and his/her caregivers.

Prevalence

Prevalence estimates of feeding problems are alarmingly high, estimated to occur in as many as 25% to 45% of children in the general population [17, 18], approximately one-third of children with developmental disabilities [19] and up to 80% of children with severe or profound mental retardation [20, 21]. Feeding disorders occur in 46% to 89% of children with autism spectrum disorder [22] and 40% to 70% of children with chronic medical conditions [1, 10, 23, 24]. Approximately half to two-thirds of children with feeding disorders present with mixed etiologies that include behavioral, physiological, and developmental factors [5, 25]. Problems may also originate from outside of the child, such as caregiver-child interaction problems, caregiver competence with feeding tasks (e.g., misinformed understanding of childhood nutrition, caregiver mental health issues), and, more broadly, other societal problems such as food scarcity or poverty [26].

Generally, younger children have more feeding problems than older children, with most children receiving their diagnoses between the ages of 1–3 years [24, 27, 28]. This typically corresponds to the time by which an affected child does not advance through developmentally appropriate feeding stages (e.g., pureed baby food to chewable solid foods) and/or their weight falters [29]. Feeding disorders can persist into adolescence and adulthood, but the occurrence rate is unknown [14]. However, the general trend is for early feeding problems to persist over time [24, 30]. Untreated, feeding problems may evolve into eating disorders in adolescence and adulthood [27]. The prevalence of feeding disorders is expected to rise as the survival rates of children with significant disease and/or developmental disabilities increase [16].

Eating disorders are distinguished from feeding disorders by the distinct characteristic of restriction of calories to intentionally control body mass, the development of abnormalities of food intake habits to control body mass (e.g., binge and purge), and persistent negative perceptions of body image [11]. Differential diagnoses that should be considered include diagnoses of anorexia nervosa, bulimia, and eating disorder NOS. Other nutrition disorders should also be excluded, including pica, rumination syndrome, choking phobia, and cyclic vomiting syndrome. Feeding problems should also be differentiated from failure to thrive (FTT), a condition that occurs when a young child's weight gain is so low that it is below the standard growth chart, leading to malnutrition. FTT affects up to 10% of children in outpatient clinics and accounts for 3–5% of pediatric hospital admissions [31]. FTT can stem from organic or social factors or from a combination of factors. Children with FTT often have long-term growth deficits with poor height and weight that can lead to problems in behavior, cognition, and academics. While FTT is a frequently occurring co-condition, it is distinctively different from a feeding disorder as FTT may occur exclusively due to social factors (e.g., poverty and lack of access to food), whereas this would be an exclusion for feeding problems [32].

Etiology

Behavioral feeding issues are typically not the origin of the feeding problem but are often the result of other factors experienced earlier in life. A history of medical, developmental, oral sensory-motor deficits, and social challenges generally precede behavioral feeding concerns [5].

Behavior problems following illness or chronic medical conditions are quite common. Often, these factors include a history of a medical concern such as cardio-respiratory problems (e.g., cardiac, premature birth, lung/breathing problems), gastrointestinal illnesses or pain (e.g., frequent vomiting, eosinophilic esophagitis, gastroesophageal reflux disease), repeated or painful instances of strep throat, and negative reactions to food allergies [33]. Children may also associate medical procedures that are aversive and/or painful (e.g., upper GI endoscopy, chemotherapy, cardiac surgery) with feeding-related difficulties. Some medications children need for other conditions may negatively impact the child's feeding (e.g., stimulant medications used to treat attention deficit/hyperactivity disorders dampen the hunger drive) decreasing the child's internal motivation to eat and drink more, often increasing negative feeding behaviors or challenges at mealtimes. Other medications can result in gastrointestinal discomfort or constipation. Consultation with medical professionals is needed when physiological or medication concerns are present.

Behavior problems associated with developmental delays and/or skills deficits occur when children have cognitive, motor, and/or oral motor delays affecting their ability to eat developmentally appropriate food [24]. These children may miss critical feeding periods in their development when they are biologically predisposed to learn to eat and drink. Many times, well-intentioned caregivers will attempt to feed these children the foods that are recommended at their chronological age, not correcting for the degree of developmental delay, resulting in food offerings that are beyond the child's skill set [34]. This may result in aversive feeding experiences like gagging, choking, and vomiting, and ultimately these children learn to resist efforts to take any foods outside of their comfort zone. This leads to delaying their advancement of diet to developmentally appropriate feeding [14]. For example, a child who is 3 years old but has cognitive and gross motor delays resulting in a developmental age of 18 months may self-limit textures to pureed food, easily dissolvable textures, and soft solids (e.g., canned fruit). Those that do not know this child would expect him to eat regular table food that would be consumed by other 3-year-old children. This problem is due in part to strictly following the American Academy of Pediatrics feeding guidelines [35] which are based only on chronological age, not on developmental age. There are some systems that take developmental status into account (e.g., Gerber Feeding Milestones) [36], but little scientific research has been conducted to determine the validity and usefulness of such systems presently.

Social and cultural factors are among the most influential components of general development and more specifically of the development of feeding habits and feeding problems. Culture influences the child, the family feeding system, and the community norms in which children feed [37]. For example, cultural norms affect aspects of choosing breast or bottle feeding, which foods to offer, at what age to offer the foods, how much the child should eat, and who feeds the child. Cultures vary on these feeding norms, and these cultural differences may contribute to the manifestation of feeding problems as some cultures prioritize individuality, whereas others value collectivistic ideals. For example, a culture that focuses on individuality may grant too much control to the child resulting in extreme food selectivity, whereas a collectivist culture may result in group expectations that result in power struggles between the caregiver and child. It is important to understand and be sensitive to cultural expectations such that treatment recommendations are provided in culturally sensitive manner. Regardless of the constellation of underlying etiologies, behavioral feeding disorders are ultimately about the interaction between the child and the adult caregivers who attempt to feed that child. The behavioral specialist must accurately identify the etiological factors and develop management strategies to help the family to successfully overcome the problems associated with the feeding disorder.

Psychological Factors

Feeding a child is an interactive process in which caregiver(s) and the child share in the responsibilities of the interaction. In an ideal feeding relationship, the caregiver selects and presents developmentally appropriate foods to the child [38]. The child must then accept the foods offered and respond appropriately to their own internal hunger and satiety cues to ensure adequacy of intake to support good nutrition. Meals are successful and more positive when caregivers and children both fulfill their responsibilities in this interactive process.

For many families, however, feeding can become stressful or a chore. There is ample evidence associating high parental stress in the presence of feeding problems [3, 26]. As feeding problems develop, caregivers become increasingly desperate to nourish their children, altering their behaviors, and deviating from the shared responsibilities and roles as described above. As the feeding problems worsen, especially when the child has poor growth, caregivers' feeding interactions can become overly controlling (e.g., long mealtimes), or caregivers may resort to force feeding, which results in children mistrusting caregivers [39]. Other caregivers may become disengaged, allowing children to have too much control at mealtimes. In such instances caregivers allow the child to graze throughout the day which diminishes their appetite at mealtimes. Caregivers may also allow their children to self-select their food choices resulting in restriction of only their most preferred foods at meal and snack times. These laissez-faire caregiver strategies result in poor child nutritional status due to limited variety of accepted foods in the diet.

There are also social costs associated with these conditions [2]. Caregivers may have emotional struggles such as guilt, shame, and frustration that are due to pressure or judgment they feel from friends, family members, or from their community. This in turn negatively affects their social support network and isolates the caregivers further resulting in great caregiver-related stress [3, 4]. Similarly, children with feeding difficulties are at an increased risk of social isolation, especially during school age years, due to odd eating habits. These eating differences may result in increased risks of bullying and exclusion from social events such as birthday parties, holiday celebrations, and sleepovers. Affected children may also isolate themselves by avoiding these social situations due to their self-awareness of their unusual eating habits and feeding difficulties. Over time the social isolation may contribute to delays in the affected child's social development [2].

Given these concerns it is important for families to not only address the feeding disorder directly but to also seek consultation regarding the variety of other psychological risk factors described above. Fortunately for these families, psychologists who treat these concerns are typically trained in general clinical child psychology or pediatric psychology making them well suited to provide such assessments and care.

Behavioral Conceptualization

The heterogeneity of feeding problems necessitates that clinicians carefully consider a broad range of factors including the medical history, developmental history, family variables, and caregiver resources when designing an individualized treatment approach [40].Treatment is often provided by a variety of healthcare professionals including physicians, psychologists, speech-language pathologists, dietitians, and other specialists [41, 42]. The assessment of feeding problems should clarify a family's treatment objectives, determine if the family's goals are appropriate and achievable, and identify components of the feeding problem. Typically, the assessment is comprised of a medical record review, caregiver-completed questionnaires, a clinical interview, and behavioral observation of the child while being fed [33]. Interdisciplinary assessments, including those completed by a physician, speech and language pathologist and/or occupational therapist, dietitian, and pediatric psychologist, are particularly well suited to achieving this objective (see Table 22.1 – Interdisciplinary feeding team members' role in assessment).

The role of the psychologist is to provide a behavioral perspective on feeding disorders, assess for comorbid behavioral or psychiatric conditions within the child or within the broader family system, and provide intervention or facilitate referrals when appropriate [42]. Given that up to 85% of feeding problems have a mixed etiology which includes a behavioral component [41, 43], a pediatric psychologist is best suited to work with feeding problems. Common behavioral concerns include comorbid psychiatric diagnoses, missed or delayed stages of feeding development, learned feeding avoidance due to aversive conditioning (e.g., choking event, force feeding history), frequency and severity of inappropriate mealtime interactions, behavioral refusals which may have been inadvertently reinforced by caregivers (allowing child to self-select diet), and inappropriate family or cultural expectations for feeding.

Behavioral Treatment Planning

The objective of a behavioral feeding assessment is to identify behavioral and/or mental health etiologies of the affected child, caregivers, and within the feeding dyad. After the assessment, a behavioral treatment plan with specific treatment

Table 22.1 Interdisciplinary feeding team members' role in assessment

Registered dietitian	Provides targeted nutrition interventions. Common goals for dietary interventions consist of improved growth (weight at or above 90% ideal body weight for length); improved growth velocity; increased nutrient intake; improved nutrient balance; redistribution of calories from protein, carbohydrate, and fat; and help for families to avoid harmful foods/supplements
Speech and language pathologist	May take an active role in treatment to facilitate development of oral motor skills for the advancement of the family's feeding goals. Interventions often include therapies to improve chewing and swallowing coordination, strengthen oral musculature, and improve oral tolerance to a broad range of flavors, textures, and temperatures of foods
Pediatric psychologist	Provides a behavioral perspective on feeding disorders, assesses for comorbid behavioral or psychiatric conditions within the child or within the broader family system, and provides interventions or facilitates referrals as appropriate. Behavioral treatment strategies generally include implementation of mealtime structure and a feeding schedule, appetite manipulation, behavior management, and parent training
Physician	Monitors overall medical well-being of the child and provides medical oversight and support as needed while the child is in treatment. Common tasks include completing medical studies to identify and treat various physiological causes (e.g., endoscopy, food allergy testing), managing various conditions through medication (e.g., medications for appetite stimulation, acid suppression therapy), and coordinating the broader treatment team

recommendations along with measurable treatment goals should be expected to guide care. Ideally, the behavioral feeding concerns are considered within the context of a multifaceted evaluation. Once the feeding problems are well-defined and the family and treatment team have agreed upon goals, then the treatment plan may be developed. One strategy to help ensure that goals are appropriate and achievable focuses on applying "SMART" criteria, which stands for S, specific; M, measureable; A, action-oriented; R, realistic; and T, timely (see Fig. 22.1 – SMART goals). Typically, behavioral treatment plans will draw from a variety of methods and techniques to achieve the stated objectives [6, 22, 44]. Generally, behavioral feeding interventions can be grouped into several categories: (1) environmental and schedule interventions, (2) increasing desirable feeding behaviors, (3) decreasing negative feeding behaviors, and (4) caregiver training (see Fig. 22.2 – Behavioral interventions). Treatment providers should ensure that adult caregivers are competent and comfortable with their own implementation of some of these techniques at home. Many programs emphasize skills training and demonstration of skills before discharging families from care. Overall, each child has their own unique and distinctive set of feeding difficulties which necessitate individual treatment plans. Fortunately, these methods are well suited and adaptable to the individual needs of the family. The majority of behavioral treatment plans use a combination of these methods to achieve treatment objectives [44] (see Table 22.2 – Behavioral intervention definitions and examples chart).

(I)   The best goals are SMART

Specific – What will you do, when, where, and with whom?

Measurable – How will you know when you meet your goal?

Action focus – What will you do? (Not what you want to change).

Realistic – Can you really do this? Can you do it at this time?

Timely – Are you ready to do this NOW?

My feeding goal is:

____

(II)   Pick a reward

Changing eating habits is hard work! It is easier for kids to achieve their goals if they get a reward for doing it. Choose something that you and your child can do together immediately after the goal is reached (e.g. give a hug or a kiss, a sticker to track progress on a chart, blow bubbles for each successful bite, or consider something after the meal that doesn't involve food such as playing a favorite game together or going to the park together).

My feeding rewards will be:

(III)   Extinguishing strategies

If rewards are not working, consider techniques to reduce problem feeding behaviors. Remember these techniques must be used consistently to work best (e.g. ignore fussing about foods, present the food until accepted and once accepted give your child a 30-second break).

My extinguishing strategies will be:

 Now track your child's progress over the next few days keeping in mind that it may take several attempts to see progress! Try combining these techniques to have the greatest effect! Call your treatment team if you have any questions.

Fig. 22.1 SMART goals

Behavioral Treatment

Environmental and Schedule Interventions

Environmental and schedule interventions are intended to minimize child distractions while focusing the child's attention on food offerings and on the adult caregivers who are overseeing the meal [15]. Schedule interventions are used to promote hunger through periods of fasting. Appropriate food offerings and seating for the child are also important considerations to maximize treatment success. These strategies are highly effective and easily implemented and thus are obvious choices to begin treatment [16]. Occasionally, these interventions in isolation of other techniques are adequate to make sufficient changes to a child's feeding negating the need for more complex care.

A *developmentally appropriate diet* should be offered to the child that matches the child's feeding skills with the appropriate volumes and textures of foods offered.

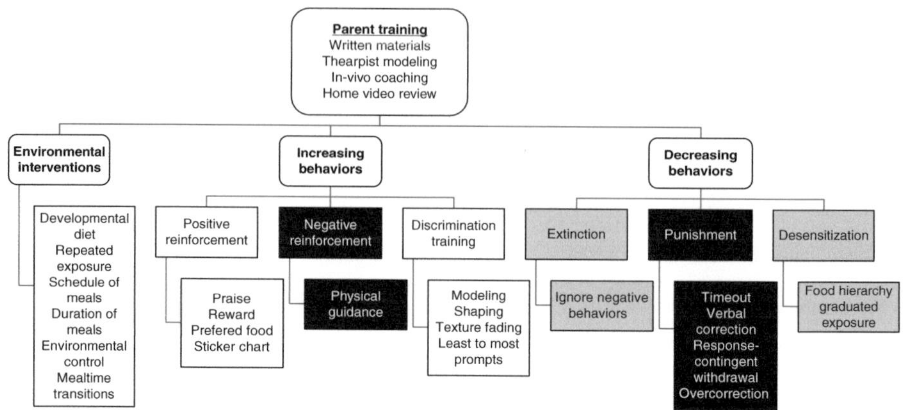

Fig. 22.2 Behavioral interventions. Note: Methods in white are suitable for families to implement at home with education and ongoing consultation. Methods in gray are suitable for families to implement at home with regular contact with treatment team. Methods in black may not be suitable for home use and require close contact with the treatment team for any use

Guidelines for recommended textures by age are published by the American Academy of Pediatrics [35]. Children who have oral motor delays, however, due to any underlying developmental disability (e.g., structural abnormalities or oral motor delays) may be at increased risk for feeding problems. Children who present with skills concerns should be evaluated by a speech and language pathologist or other well-qualified professional who is competent to determine the child's feeding skills and safety limitations. This specialist should provide guidance on the child's ability to safely manage various textures and appropriate pacing while eating [16].

The feeding environment should promote that all meals and snacks are offered at a table, with the child sitting in an appropriate chair or high chair matched to their developmental level [14]. Appropriate seating ensures that the child is well supported. For children who tend to get up from the table or flee from the meal, use of a securing strap is recommended. The feeding environment should limit distractions present at mealtimes to focus the child's attention on eating and drinking. Distracting items such as toys, television, and even family pets should be out of the child's sight. In distraction-free environments, caregivers will not compete with other factors that diminish their ability to manage the meal.

The mealtime schedule is intended to promote hunger within the child, thus increasing their motivation to eat a broader variety of foods and/or increasing their overall intake [15]. Meals should be offered at fixed intervals of every 2 to 4 h to promote hunger without causing the child to experience excessive hunger and frustration. During fasting periods, the child is to refrain from eating and drinking any items that contain calories. However, water should be encouraged for hydration and to promote good metabolism. Meals should be on a fixed duration to teach children to attend to eating while foods are available and to establish the hunger and satiation cycle. Generally, children under the age of 5 years have shorter attention spans and

Table 22.2 Behavioral intervention definitions and examples chart

	Definition	Examples of interventions
Environmental and schedule strategies		
Developmentally appropriate diet	Matching a child's developmental and oral motor skills with appropriate textures well suited to facilitate the child's ability to eat a well-balanced diet	Referring to the American Academy of Pediatrics recommendations for textures Evaluation of developmental delays which may necessitate adaptation to match developmental ability of child
Repeated exposure	Repeated offerings of new/non-preferred foods at challenge meals and snacks	Attempting to complete 10 or more exposures to a food before changing to a new challenge Children must taste challenge foods at specified meals and snacks
Schedule and duration of meals	Feeding a child on a fixed schedule of meals and snacks with periods of no caloric intake between scheduled feedings to induce hunger	Meals and snacks scheduled at least 3 h apart Meal duration not to exceed 30 min
Stimulus control	Manipulation of mealtime environmental factors known to increase desirable behaviors and reduce problem behaviors within the meal. These techniques do not require specific training in applied behavioral strategies but do require nutritional monitoring to ensure safety of use	All meals at the table Child securely seated in appropriate chair Rigid meal time schedule Meal free from distractions (e.g., TV, toys) Elimination of grazing between meals Decrease in supplemental feedings Allow child to "fail" a meal to experience natural consequence of increased hunger
Mealtime transition	Strategies which facilitate a child's transition to the mealtime environment. Typically, families are advised to avoid active or strongly preferred activities just before the meal as this may contribute to a child's resistance to the transition	Quiet or less desirable activities preceding the meal Ritual activities preceding the meal (e.g., washing hands, giving thanks) Pleasant activity planned if the child reaches meal objectives
Interventions to increase behaviors		

(continued)

Table 22.2 (continued)

	Definition	Examples of interventions
Stimulus control	Manipulation of mealtime environmental factors known to increase desirable behaviors and reduce problem behaviors within the meal. These techniques do not require specific training in applied behavioral strategies but do require nutritional monitoring to ensure safety of use	All meals at the table Child securely seated in appropriate chair Rigid meal time schedule Meal free from distractions (e.g., TV, toys) Elimination of grazing between meals Decrease in supplemental feedings Allow child to "fail" a meal to experience natural consequence of increased hunger
Positive reinforcement	Increases the frequency of a desirable feeding behavior due to the addition of a reward immediately following the desired feeding response	Cheering for a child who tastes a new food Giving a sticker as a reward for reaching a food volume goal Offering a preferred food after the child accepts a new or non-preferred food Punishment: Withholding a preferred toy when a child refuses to taste a new food Extinction: Withholding attention from a child's complaints about foods
Negative reinforcement	Increase the frequency of a desirable feeding behavior when the consequence is the removal of an aversive stimulus immediately following the desired feeding response	Avoidance conditioning occurs when a behavior prevents an aversive stimulus from starting or being applied (e.g., if a new food is accepted, the child will not have an increase in the total number of bites needed to reach the bite goal Escape conditioning occurs when behavior removes an aversive stimulus that has already started (e.g., release of a physical restraint when the child accepts the food presented)

Interventions to decrease behaviors

	Definition	Examples of interventions
Extinction	Reduces the frequency of an undesired feeding behavior due to the removal of a reward immediately following the undesired feeding response	Ignoring inappropriate feeding behaviors Continuing to prompt desired feeding behavior

Table 22.2 (continued)

	Definition	Examples of interventions
Punishment	Reduces the frequency of an undesired feeding behavior by presenting an aversive stimulus or removing a rewarding stimulus because of undesired behavior	The child receives a verbal rebuke for non-compliance The child is given a time-out Preferred activities or toys are withheld after the meal
Desensitization	The negative behavior is reduced by pairing repeated exposures to the aversive stimulus (e.g., new or non-preferred food) in the absence of an aversive event or with the presence of a positive reinforcer	The child's physiological anxiety response is reduced after numerous exposures Distraction techniques may be paired with the exposures (e.g., plays with preferred toy) Relaxation techniques may be used to reduce or eliminate anxiety response when child is presented with feared stimulus

should complete meals in under 20 min. Older children may take longer and have greater attention spans; therefore up to 30 min for meals is permissible. Children with known feeding and swallowing skill difficulties may require additional time to eat. However, such children are at an increased risk of becoming fatigued and frustrated resulting in more difficult behavioral interactions. Close consultation with interdisciplinary care providers is recommended in such cases [39].

Increasing Desirable Feeding Behaviors

Increasing desirable feeding behavior strategies are used to promote target behaviors that caregivers desire from their children within a feeding context [40]. Common examples of target behaviors include increased volume consumed, increased variety of foods and/or beverages consumed, increased willingness to work therapeutically to advance textures, and increased self-feeding. To maximize the effectiveness of these strategies, consistent application is essential. It is also important for caregivers to be aware of what is most reinforcing to the child at any given time due to children frequently changing their level of interest in items. This will help to determine what strategy is most effective. For example, a child may enjoy receiving stickers for accepting bites, but over time, the level of motivation for yet another sticker may decline necessitating a change.

Positive reinforcement is defined as adding something to the environment immediately after the behavior occurs which then leads to an increase in the probability of the behavior occurring in the future [15]. Examples of positive reinforcement in feeding include contingent use of social praise, positive attention, preferred food or drink, physical affection, and granting a tangible reward or item (e.g., stickers, bubbles). Among these methods of reinforcement, contingent social attention is widely considered to be the easiest and most useful form of positive reinforcement [39]. For example, a child who tries a new food for the first time may receive verbal praise and a hug from his mother. The primary advantage to this technique is its simplicity as it is available to everyone and takes minimal effort to use.

Negative reinforcement involves removing an aversive stimulus following a desired behavior, which in turn increases the probability of the desired behavior occurring in the future [40]. An example of negative reinforcement is nonremoval of the spoon. In this method, a spoon with a non-preferred food is presented about 1 inch from the child's mouth and maintained until the bite is accepted. In this scenario, the child learns that avoidance of the spoon merely prolongs the undesirable condition. Once the child accepts the bite (desirable behavior), the child receives a short break from the spoon (reinforcement).

Differential reinforcement, or the simultaneous use of attending to positive behaviors while ignoring negative behaviors, is well supported in the literature and is commonly used in behavioral therapy [45].For example, a child may verbally refuse to eat a non-preferred food. In this scenario, the caregiver should ignore refusals and wait for a desirable behavior that can be reinforced. In time, the child learns verbal refusals are ignored, but that acceptance will be rewarded.

Discrimination refers to a pairing of an antecedent stimulus with either positive or negative reinforcement that then increases the probability of a specific behavior occurring [22]. In feeding, the child's caregiver learns to present a utensil with a specific prompt such as "take a bite" (antecedent stimulus). The child has learned through repeated experiences that the acceptance of the spoon after the prompt means positive reinforcement will be issued with compliance. Similarly, non-compliance will be followed by punishment or withdrawal of attention to the child. Based upon this operant conditioning paradigm, the child then opens and accepts the bite and receives praise [45].

Progressive training techniques, such as shaping and fading, are commonly used behavioral strategies that are employed to develop more complex feeding behaviors [34]. These strategies involve reinforcement of incremental steps that gradually build to form a more complex and desirable feeding behavior [40]. *Shaping* involves providing reinforcement for successive approximations to a desired behavior that is the end goal. This breaks down the behavior into smaller, easier steps for the child and reinforces each behavior along the way to guide the child toward the final goal. For example, a family of a child who only eats pureed foods may have a goal to get their child to eat solid food. To achieve this goal, reinforcement of systematic texture advancement is planned as follows: (1) accepting thicker puree, (2) accepting lumpy puree, (3) accepting soft solid foods, (4) accepting easily dissolvable textures, and, (5) finally, chewing table foods. *Fading* is a technique used to establish independent behavior with the gradual removal of prompting, assistance, and reinforcement [40]. For example, teaching self-feeding skills would include the child holding the spoon with the feeder's hand over the child's hand then gradually removing support and guidance as the child increasingly feeds with success.

Desensitization is the repeated exposure of new foods and textures. It is essential to familiarize a child and desensitize them to unfamiliar flavors and textures to expand their diet gradually [15]. Neophobia, or preference for familiar instead of new foods, is common by the age of 2 and often thought to be adaptive for children such that unfamiliar foods (and non-edible items) may be dangerous so should be avoided [46]. When a child initially rejects new foods, however, parents often respond to the child by withdrawing the demand, immediately removing the food and allowing escape. In such situations, the caregiver is reinforcing the negative feeding behavior.

Decreasing Problem Feeding Behaviors

In addition to promotion of desirable feeding behaviors, elimination of behaviors that interfere with feeding must also be managed. Behavioral techniques to manage these problems include extinction, punishment, response contingent withdrawal of positive reinforcement, and overcorrection techniques.

Extinction is the systematic withholding of a reward following a problem feeding behavior which has been targeted for elimination. The most common example of extinction, in a feeding disorder treatment context, is to ignore undesired child behaviors such as verbal refusals or tantrums [6, 45]. Often, extinction techniques are difficult for caregivers to implement due to longstanding habits of attending to food avoidant behaviors exhibited by the child. Thus, learning these techniques frequently involves in vivo training for caregivers [33].

Punishment is the delivery of an aversive stimulus (or the removal of a rewarding stimulus), weakening the probability that the undesirable feeding behavior will occur. Punishment procedures involving highly aversive stimuli are recommended only when less intrusive procedures are ineffective and when the target behavior is damaging to the child or others (e.g., child displays physical aggression) and should only be used when the family is carefully monitored by trained personnel [14]. Perhaps the most commonly used punishment technique is *time-out* from positive reinforcement. In a feeding context, the child may be turned or moved away from the table to eliminate any reinforcement from the child's refusals. Timeout at the table is commonly used because it is safe and highly effective and takes less time away from the meal and momentum of the feeding. Another form of punishment is *verbal correction* in which a firm "NO" is paired with the problem feeding behavior [14]. This is typically followed by several seconds of attention withdrawal. While this technique can be effective, verbal correction should be used cautiously, as in some cases, negative verbal attention may actually serve as a positive reinforcement. Therefore, it is essential to continually monitor the effects of delivering punishment to determine whether the technique is effectively decreasing the target behavior.

Response-contingent withdrawal of positive reinforcement and *response cost for refusal* [22, 34, 45] are other forms of punishment for undesired behaviors. Typically, these techniques involve the withdrawal of toys or other preferred stimuli during a meal or at the end of a meal because of misbehavior. To be most effective, the child should have the opportunity to regain access to the preferred stimuli by engaging in cooperative behavior either at the meal or at a subsequent meal.

Finally, *overcorrection*, a procedure in which the child is physically directed through a series of repetitive, presumably unpleasant acts, has also been used as another form of punishment [40]. This technique is frequently used for children who intentionally throw foods or spit up during meals. For example, if a child throws food during the meal as a refusal behavior, overcorrection would involve the caregiver directing the child to clean up all the food the child threw during the meal and additional food put on the ground as a deterrent for throwing food in the future.

Caregiver Training

Awareness of *caregiver stress* is a vital component of treatment [44]. Caregiver-child interactions are often strained when a child has a feeding disorder. This may be particularly pronounced by the time the family seeks treatment. Past research has shown elevated levels of caregiver stress beyond expected levels [3, 4, 18, 26] among caregivers of children with a feeding disorder. Normalizing the caregiving experience within a feeding context is a goal that is too often overlooked, especially since families often express that improvement in mealtime interactions is a primary goal for treatment. Fortunately, caregiver training and support has been shown to significantly decrease caregiver stress [4].

Caregiver skill mastery is a crucial component of behavioral management ensuring that treatment gains generalize to the home environment. Educating caregivers about behavioral theory and applications of behavioral strategies further enhances the probability of success [22, 44]. Caregiver training typically involves a combination of written materials, modeling, in vivo coaching, and reviewing caregiver recorded meals from the child's home environment. Building caregiver mastery of techniques should result in greater caregiver confidence executing the feeding plan at home with their child. Frequently, caregiver training teaches families to focus on understanding how adaptive and maladaptive behaviors develop and how they are maintained, how to assess antecedents and consequences as they affect behavior, and how to select and use behavioral techniques to affect desirable changes within the child at mealtimes [16]. Parent training often includes (1) the provision of written information including descriptions of intervention techniques to be used, (2) therapist modeling intervention techniques during a simulated meal, (3) in vivo coaching – directly with the child in the room or through remote coaching (e.g., behind a one-way mirror) – to refine parent skills, and (4) review of home video to refine treatment plans specific to the home environment and the individual family needs.

Treatment Settings

Treatment of feeding disorders is most commonly conducted by an individual provider from within the patient family's community. Other treatment approaches include multidisciplinary treatment and interdisciplinary treatment models.

Treatment of intractable or severe feeding problems may require more intensive approaches such as day treatment or inpatient care [22, 44].

Individual Outpatient

Treatment of feeding disorders often starts with an individual community provider in an outpatient setting. According to this model of care, one provider treats the child adopting a transdisciplinary approach managing all the medical, dietary, skills and safety, and behavioral concerns [16]. Treatment sessions typically occur weekly to every other week. Frequently, the provider will be a speech and language pathologist or an occupational therapist. This model of treatment has the advantages of being widely available in the local community. For patients with low severity, this model of treatment is generally adequate. The disadvantage of this treatment model is that local providers may have limited skills for management of severe behavioral problems. When the underlying etiology of the child is complex or more severe, other treatment models should be considered.

Multidisciplinary Treatment

Feeding problems that are complex may necessitate the expertise of more than one provider discipline [16]. For example, a child may present with both behavioral and feeding skill problems necessitating consultation with a speech and language pathologist and a psychologist. In such cases multidisciplinary treatment models may be effective. Multidisciplinary care involves two or more disciplines working in a coordinated manner. Each of the treatment disciplines shares assessment and treatment planning information and attempts to coordinate treatment with the family. Families benefit from the perspective of multiple specialists, but the primary responsibility for coordination of care falls to the family. Advantages of this treatment approach include greater access to essential disciplines. Disadvantages may include disjointed care and the possibility of conflicting recommendations across providers.

Interdisciplinary Treatment

Treating a child who presents with a complex etiology is best managed within an interdisciplinary clinic. According to this model of care, patients are evaluated and treated by multiple disciplines simultaneously [16]. Patient families benefit from teams working together in real time in a highly coordinated fashion. Families benefit from being able to discuss their child's treatment needs in a complex manner and receiving a synthesized response from the entire treatment group. Ideally, interdisciplinary treatment teams combine medical, dietary, skills and safety, and behavioral specialists. The primary disadvantage to interdisciplinary care is the relative lack of available teams with very few communities having this resource available locally.

Intensive Outpatient and Day Treatment

When a feeding disorder is too severe or requires close medical management, a more intensive treatment setting is needed. One option is day treatment or intensive outpatient care which is particularly well suited to patients who need greater frequency of treatment sessions and to families who need greater support for caregiver training [22, 44]. Day treatment typically involves the child and family coming to the treatment clinic daily for multiple feeding sessions for 5 or more consecutive days. This model of care is frequently used to help families reach their feeding goals more rapidly, but is not intended for patients who require close medical monitoring. In a recent review by Lukens and Silverman [44], day hospital settings were shown to have an average length of stay of more than 30 days. These programs primarily used behavioral interventions with contingency management components [22, 47, 48]. Day treatment programs typically employ a three-phase model with education, modeling, in vivo, and then remote caregiver coaching as the key component to treatment [44].

Inpatient Treatment

Intensive inpatient feeding programs are reserved for the most severe and complicated feeding cases. Often these are children with complex medical issues and dependence on supplementary feedings (e.g., gastrostomy tubes), and/or they have needs for nutritional and/or medical monitoring during treatment. Inpatient program duration ranges from 2 to 8 weeks with treatment session frequency ranging from 3 to 6 sessions daily dependent upon the individual program specifics [22, 44]. Intensive treatment programs offer repeated behavioral feeding therapy sessions with a behavior therapist while providing ongoing assessments by other interdisciplinary treatment team members (e.g., medical, nutrition, speech and language, occupational therapy). Caregiver training with the three-phase model is also a key component to this intensive program as well.

Potential advantages to intensive feeding programs over traditional outpatient care include (1) increased environmental control; (2) varying degrees of daily medical and nutritional monitoring, thus ability to manipulate appetite; (3) more frequent treatment sessions; and (4) repeated parent training [16, 22, 44, 47]. While intensive feeding programs are recommended for more complex and challenging feeding disorders, there are also important possible disadvantages [49]. Not only can intensive inpatient programs be very expensive, the costs may not be fully covered or authorized by third-party payers [47]. The length and intensity of the program can also be disruptive to the rest of the family's lives and schedules, especially if the program is not located close to home. Finally, inpatient treatment programs are also few in number, and thus it can be difficult for families to access such care [44].

Conclusion

Pediatric feeding disorders are common. These conditions stem from a broad array of conditions that impact the physical functioning of the child, skills and safety with feeding, and the nutritional well-being of the affected child. Thus, pediatric feeding disorders are best managed by interdisciplinary treatment teams. Once the underlying etiological condition(s) are effectively managed, behavioral difficulties often linger. Fortunately, behavioral interventions have been shown to be highly effective and safe. Treatment setting can be tailored to meet the individual needs of patients, but unfortunately, access to intensive treatment programs is limited. Regardless of the treatment modality, effective caregiver training is essential to generalizing treatment gains to the home to ensure long-term treatment success.

References

1. Burklow KA, Phelps AN, Schultz JR, McConnell K, Rudolph C. Classifying complex pediatric feeding disorders. J Pediatr Gastroenterol Nutr. 1998;27(2):143–7. PubMed PMID: 9702643.
2. Silverman AH. Feeding disorders: social factors. In: Wenzel A, editor. Abnormal and clinical psychology. Thousand Oaks: SAGE; 2017. p. 1451–2.
3. Garro A, Thurman SK, Kerwin ME, Ducette JP. Parent/caregiver stress during pediatric hospitalization for chronic feeding problems. J Pediatr Nurs. 2005;20(4):268–75. PubMed PMID: 16030506.
4. Greer AJ, Gulotta CS, Masler EA, Laud RB. Caregiver stress and outcomes of children with pediatric feeding disorders treated in an intensive interdisciplinary program. J Pediatr Psychol. 2008;33(6):612–20. PubMed PMID: 18056140.
5. Rommel N, De Meyer AM, Feenstra L, Veereman-Wauters G. The complexity of feeding problems in 700 infants and young children presenting to a tertiary care institution.[see comment]. J Pediatr Gastroenterol Nutr. 2003;37(1):75–84.
6. Kerwin ME. Empirically supported treatments in pediatric psychology: severe feeding problems. J Pediatr Psychol. 1999;24(3):193–214; discussion 5–6. PubMed PMID: 10379133.
7. Malas K, Trudeau N, Chagnon M, McFarland DH. Feeding-swallowing difficulties in children later diagnosed with language impairment. Dev Med Child Neurol. 2015;57(9):872–9. PubMed PMID: 25809143.
8. Malas K, Trudeau N, Giroux MC, Gauthier L, Poulin S, McFarland DH. Prior history of feeding-swallowing difficulties in children with language impairment. Am J Speech Lang Pathol. 2017;26(1):138–45. PubMed PMID: 28166549.

9. Gorman J, Leifer M, Grossman G. Nonorganic failure to thrive: maternal history and current maternal functioning. J Clin Child Psychol. 1993;22(3):327–36.

10. Manikam R, Perman JA. Pediatric feeding disorders. J Clin Gastroenterol. 2000;30(1):34–46. PubMed PMID: 10636208.

11. American Psychiatric Association. DSM-5 Task Force. Diagnostic and statistical manual of mental disorders : DSM-5. 5th ed. Washington, DC: American Psychiatric Association; 2013. xliv, 947 p.

12. Organization WH. International statistical classification of diseases and related health problems. Geneva: World Health Organization; 2015.

13. Chatoor I, Ganiban J, Harrison J, Hirsch R. Observation of feeding in the diagnosis of posttraumatic feeding disorder of infancy. J Am Acad Child Adolesc Psychiatry. 2001;40(5):595–602. PubMed PMID: 11349705.

14. Silverman AH. Behavioral management of feeding disorders of childhood. Ann Nutr Metab. 2015;66(Suppl 5):33–42. PubMed PMID: 26226995.

15. Linscheid TR. Behavioral treatments for pediatric feeding disorders. Behav Modif. 2006;30(1):6–23. PubMed PMID: 16332643.

16. Silverman AH. Interdisciplinary care for feeding problems in children. Nutr Clin Prac. 2010;25(2):160–5. PubMed PMID: 20413696.

17. Bentovim A. The clinical approach to feeding disorders of childhood. J Psychosom Res. 1970;14:267–76.

18. Forsyth BWC, Leventhal JM, McCarthy PL. Mothers' perceptions of problems of feeding and crying behaviors: a prospective study. Am J Dis Child. 1985;139:269–72.

19. Gouge AL, Ekvall SW. Diets of handicapped children: physical, psychological, and socioeconomic correlations. Am J Ment Defic. 1975;80(2):149–57.

20. Manikam R, Perman JA. Pediatric feeding disorders. J Clin Gastroenterol. 2000;30(1):34–46.

21. Perske R, Clifton A, McLean BM, Stein JE, editors. Mealtimes for severely and profoundly handicapped persons: new concepts and attitudes. Baltimore: University Park Press; 1977.

22. Sharp WG, Volkert VM, Scahill L, McCracken CE, McElhanon B. A systematic review and meta-analysis of intensive multidisciplinary intervention for pediatric feeding disorders: how standard is the standard of care? J Pediatr. 2017;181:116–24 e4. PubMed PMID: 27843007.

23. Carruth BR, Ziegler PJ, Gordon A, Barr SI. Prevalence of picky eaters among infants and toddlers and their caregivers' decisions about offering a new food. J Am Diet Assoc. 2004;104(1 Suppl 1):s57–64. PubMed PMID: 14702019.

24. Dahl M, Sundelin C. Feeding problems in an affluent society. Follow-up at four years of age in children with early refusal to eat. Acta Paediatr. 1992;81(8):575–9.

25. Budd KS, McGraw TE, Farbisz R, Murphy TB, Hawkins D, Heilman N, et al. Psychosocial concomitants of children's feeding disorders. J Pediatr Psychol. 1992;17:81–94.

26. Davies WH, Satter E, Berlin KS, Sato AF, Silverman AH, Fischer EA, et al. Reconceptualizing feeding and feeding disorders in interpersonal context: the case for a relational disorder. J Fam Psychol. 2006;20(3):409–17.

27. Marchi M, Cohen P. Early childhood eating behaviors and adolescent eating disorders. J Am Acad Child Adolesc Psychiatry. 1990;29:112–7.

28. Babbitt RL, Hoch TA, Coe DA, Cataldo MF, Kelly KJ, Stackhouse C, et al. Behavioral assessment and treatment of pediatric feeding disorders. J Dev Behav Pediatr. 1994;15(4):278–91. PubMed PMID: 7798374.

29. Arvedson JC, Brodsky L. Pediatric swallowing and feeding: assessment and management. 2nd ed. Australia/Albany, NY: Singular Publishing Group; 2002. x, 644 p.

30. Babbitt RL, Hoch TA, Coe DA. Behavioral feeding disorders. In: Tuchman DN, Walters RS, editors. Disorders of feeding and swallowing in infants and children. San Diego: Singular; 1994. p. 77–95.

31. Bithoney WG, Rathbun JM. Failure to thrive. In: Levine M, Carey W, Crocker A, Gross R, editors. Developmental-behavioral pediatrics. Philadephia: Saunders; 1983. p. 557–72.

32. Frank DA, Drotar D, Cook JT, Bleiker JS, Kasper D. Failure to thrive. In: Reece M, Ludwig S, editors. Child abuse: medical diagnosis and management. Philadelphia: Lea & Freiber; 2001. p. 307–38.
33. Silverman AH, Tarbell S. Feeding and vomiting problems in pediatric populations. In: Roberts MC, Steele RG, editors. Handbook of pediatric psychology. New York: Guilford Press; 2009. p. 429–45.
34. O'Brien S, Repp AC, Williams GE, Christophersen ER. Pediatric feeding disorders. Behav Modif. 1991;15(3):394–418. PubMed PMID: 1953626.
35. Pediatics AAP. Infant food and feeding. https://www.aap.org/en-us/advocacy-and-policy/aap-health-initiatives/HALF-Implementation-Guide/Age-Specific-Content/pages/infant-food-and-feeding.aspx. 2017 [cited 2017 Oct. 31, 2017].
36. Briefel RR. New findings from the feeding infants and toddlers study: data to inform action. J Am Diet Assoc. 110(12):S5–7.
37. Silverman AH. Feeding disorders: cultural factors. In: Wenzel A, editor. Abnormal and clinical psychology, vol. 3. Thousand Oaks: SAGE; 2017. p. 1441.
38. Satter E. How to get your kid to eat – but not too much. Palo Alto/Emeryville: Bull Pub. Co./Distributed in the U.S. by Publishers Group West; 1987. p. 396.
39. Silverman AH. Feeding and vomiting problems in pediatric populations. In: Roberts MC, Steele RG, editors. Handbook of pediatric psychology. 5th ed. New York: Guilford Press; 2017. p. 401–15.
40. Kedesdy JH, Budd KS. Childhood feeding disorders: biobehavioral assessment and intervention. Baltimore: Paul H. Brookes Pub. Co.; 1998. xi, 402 p.
41. Burklow KA, Phelps AN, Schultz JR, McConnell K, Rudolph C. Classifying complex pediatric feeding disorders. J Pediatr Gastroenterol Nutr. 1998;27(2):143–7.
42. Fischer EA, Silverman AH. Behavioral conceptualization, assessment, and treatment of pediatric feeding disorders. Semin Speech Lang. 2007;28(3):223–31.
43. Linscheid TJ, Budd KS, Rasnake LK. Pediatric feeding problems. In: Roberts MC, editor. Handbook of pediatric psychology. New York: Gulford; 2003. p. 481–98.
44. Lukens CT, Silverman AH. Systematic review of psychological interventions for pediatric feeding problems. J Pediatr Psychol. 2014;39(8):903–17. PubMed PMID: 24934248.
45. Piazza CC, Patel MR, Gulotta CS, Sevin BM, Layer SA. On the relative contributions of positive reinforcement and escape extinction in the treatment of food refusal. J Appl Behav Anal. 2003;36(3):309. PubMed PMID: 2003-08852-002. English.
46. Birch LL, McPhee L, Steinberg L, Sullivan S. Conditioned flavor preferences in young children. Physiol Behav. 1990;47(3):501–5. PubMed PMID: 2359760.
47. Williams KE, Riegel K, Gibbons B, Field DG. Intensive behavioral treatment for severe feeding problems: a cost-effective alternative to tube feeding? J Dev Phys Disabil. 2007;19(3):227. PubMed PMID: 2008-00558-006. English.
48. Clawson EP, Kuchinski KS, Bach R. Use of behavioral interventions and parent education to address feeding difficulties in young children with spastic diplegic cerebral palsy. NeuroRehabil. 2007;22(5):397–406. PubMed PMID: 2008-00354-006. English.
49. Silverman AH, Kirby M, Clifford LM, Fischer E, Berlin KS, Rudolph CD, et al. Nutritional and psychosocial outcomes of gastrostomy tube-dependent children completing an intensive inpatient behavioral treatment program. J Pediatr Gastroenterol Nutr. 2013;57(5):668–72. PubMed PMID: 23783012.

Chapter 23
The Role of a Multidisciplinary Aerodigestive Program

Julina Ongkasuwan and Eric H. Chiou

Introduction

One of the biggest developments to occur in the realm of pediatric dysphagia in recent years has been the rise of the multidisciplinary aerodigestive program. Children with complex congenital or acquired conditions affecting swallowing, breathing, digestion, and growth, often referred to collectively as aerodigestive disorders, frequently require the services of multiple pediatric specialists and allied health providers, both in terms of diagnosis and for long-term management. Indeed, the number of children with such medical complexity has increased over the years – largely as the result of medical advancements in diagnosis and treatment which have led to improved survival of premature infants, as well as children with congenital anomalies and chronic disease. Furthermore, due to the complex nature of many aerodigestive conditions, the concept of coordinated, multidisciplinary care has become particularly relevant and sought-after.

J. Ongkasuwan
Department of Otolaryngology Head and Neck Surgery,
Baylor College of Medicine/Texas Children's Hospital, Houston, TX, USA
e-mail: julinao@bcm.edu

E. H. Chiou (✉)
Department of Pediatrics, Baylor College of Medicine/Texas Children's Hospital,
Houston, TX, USA
e-mail: ehchiou@bcm.edu

© Springer International Publishing AG, part of Springer Nature 2018
J. Ongkasuwan, E. H. Chiou (eds.), *Pediatric Dysphagia*,
https://doi.org/10.1007/978-3-319-97025-7_23

The Start of a Movement

The term "aerodigestive" in reference to the combination of the upper airway, respiratory, and digestive tracts has actually been in use for decades. The earliest PubMed citation containing the term "aerodigestive" comes from a French publication in 1955 reporting on myoclonic syndrome of the aerodigestive tract [1]. A survey of the number of aerodigestive citations by year reveals a significant increase in the use of the term starting in the 1990's with steady growth to present day. On the other hand, coordinated aerodigestive medicine is a relatively new concept which has seemingly grown exponentially just within the past 10 years. The exact prevalence of complex aerodigestive disorders in children is difficult to estimate but is likely more common than previously thought, as suggested by the rapid rise of multidisciplinary aerodigestive programs. The first pediatric aerodigestive program was established at Cincinnati Children's Hospital Medical Center in 1999. Since then an additional 50 such centers have been established in 32 states at last count [2]. Along with the increase of these programs, typically based at tertiary and quaternary pediatric care facilities and children's hospitals, there has been a growing presence of aerodigestive-focused sessions at pediatric subspecialty conferences, the development of an annual multidisciplinary aerodigestive conference, and more recently the formation of a formal, independent aerodigestive society aimed at advancing clinical care, research, advocacy, and educational endeavors.

The rapid growth of pediatric aerodigestive programs speaks volumes toward the desire from patients and families, primary care physicians, as well as hospital administrations to improve the care provided to patients with complex swallowing, breathing, and digestive problems. The spectrum of conditions which potentially fall within the scope of aerodigestive disorders is broad and includes structural or physiologic airway disease, chronic lung disease, lung injury from aspiration or infection, gastroesophageal reflux, eosinophilic esophagitis, esophageal dysmotility, congenital anomalies of the upper digestive tract, dysphagia, and behavioral feeding problems. In addition to often having multiple chronic medical problems and frequent hospital admissions, it is the intersection and potential interaction between conditions that can make patients with aerodigestive disorders particularly difficult for pediatricians to manage alone. Aerodigestive programs therefore have sought to fill a significant void in the medical landscape, but until recently there was little by way of definition or minimum requirements.

What Makes an Aerodigestive Program?

Even among aerodigestive programs, there is a fair amount of variability when it comes to clinical scope, structure, and components. Some programs focus on the diagnosis and management of feeding disorders, including risk of aspiration, in medically complex children. In other cases, there is an emphasis on optimization of patients undergoing complex airway surgery or reconstruction. The strengths and limitations and availability of resources of the parent institution may also influence how an aerodigestive program operates.

Through an iterative, questionnaire-based Delphi method, Boesch and colleagues sought to define the essential components of an aerodigestive program. Among thirty-three specialists from well-established aerodigestive programs across the country, there was consensus that the core components of an aerodigestive program should include the following: care coordinator/nursing, gastroenterology, otolaryngology, pulmonology, and speech language pathology. Ancillary members of an aerodigestive program might include a sleep specialist, respiratory therapist, dietitian, and social worker. Finally, because swallowing and feeding problems are so prevalent among children with aerodigestive disorders, the availability of clinical assessment of swallowing, videofluoroscopic swallow study (VFSS), fiber-optic endoscopic evaluation of swallowing (FEES), and provision of feeding therapy were all felt to be essential [2].

Most aerodigestive programs are structured so that patients are seen by multiple specialists as part of a single visit to the clinic. In addition to facilitating interdisciplinary discussion and collaboration among providers, there are practical advantages for the patient and family to this shared clinic approach as well – reducing the need for multiple trips to the medical center and potentially shortening the time required to complete the evaluation. In order to orchestrate these multiple consultations and diagnostic tests to occur smoothly in a short span of time, there is usually a significant amount of preparation, planning, and coordination that goes on behind the scenes. Most programs have adopted a team meeting structure where new referrals are reviewed, and a plan for evaluation is developed. After patients have been seen in the aerodigestive program, the team meeting is also the venue for summarizing results from diagnostic testing as well as formulating a cohesive care plan and recommendations to be communicated back to the patient, family, and primary care provider. Many programs also use a care coordinator, often a nurse, nurse practitioner, or physician assistant, to serve as the primary conduit of information between the patient/family, primary care provider, and the aerodigestive team. This helps to facilitate clear communication and ensure that the care plan is carried out as intended and adjusted as needed depending on feedback from the patient/family.

Another primary advantage of an aerodigestive program is the ability to coordinate diagnostic and therapeutic endoscopic procedures under a single general anesthesia episode. In most cases, this is comprised of direct laryngobronchoscopy, flexible bronchoscopy with bronchoalveolar lavage, and esophagogastroduodenoscopy with biopsy – also known as a "triple endoscopy." Performing these procedures together allows all providers to directly observe findings in real time, facilitating discussion, and development of a collaborative plan with each other. Combining procedures also reduces the potential risks associated with multiple episodes of general anesthesia, especially for young children and infants – the age groups with the highest prevalence of swallowing and feeding difficulties and who may be most vulnerable to the neurotoxic effects of anesthetic agents on the developing brain [3, 4].

Although there is general consensus on many of the theoretical benefits of a coordinated approach with an aerodigestive program, evidence to support these hypotheses are still relatively limited. As the field of aerodigestive medicine matures, further research and data will help to document improvements in outcomes and hopefully lead to the development of evidence-based clinical guidelines. Eventually, the identity of aerodigestive programs may expand beyond serving as centers for primarily diagnostic or therapeutic procedures, with some proposing to redefine the medical home for complex patients [5].

It's a Great Idea: Now What?

The primary goal of a coordinated multidisciplinary program is to improve patient care; however, in order to be sustainable, the program must also work financially. Institutional "buy-in" is essential. Developing an aerodigestive program requires the commitment of dedicated personnel, time, space, and equipment. Now that programs across the country are maturing, the next challenge is to determine if patient care is improving. Primary outcome measures must be twofold: patient-based clinical outcomes and impact on healthcare costs.

Aerodigestive patients are often medically complex with numerous previous records, thus they require more time than a routine visit. Clinicians may see a corresponding drop in outpatient and operative volume when compared to a general clinic for their specialty. In 2017 Mudd et al. at Children's National found that their multidisciplinary program operated at a net-positive margin [6]. A clinical coordinator, while nonrevenue generating, is essential for the structure and flow of an aerodigestive program. He or she also acts as a communication interface between the clinicians and patients by screening referrals, triaging phone calls, and relaying recommendations.

If the patients are going to be seen jointly by multiple team members, there needs to be a large enough clinic space to accommodate the team. For some aerodigestive programs, in addition to the otolaryngologist, pulmonologist, and gastroenterologist, there may be an anesthesiologist, speech pathologist, respiratory technician, dietitian, social worker, advanced practice provider, clinical coordinator, and an array of learners streaming through the clinic. In addition, the clinic should have the capability of performing flexible endoscopic laryngoscopies and flexible endoscopic evaluations of swallow as needed. In 2017, Rotsides et al. at Children's National reported that the multidisciplinary team resulted in clinical improvement in 73% of patients who had seen only a single specialist previously [7].

If the team plans on performing joint endoscopies back to back in the operating room, the institution has to have enough equipment and personnel to support the patient flow. Dedicated anesthesiologists can also help increase efficiency. In 2015 Collaco et al. at Johns Hopkins found that with a multidisciplinary approach, they were able to reduce the number of anesthetics for these children by 41% [8].

What Is the Return on Investment?

In 2016, Skinner et al. at Johns Hopkins reported that enrollment in their multidisciplinary aerodigestive program resulted in a shift from inpatient to outpatient care with a 20% reduction in patient charges [9]. In 2017 Appachi et al. at Cleveland clinic found that by acting as a medical home for aerodigestive patients, they were able to decrease technical direct costs by 70% and hospital days by 1 week per year [10]. Also in 2017, Garcia et al. at Harvard used time-driven activity-based costing to look at children with laryngeal clefts and found that the multidisciplinary team potentially had a costs savings of 20% to 40% [11].

Where Do We Go Next?

Clearly the results are just starting to trickle in regarding the clinical and financial impacts of aerodigestive programs across the country. As programs mature and collect data, a clearer picture should emerge regarding the role of aerodigestive programs in the management of patients with dysphagia.

Aerodigestive programs are uniquely positioned to help develop guidelines for the evaluation of children with dysphagia. In addition, specific populations such as laryngeal cleft, eosinophilic esophagitis, and tracheoesophageal fistula can be studied systematically. The field of pediatric aerodigestive medicine is poised for new research and discoveries, including better understanding the role of diagnostic testing and endoscopic evaluation, the significance of gastroesophageal reflux and optimal management, as well as long-term outcomes for children with aerodigestive disorders.

Conclusion

The intersection of medical specialties and the cross-fertilization of ideas in the field of aerodigestive medicine are invigorating. Nationally, groups interested in studying children with complex aerodigestive disorders are organizing to share and disseminate information, protocols, and research. What we learn can then be brought back to our colleagues within our specialties and those on the front line in primary care.

References

1. Camps F, Terracol J. Myoclonic syndrome of the aerodigestive tract. Rev Otoneuroophtalmol. 1955;27(7):392–4.
2. Boesch RP, Balakrishnan K, Acra S, Benscoter DT, Cofer SA, Collaco JM, Dahl JP, Daines CL, DeAlarcon A, DeBoer EM, Deterding RR, Friedlander JA, Gold BD, Grothe RM, Hart

CK, Kazachkov M, Lefton-Greif MA, Miller CK, Moore PE, Pentiuk S, Peterson-Carmichael S, Piccione J, Prager JD, Putnam PE, Rosen R, Rutter MJ, Ryan MJ, Skinner ML, Torres-Silva C, Wootten CT, Zur KB, Cotton RT, Wood RE. Structure and functions of pediatric aerodigestive programs: a consensus statement. Pediatrics. 2018;141(3):e20171701.

3. Wilder RT, Flick RP, Sprung J, et al. Early exposure to anesthesia and learning disabilities in a population-based birth cohort. Anesthesiology. 2009;110:796–804.

4. Ikonomidou C, Bosch F, Miksa M, et al. Blockade of NMDA receptors and apoptotic neurodegeneration in the developing brain. Science. 1999;283:70–4.

5. Galligan MM, Bamat TW, Hogan AK, Piccione J. The pediatric aerodigestive center as a tertiary care-based medical home: a proposed model. Curr Probl Pediatr Adolesc Health Care. 2018;48(4):104–10. pii: S1538-5442(18)30033-6.

6. Mudd PA, Silva AL, Callicott SS, Bauman NM. Cost analysis of a multidisciplinary aerodigestive clinic: are such clinics financially feasible? Ann Otol Rhinol Laryngol. 2017;126(5):401–6.

7. Rotsides JM, Krakovsky GM, Pillai DK, Sehgal S, Collins ME, Noelke CE, Bauman NM. Is a multidisciplinary aerodigestive clinic more effective at treating recalcitrant aerodigestive complaints than a single specialist? Ann Otol Rhinol Laryngol. 2017;126(7):537–43.

8. Collaco JM, Aherrera AD, Au Yeung KJ, Lefton-Greif MA, Hoch J, Skinner ML. Interdisciplinary pediatric aerodigestive care and reduction in health care costs and burden. JAMA Otolaryngol Head Neck Surg. 2015;141(2):101–5.

9. Skinner ML, Lee SK, Collaco JM, Lefton-Greif MA, Hoch J, Au Yeung KJ. Financial and health impacts of multidisciplinary aerodigestive care. Otolaryngol Head Neck Surg. 2016;154(6):1064–7.

10. Appachi S, Banas A, Feinberg L, Henry D, Kenny D, Kraynack N, Rosneck A, Carl J, Krakovitz P. Association of enrollment in an aerodigestive clinic with reduced hospital stay for children with special health care needs. JAMA Otolaryngol Head Neck Surg. 2017;143(11):1117–21.

11. Garcia JA, Mistry B, Hardy S, Fracchia MS, Hersh C, Wentland C, Vadakekalam J, Kaplan R, Hartnick CJ. Time-driven activity-based costing to estimate cost of care at multidisciplinary aerodigestive centers. Laryngoscope. 2017;127(9):2152–8.

Index

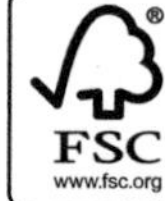

MIX
Papier aus verantwortungsvollen Quellen
Paper from responsible sources
FSC® C105338

If you have any concerns about our products,
you can contact us on
ProductSafety@springernature.com

In case Publisher is established outside the EU,
the EU authorized representative is:
**Springer Nature Customer Service Center GmbH
Europaplatz 3, 69115 Heidelberg, Germany**

Printed by Libri Plureos GmbH
in Hamburg, Germany